Abernathy's
SURGICAL SECRETS
Fourth Edition

ALDEN H. HARKEN, M.D.
Professor and Chairman
Department of Surgery
University of Colorado Health Sciences Center
Denver, Colorado

ERNEST E. MOORE, M.D.
Professor and Vice-Chairman
Department of Surgery
University of Colorado Health Sciences Center
Chief of Surgery
Denver Health Medical Center
Denver, Colorado

D1287219

HANLEY & BELFUS, INC./ Philadelphia

Publisher: HANLEY & BELFUS, INC.
Medical Publishers
210 South 13th Street
Philadelphia, PA 19107
(215) 546-7293; 800-962-1892
FAX (215) 790-9330
Web site: http://www.hanleyandbelfus.com

Note to the reader: Although the information in this book has been carefully reviewed for correctness of dosage and indications, neither the authors nor the editors nor the publisher can accept any legal responsibility for any errors or omissions that may be made. Neither the publisher nor the editors make any warranty, expressed or implied, with respect to the material contained herein. Before prescribing any drug, the reader must review the manufacturer's current product information (package inserts) for accepted indications, absolute dosage recommendations, and other information pertinent to the safe and effective use of the product described.

Library of Congress Cataloging-in-Publication Data

Abernathy's Surgical Secrets / edited by Alden H. Harken, Ernest E. Moore.—4th ed.
    p. ; cm.—(The Secrets Series®)
   Includes bibliographical references and index.
   ISBN 1-56053-363-3 (alk. paper)
     1. Surgery—Examinations, questions, etc. I. Title: Surgical Secrets.
  II. Harken, Alden H. III. Moore, Ernest Eugene. IV. Abernathy, Charles. V. Series.
  |DNLM: 1. Surgical Procedures, Operative—Examination Questions.
WO 18.2 A146 2000|
RD37.2.S975 2000
617'.0076—dc21

                                      99-050332

SURGICAL SECRETS, 4th Edition   ISBN 1-56053-363-3

Last digit is the print number: 9 8 7 6 5 4 3 2 1

CONTENTS

CONTRIBUTORS

Brett B. Abernathy, M.D.
Clinical Instructor, Division of Urology, University of Colorado Health Sciences Center, Denver, Colorado

Benjamin O. Anderson, M.D., FACS
Associate Professor, Department of Surgery, and Medical Director, Breast Care Program, University of Washington School of Medicine, Seattle, Washington

Thomas E. Bak, M.D.
Instructor Surgeon, Division of Transplant Surgery, Department of Surgery, University of Colorado Health Sciences Center, Denver, Colorado

Carlton C. Barnett, Jr., M.D.
Junior Faculty Associate, Department of Surgical Oncology, The University of Texas M.D. Anderson Cancer Center, Houston, Texas

James Bascom, M.D.
Assistant Professor (Ret.), Department of Surgery, University of Colorado Health Sciences Center, Denver, Colorado

Paul Bauling, M.D.
Assistant Professor, Department of Surgery, University of Colorado Health Sciences Center, Denver, Colorado

B. Timothy Baxter, M.D.
Professor, Department of Surgery, University of Nebraska College of Medicine, Omaha, Nebraska

Allen T. Belshaw, M.D.
Assistant Clinical Professor, Department of Surgery, University of Colorado Health Sciences Center, Denver, Colorado

Denis D. Bensard, M.D.
Assistant Professor of Surgery and Pediatrics, Division of Pediatric Surgery, Department of Surgery, University of Colorado Health Sciences Center, Denver, Colorado

Walter L. Biffl, M.D.
Assistant Professor, Department of Surgery, University of Colorado Health Sciences Center, Denver, Colorado

James M. Brown, M.D.
Associate Professor, Division of Thoracic and Cardiovascular Surgery, University of Maryland School of Medicine, Baltimore, Maryland

Kerry Brega, M.D.
Assistant Professor, Division of Neurosurgery, Department of Surgery, University of Colorado Health Sciences Center, Director of Neurosurgery, Denver Health Medical Center, Denver, Colorado

Elizabeth C. Brew, M.D.
Exempla Lutheran Medical Center, Wheat Ridge, Colorado

Jon M. Burch, M.D.
Professor, Department of Surgery, University of Colorado Health Sciences Center, and Chief, General and Vascular Surgery, Denver Health Medical Center, Denver, Colorado

Mark P. Cain, M.D.
Assistant Professor of Pediatric Urology, Indiana University School of Medicine, Indianapolis, Indiana

David. N. Campbell, M.D.
Professor, Divisions of Cardiothoracic Surgery and Vascular Surgery, Department of Surgery, University of Colorado Health Sciences Center, Denver, Colorado

Sandra C. Carr, M.D.
Fellow in Vascular Surgery, Department of Surgery, Northwestern University Medical School, Chicago, Illinois

Karin Cesario, M.D.
Resident, Department of Surgery, University of Colorado Health Sciences Center, Denver, Colorado

David J. Ciesla, M.D.
Resident in General Surgery, Department of Surgery, University of Colorado Health Sciences Center, Denver, Colorado

Frank H. Chae, M.D.
Assistant Professor, Department of Surgery, University of Colorado Health Sciences Center, Denver, Colorado

Joseph C. Cleveland, Jr., M.D.
Resident, Division of Cardiothoracic Surgery, Department of Surgery, University of Colorado Health Sciences Center, Denver, Colorado

Clay Cothren, M.D.
Resident, Department of Surgery, University of Colorado Health Sciences Center, Denver, Colorado

Jeff Cross, M.D.
Assistant Clinical Professor, Department of Surgery, University of Colorado Health Sciences Center, Denver, Colorado

Firouz Daneshgari, M.D.
Assistant Professor, Division of Urology, University of Colorado Health Sciences Center, Denver, Colorado

Kirstan K. Donnahoo, M.D.
Resident, Department of Urology, Indiana University School of Medicine, Indianapolis, Indiana

J. Paul Elliott, M.D.
Assistant Professor, Division of Neurosurgery, Department of Surgery, University of Colorado Health Sciences Center, Denver, Colorado

Michael E. Fenoglio, M.D.
Associate Clinical Professor, Department of Surgery, University of Colorado Health Sciences Center, Denver, Colorado

Christina A. Finlayson, M.D.
Assistant Professor, Department of Surgery, University of Colorado Health Sciences Center, Denver, Colorado

Reginald J. Franciose, M.D.
Assistant Professor, Department of Surgery, University of Colorado Health Sciences Center, and Attending Trauma Surgeon, Denver Health Medical Center, Denver, Colorado

David A. Fullerton, M.D.
Professor, Division of Cardiothoracic Surgery, Department of Surgery, Northwestern University Medical School, and Attending Surgeon, Northwestern Memorial Hospital, Chicago, Illinois

Glenn W. Geelhoed, M.D., M.P.H., FACS
Professor of Surgery and Professor of International Medical Education, Office of the Dean, George Washington University Medical Center, Washington, DC

Doru I.E. Georgescu, M.D., FACS
Private Practice, Thornton, Colorado

Ricardo J. Gonzalez, M.D.
Resident, Department of Surgery, University of Colorado Health Sciences Center, Denver, Colorado

Michael J.V. Gordon, M.D.
Associate Professor, Director of Hand Surgery, Division of Plastic Surgery, Department of Surgery, University of Colorado Health Sciences Center, and Chief of Plastic Surgery, Veterans Administration Medical Center, Denver, Colorado

Michael Grosso, M.D.
Associate Professor, Department of Surgery, Jefferson Medical College of Thomas Jefferson University, Philadephia, Pennsylvania; Attending Surgeon, Deborah Heart and Lung Center, Browns Mills, New Jersey

James B. Haenel, R.R.T.
Clinical Instructor, Department of Surgery, Denver Health Medical Center, Denver, Colorado

Alden H. Harken, M.D.
Professor and Chairman, Department of Surgery, University of Colorado Health Sciences Center, Denver, Colorado

Gilbert Hermann, M.D.
Clinical Professor, Department of Surgery, University of Colorado Health Sciences Center, and Chairman, Department of Surgery, Rose Medical Center, Denver, Colorado

Gwendolyn J. Hewitt, M.D.
University of Colorado Health Sciences Center, Denver, Colorado

Jeffrey L. Johnson, M.D.
Chief Resident in General Surgery, Department of Surgery, University of Colorado Health Sciences Center, Denver, Colorado

Darrell N. Jones, Ph.D.
Associate Director, Vascular Diagnostic Laboratory, Vascular Surgery Section, Department of Surgery, University of Colorado Health Sciences Center, Denver, Colorado

Igal Kam, M.D.
Chief of Transplantation, Associate Professor, Division of Transplant Surgery, Department of Surgery, University of Colorado Health Sciences Center, Denver, Colorado

Frederick M. Karrer, M.D.
Assistant Professor, Division of Pediatric Surgery, Department of Surgery, University of Colorado Health Sciences Center, Denver, Colorado

Lawrence L. Ketch, M.D.
Head, Plastic, Hand, and Burn Surgery, Department of Surgery, University of Colorado Health Sciences Center, and Chairman, Pediatric Plastic Surgery, Children's Hospital, Denver, Colorado

G. Edward Kimm, Jr., M.D.
Assistant Clinical Professor, Department of Surgery, University of Colorado Health Sciences Center, Denver, Colorado

William C. Krupski, M.D.
Professor, Vascular Surgery Section, Department of Surgery, University of Colorado Health Sciences Center, Denver, Colorado

Kathleen Liscum, M.D.
Assistant Professor, Department of Surgery, Baylor College of Medicine, Houston, Texas

Joyce A. Majure, M.D., FACS
Private Practice, Lewiston, Idaho

Stephen D. Malley, M.D.
Staff Surgeon, Department of General Surgery, Memorial Hospital West Volusia, Deland, Florida

James R. Mault, M.D.
Assistant Professor, Division of Cardiothoracic Surgery, Department of Surgery, University of Colorado Health Sciences Center, Denver, Colorado

Patrick L. McConnell, M.D.
Department of Surgery, University of Utah School of Medicine, Salt Lake City, Utah

Robert C. McIntyre, Jr., M.D.
Associate Professor, Division of GI, Tumor, and Endocrine Surgery, Department of Surgery, University of Colorado Health Sciences Center, Denver, Colorado

Margaret M. McQuiggan, M.S., R.D., C.S.M.
Clinical Dietitian Specialist, Department of Food and Nutrition, Hermann Hospital, Houston, Texas

Randall B. Meacham, M.D.
Associate Professor, Division of Urology, University of Colorado Health Sciences Center, Denver, Colorado

Daniel R. Meldrum, M.D.
Instructor and Fellow, Division of Cardiac Surgery, The Johns Hopkins University Hospital, Baltimore, Maryland

Ernest E. Moore, M.D.
Professor and Vice-Chairman, Department of Surgery, University of Colorado Health Sciences Center, and Chief of Surgery, Denver Health Medical Center, Denver, Colorado

Frederick A. Moore, M.D.
Professor and Vice-Chairman, Department of Surgery, University of Texas–Houston Medical School, and Chief, General Surgery and Trauma/Critical Care, Hermann Hospital, Houston, Texas

John B. Moore, M.D., FACS
Associate Clinical Professor, Department of Surgery, University of Colorado Health Sciences Center, Denver, Colorado

Mark R. Nehler, M.D.
Assistant Professor, Vascular Surgery Section, Department of Surgery, University of Colorado Health Sciences Center, Denver, Colorado

William R. Nelson, M.D.
Clinical Professor, Department of Surgery, University of Colorado Health Sciences Center, Denver, Colorado

Lawrence W. Norton, M.D.
Emeritus Professor, Department of Surgery, University of Colorado Health Sciences Center, Denver, Colorado

Patrick. J. Offner, M.D., M.P.H., FACS
Assistant Professor, Department of Surgery, University of Colorado Health Sciences Center, and Chief, Surgical Critical Care, Denver Health Medical Center, Denver, Colorado

David A. Partrick, M.D.
Instructor and Fellow, Division of Pediatric Surgery, Department of Surgery, University of Colorado Health Sciences Center and Resident, Department of Pediatric Surgery, The Children's Hospital, Denver, Colorado

William H. Pearce, M.D.
Professor, Department of Surgery, Northwestern University Medical School, Chicago, Illinois

Nathan W. Pearlman, M.D.
Professor, Department of Surgery, University of Colorado Health Sciences Center, Denver, Colorado

Jeffery Pence, M.D.
Assistant Professor of Surgery and Pediatrics, Division of Pediatric Surgery, East Carolina University School of Medicine, Greenville, North Carolina

Norman E. Peterson, M.D.
Professor, Division of Urology, University of Colorado Health Sciences Center, and Associate Director of Surgery and Chief of Urology Division, Denver Health Medical Center, Denver, Colorado

Steven L. Peterson, D.V.M., M.D.
Assistant Professor, Division of Plastic Surgery, Department of Surgery, University of Colorado Health Sciences Center, and Chief of Plastic and Reconstructive Surgery, Denver Health Medical Center, Denver, Colorado

Marvin Pomerantz, M.D.
Professor, Division of Cardiothoracic Surgery, Department of Surgery, University of Colorado Health Sciences Center, Denver, Colorado

John Ridge, M.D., Ph.D.
Chief, Head and Neck Surgery Section, Fox Chase Cancer Center, Philadelphia, Pennsylvania

Laurel H. Saliman, M.D.
Resident in Orthopedic Surgery, University of Colorado Health Sciences Center, Denver, Colorado

Peter A. Seirafi, M.D.
Chief Resident, Division of Cardiothoracic Surgery, Department of Surgery, University of Colorado Health Sciences Center, Denver, Colorado

Craig H. Selzman, M.D.
Chief Resident, Department of Surgery, University of Colorado Health Sciences Center, Denver, Colorado

Wade R. Smith, M.D.
Assistant Professor of Orthopedic Surgery, University of Colorado Health Sciences Center, and Chief, Orthopedic Trauma, Denver Health Medical Center, Denver, Colorado

Douglas Y. Tamura, M.D.
Chief Resident, Department of Surgery, University of Colorado Health Sciences Center, Denver, Colorado

Greg Van Stiegmann, M.D.
Professor, Department of Surgery, University of Colorado Health Sciences Center, Denver, Colorado

Michael E. Wachs, M.D.
Assistant Professor, Division of Transplant Surgery, Department of Surgery, University of Colorado Health Sciences Center, Denver, Colorado

Thomas A. Whitehill, M.D.
Assistant Professor, Vascular Surgery Section, Department of Surgery, University of Colorado Health Sciences Center, Denver, Colorado

Glenn J.R. Whitman, M.D.
Professor of Surgery and Chief of Cardiothoracic Surgery, Medical College of Pennsylvania, Philadelphia, Pennsylvania

Garret Zallen, M.D.
Department of Surgery, University of Colorado Health Sciences Center, Denver, Colorado

PREFACE TO THE FIRST EDITION

Surgical Secrets is not intended as a textbook in the traditional sense. It is a pathway of questions from diagnosis to recovery. We first discovered the need for this approach when our students were assigned chapters in a major surgical textbook and then on discussion could not "pull out" the key information. The way we solve this as surgeons is by a series of key questions.

The editors gave the contributing authors wide latitude in style (some are long, some are short) and encouraged them to duplicate the verbal teaching process they use on rounds, in the OR, and on oral exams.

We teach students by asking questions. Knowing "the right question" and its answers is the key to clinical surgery for both a student and the most experienced practitioner. Of the two components of learning surgery, one is experiential and the other didactic, the part that can be written. The only way to learn the experiential component is by long hours of watching, trying and trying again. It takes a *long* time.

But the other part of learning surgery, the "book knowledge," can and should be learned rapidly. A student should learn surgery 101, 202 . . . 606 all simultaneously, for a patient problem is almost always a complex constellation of decisions, questions, and judgments. To suggest that a student should not learn the ins and outs of aortic grafts, and instead be exposed only to fundamental wound healing concepts, is to belittle the student's ability to handle complicated concepts. Surgery, unlike calculus, is not abstract and can be learned (insofar as the didactic information is concerned) in full breadth at an early stage.

This volume is designed to be carried in a coat pocket. We hope it will also be carried in the coat pockets of many experienced surgeons as they ask the "questions of surgical practice" in their daily work.

Surgical Secrets is *not* intended only to be a guide to help pass an examination. Rather, the questions here teach the knowledge a surgeon must know in order to take care of a patient with a particular problem.

Socrates was correct. The best way to teach is to question. We hope we have followed his precepts, perhaps providing even more help in finding answers.

Charles M. Abernathy, M.D.
Brett B. Abernathy, M.D.

PREFACE TO THE SECOND EDITION

We estimate that over one half of *all* medical students over the last five years have bought *Surgical Secrets* (we assume the other half either borrowed it or stole it!). This confirms our notion that learning medical information in a question-and-answer format is a preferred method for many students. Somehow, reading a chapter in *Surgical Secrets* seems to "set the glue" on the information in a different way from reading a similar chapter in a large textbook.

We were amazed as we reviewed and revised the book at how much information it contains. Although we editors and the authors have edited and read the chapters many times, we are frequently asked questions from *Surgical Secrets* that even we can't answer!

This edition features a new "Atlas of Technical Tips." Original line drawings depict methods of tying sutures, holding needles, and other basic techniques. This Atlas is not intended to be comprehensive, but instead represents a starting point for the use of surgical instruments. We also believe that it lends a sense of "completeness" to *Surgical Secrets*.

Enjoy the book and learn from it, and don't hesitate to send us notes about its content (a suggestion form is provided on page 318). Like all good surgeons, we are constantly striving for improvement.

Charles M. Abernathy, M.D.
Alden H. Harken, M.D.

PREFACE TO THE THIRD EDITION AND DEDICATION TO CHARLIE ABERNATHY

Charlie Abernathy never had a neutral effect on anyone. Charlie's effervescent enthusiasm for education, medicine, books, students, innovation, cattle, DNA, old cars, skiing, critical care, and his patients will sustain happy and rewarding memories for all of us lucky enough to have known him. Charlie challenged us all. Most of us feel pretty good if we have one or two good ideas each decade. Charlie sparked an idea a minute—and most of them were pretty good.

After medical school at Northwestern and surgical training in Boston and Colorado, Charlie joined Ted Dickinson to practice surgery in Montrose, Colorado. Charlie was a superb surgeon, gifted internist, sensitive psychiatrist, compassionate pediatrician, imaginative urologist/gynecologist, and practical family physician ("specialization" Charlie would have said "is for insects").

Charlie's loyalty and love for the University of Colorado prompted him to run for university Regent. The Regents are the nine folks who run our university, and in state-wide campaigns frequently pull more voters than the governor's race. Predictably, Charlie was elected. Soon thereafter, we successfully recruited Charlie and Martha back to the Department of Surgery at Denver General and the University Hospitals. With Charlie around, we "red-lined" excitement and the "fun-meter was always in the green zone." Charlie challenged everything and everyone.

While perusing a stand of black walnut trees (Charlie planned to make them into capnometers that could induce the "diving seal reflex" in trauma victims, thus redistributing limited blood flow toward metabolically downregulated vital organs), Charlie thought: "You know, medical education is all backwards. Medical students read textbooks to discover the answers. We faculty members don't fool with the answers—we simply change the questions. In order to conceptualize surgical biology (and to thrive on ward rounds), students need to know the right questions."

Thus originated the concept for *Surgical Secrets*, which later blossomed into *The Secrets Series®*, Q & A books in over 20 medical disciplines designed to make the subject interesting to medical students, residents, and even practitioners. Characteristically, Charlie identified a way to make medical education stimulating, rewarding, and fun.

In this third edition of *Surgical Secrets*, we hope to have captured some vintage Abernathy—his irreverence, challenge, humor, dignity, erudition, and "working model" doctor practicality. You will note that the questions have been thoroughly updated or completely changed. New authors have written a number of the chapters in order to give a new perspective on the material. Chapters new to this edition include tuberculosis, heart and lung transplantation, antibiotics, penetrating thoracic trauma, urinary tract trauma, and health care management.

If we have been able to impart even just a little Abernathy in the following pages, we are convinced that the "questions" of surgical biology will live for another group of surgical students and residents.

With affection, admiration, and respect, we dedicate this edition to Charlie's enduring memory.

Alden H. Harken, M.D.
Ernest E. Moore, M.D.
Linda C. Belfus

PREFACE TO THE FOURTH EDITION

Apparently there is a town in Texas that is so tough that there are no "innocent bystanders." Charlie Abernathy could have been the mayor of that town. On rounds with students, residents, and faculty, Charlie would swing at anything that moved. Charlie's surgical rounds were so exciting that students used to go out bungee jumping afterwards just to relax. Charlie emphasized that "good education is good theatre." If you cannot keep someone's attention, you certainly cannot impart information. Similarly, it is tough to learn while you are sound asleep.

As G.K. Chesterton eloquently stated: "It isn't that they can't see the solution, it is that they can't see the problem." Charlie believed that real knowledge is always founded on a thoughtfully formulated question. In this 4th edition of *Surgical Secrets*, we have once again come up with new questions and challenged some of the answers to the old questions. That is what makes surgery gratifying, rewarding, stimulating, fun, and dynamic. Charlie was dynamic. This 4th edition is again dedicated to him and his love of dynamic dialogue. Charlie had a dog, but deep in his heart he disparaged dog owners as lightweights who don't have the courage to bite people themselves. So strap on your seat belts and let's take a cyclothymic roller-coaster ride through surgery and into the new millennium!

Alden H. Harken, M.D.
Ernest E. Moore, M.D.
Linda C. Belfus

I. General Topics

1. PREPARING FOR YOUR SURGERY ROTATION

Alden H. Harken, M.D.

Surgery is a participatory, team, and contact sport. Present yourself to patients, residents, and attendings with enthusiasm (which covers a multitude of sins), punctuality (type A people do not like to wait), and cleanliness (you must look, act, and smell like a doctor).

1. Why should you introduce yourself to each patient and ask about the chief complaint?
Symptoms are perception, and perception is more important than reality. To a patient, the chief complaint is not simply a matter of life and death—it is much more important. Patients routinely are placed into compromising, uncomfortable, embarrassing, and undignified predicaments. Patients, however, are people. They have interests, concerns, anxieties, and a story. As a student, you have an opportunity to place your patient's chief complaint into the context of the rest of his or her life. This skill is important, and the patient will *always* be grateful. You can serve a real purpose as a listener and translator for the patient and his or her family.

Patients want to trust and love you. This trust and belief in surgical therapy are formidable tools. The more a patient understands about his or her disease, the more the patient can participate in getting better. Recovery is faster if the patient helps. Similarly, the more the patient understands about his or her therapy (including its side effects and potential complications), the more effective the therapy is (this principle is not in the textbooks). You can be your patient's interpreter. This is the fun of surgery (and medicine).

2. What is scut work?
The word *scut* is derived from the Greek god Scutious Rex, who exhibited the tranquil consciousness of effortless superiority—a fundamental surgical attribute. Scut work is detail work that needs to be done. Always leap at the opportunity to shag x-rays, track down lab results, and retrieve a bag of blood from the bank. The team will recognize your enthusiasm and reward your contributions.

3. What is the best approach to surgical notes?
Surgical notes should be succinct. Most surgeons still move their lips when they read.
Admission orders
Admit to 5 West (attending's name)

Condition:	Stable
Diagnosis:	Abdominal pain; r/o appendicitis
Vital signs:	q 4 hours
Parameters:	Please call H.O. for:
	temp[erature] > 38° C
	160 < BP < 90
	120 < HR < 60
Diet:	NPO

Fluids   1000 LR w 20 mEq KCl @ 100 ml/HR
Med[ication]s: ASA 650 mg PR prn for T > 38.5
Thank you
Sign your name/leave space for resident's signature
(your beeper number)
Note: You cannot be too polite or too grateful to patients or nurses.

r/o = rule out, q = every, H.O. = house officer, BP = systolic blood pressure, HR = heart rate, NPO = nothing by mouth (this includes water and pills), ASA = aspirin, PR = per rectum, prn = as needed, T = temperature. Other useful abbreviations: OOB = out of bed, BRP = bathroom privileges.

History and physical examination (H & P)

Mrs. O'Flaherty is a 55 y/o w ♀ [white female] admitted for cc [chief complaint]: "my stomach hurts." Pt [patient] was in usual state of excellent health until 2 days PTA [prior to admission] when she noted gradual onset of crampy mid-epigastric pain. Pain is now severe (7/10—7 on a scale of 10) and recurrent q 5 minutes. Pt described + vomiting (+ bile, – blood) [with bile, without blood].

PMH [past medical history]
    Hosp[italizations]: Pneumonia (1991)
                        Childbirth (1970, 1972)
                        Surg[ery]—splenectomy for trauma (1967)
    Allergies: codeine, shellfish
    ETOH [alcohol]: social
    Tobacco: 1 ppd [pack per day] × 25 years
ROS [review of systems]
    Resp[iratory]: productive cough
    Cardiac: ō chest pain   [ō = not observed, noncontributory, or not there]
             ō MI [myocardial infarction]
    Renal: ō dysuria
           ō frequency
    Neuro[logic]: WNL [within normal limits]

Physical examination (P.E.)

BP: 140/90   H.R.: 100 (regular)
R.R. [respiratory rate]: 16 beats/min   Temp: 38.2°C

WD [well-developed], WN [well-nourished], mildly obese, 55 y/o ♀ in moderate abdominal distress.

HEENT [head, eyes, ears, nose, and throat]: WNL
Resp: Clear lungs bilat[erally]
                ō wheeze
Heart: ō m [murmur]
                RSR [regular sinus rhythm]
Abdomen: Mildly distended, crampy, mid-epigastric pain
                High-pitched rushes that coincide with crampy pain
                Tender to palpation (you do not need to hurt the patient to find this out)
                ō Rebound
Rectal: (Always do—never defer the rectal exam on your surgical rotation)
                Hematest—negative for blood
                No masses, no tenderness
Pelvic: No masses
                No adnexal tenderness
                No chandelier sign—if motion of cervix makes your patient hit the chandelier → pelvic inflammatory disease (PID: gonorrhea)
Extremities: Full ROM [range of motion]
                ō edema
                Bounding (3+) pulses

Imp[ression]:	Abdominal pain
	r/o SB [small bowel] obstruction 2° [secondary] to adhesions
Rx:	NG [nasogastric] tube
	IV fluids
	Op[erative] consent
	Type and hold
	Signature

Notes on the surgical H&P

- A surgical H&P should be succinct and focused on the patient's problem.
- Begin with the chief complaint (in the patient's words).
- Is the problem new or chronic?
- PMH: always include prior hospitalizations and medications.
- ROS: restrict review to organ systems (lung, heart, kidneys, and nervous system) that may affect this admission.
- P.E.: Always begin with vital signs (including respiration and temperature)—that is why these signs are vital.
- Rebound means inflammatory peritoneal irritation or peritonitis.

Preop[erative] note

The preoperative note is a check list confirming that both you and the patient are ready for the planned surgical procedure. Place this note in the Progress Notes:

Preop dx [diagnosis]:	SB obstruction 2° to adhesions
CXR [chest x-ray]:	Clear
ECG [electrocardiogram]:	NSR w/ST-T wave changes
Blood:	Type and cross-match × 2 units
Consent:	In chart

Operative note

The operative note should provide anyone who encounters the patient after surgery with all the needed information:

Preop dx:	SB obstruction
Postop dx:	Same, all bowel viable
Procedure:	Exp[loratory] Lap[arotomy] with lysis of adhesions
Surgeon:	Name him/her
Assistants:	List them
Anesthesia:	GEA [general endotracheal anesthesia]
I&O (in and out):	1200 ml Ringer's lactate (R/L) in
	Out: 400 ml urine
EBL [estimated blood loss]:	50 ml
Specimen:	None
Drains:	None
	Sign your name

2. CARDIOPULMONARY RESUSCITATION

Michael Grosso, M.D., and Alden H. Harken, M.D.

1. What is sudden cardiac death?

Sudden ventricular fibrillation. Numerous triggers have been postulated. Surprisingly, only 20% of patients resuscitated after an out-of-hospital episode of ventricular fibrillation exhibit electrocardiographic (EKG) evidence of a transmural myocardial infarction.

2. What is the dominant determinant of successful cardiopulmonary resuscitation (CPR)?

How soon you start. If effective CPR is initiated within 2 minutes of ventricular fibrillation, it is almost uniformly successful. If you begin CPR after 4 minutes, success plummets to 50%.

3. What are the ABCs?

Airway, breathing, and circulation. But things have changed. With a witnessed, in-hospital cardiac arrest, the most effective initial maneuver is electrical cardioversion—then proceed to secure an airway.

4. How do you electrically cardiovert (shock) a patient?

Place electrolyte (conductive) gel on the hand-held paddles. Place one paddle in the right subclavicular area and the other in the mid-axillary line at the level of the eighth intercostal space (over the apex of the heart). The cognoscenti now suggest that the first shock should be only 200 joules. When we are frightened (as we usually are), we typically crank the machine up to the top—360 joules.

5. Is there an immediate need for an oral, nasopharyngeal, or S-tube airway?

No. Although they may serve a useful function as a bite block, they also may induce vomiting or vocal cord spasm in a semiconscious patient.

6. What is the common cause of airway obstruction in an unconscious patient?

The epiglottis, not the tongue.

7. How do you establish an airway—even in a patient with suspected neck injury?

The three basic maneuvers are head tilt, chin tilt, and jaw thrust. In an unconscious patient, the jaw muscles relax. The jaw thrust actually subluxes the mandible, pulling the tongue and epiglottis anteriorly off the upper airway (with minimal cervical hyperextension).

8. Is endotracheal intubation mandatory?

No.
- Mouth-to-mouth ventilation delivers 16% inspired oxygen.
- Bag-mask ventilation delivers 21% oxygen.
- Bag-mask ventilation with an oxygen supply can deliver close to 100% oxygen.

9. What are the advantages of endotracheal intubation?

An absolutely secure airway. In addition, positive pressure breathing (mouth-to-mouth or bag-mask) can deliver significant amounts of air to the stomach. Gastric distention impairs diaphragmatic movement and may predispose to aspiration.

10. Does an endotracheal tube (even with the cuff up) prevent aspiration?

Unfortunately, no. If you place a couple of drops of methylene blue on the tongue of an intubated patient, you can suction "blue" from the other end of the tube (beyond the cuff) within 90 seconds.

11. What size endotracheal tube should you use?

Select a tube with an internal diameter equal to the width of the patient's thumbnail. For a 70-kg adult, an 8.0-mm tube is perfect.

12. Does an endotracheal tube produce significant airway resistance?

Surprisingly, no. Try it. Take a small (5.0-mm) tube, and breathe through it for a half hour. You will end up with drool all over your shirt, but otherwise you will not be uncomfortable.

13. How do you know if the endotracheal tube is in the proper position?

The quick and relatively reliable techniques to confirm appropriate endotracheal tube position are (1) to listen to both lung fields; (2) to observe symmetrical chest excursion with each tidal breath; (3) to listen over the epigastrium (you don't want to hear gurgles); and (4) to observe pink rather than cyanotic mucous membranes. Even if each of these criteria is met, you should confirm tube position as soon as possible by chest radiograph.

14. Which is preferred—oral or nasal intubation?

Oral intubation is the preferred method. The tube is visualized directly through the vocal cords, ensuring proper placement. Nasal intubation is a blind technique, relatively contraindicated in patients with maxillofacial trauma (because of the risk of intracranial placement of the tube through an anterior fossa fracture) and in patients with known or suspected coagulopathy (because nasal mucosa is well vascularized, intubation may cause major epistaxis). Conversely, in patients with suspected cervical spine injury, nasal intubation can be accomplished while maintaining cervical immobilization.

15. What is the role of an esophageal obturator airway (EOA)?

None. The EOA was adopted to eliminate the problem of gastric dilatation. The tube can be placed quickly. Successful attempts range from 96–99%. The major drawbacks are risk of esophageal perforation (low: 0.2–2%) and inadvertent tracheal placement preventing ventilation. No data indicate that the device is safe in patients with cervical spine injury; therefore, at present it is not recommended in trauma patients. In addition, the technique probably has no role in in-hospital resuscitation because other methods of airway control are accessible. At present the EOA is *not* indicated because alternative techniques (mask or endotracheal tube) are both safer and more effective.

16. What is the proper method of external chest compression?

Place the patient on a firm surface—typically the floor. The rescuer should be positioned beside the patient's chest. Both hands are placed at the compression point, which is located just above the xiphoid-sternal junction. Keep your arms straight and your shoulders directly over the patient's sternum. The compression depth should be 4–5 cm. Maintain hand position on the sternum at all times. With one rescuer: 15 compressions followed by 2 ventilations, then repeat cycle. With two rescuers: 5 compressions, 1 ventilation. Compression rates: one rescuer, 80/minute; two rescuers, 60/minute. Monitor the carotid pulse to assess effectiveness of CPR and return of spontaneous pulses.

17. What are the essentials of external chest compressions?

Effective CPR produces blood flow. Typically, one can produce a pulse and systolic blood pressure with adequate chest compression. However, to produce the blood flow and, in turn, tissue perfusion requires prolonging the compression phase. Increasing the compression phase from 30% to 50% more than *doubles* the flow. Compression rate is relatively unimportant. Rates between 40 and 80/minute produce comparable results.

18. What are the complications of external chest compressions?
   Complications of CPR are multiple and frequent. The rate of rib and sternal fracture ranges from 40–80%. Major cardiac or pericardial injuries (lacerations) are rare but may occur. Bone marrow and fat emboli are common—80% in one series. In addition, damage to intraabdominal organs (although uncommon) has been reported, including lacerations, contusions, and rupture of liver, spleen, kidneys, colon, stomach, and diaphragm. Strict attention to details of hand placement and compression depth minimizes complications.

19. Is the central line the best access to the circulation?
   Yes. Contrary to popular belief, however, large volumes of fluid can be delivered to the venous system more quickly via large-bore peripheral venous catheters. A 14-gauge, 5-cm catheter (peripheral) can deliver twice the flow of a 16-gauge, 20-cm catheter (central). Central line placement may be associated with significant complications, including pneumothorax, air embolus, and arterial puncture. In hypovolemic patients, in whom central veins are collapsed and peripheral veins are constricted, venous cannulation can be frustratingly difficult. Conversely, in the 55-year-old cigar-chomping banker in the cardiac care unit (CCU) suffering postinfarction cardiogenic shock, all of the blood volume is back up behind his heart—suffusing his veins.

20. Does a central line offer both therapeutic and diagnostic advantages?
   Yes. A central line permits direct delivery of drugs to the right side of the heart. A central line also permits blood gas sampling.

21. Is it necessary to monitor arterial blood gases during resuscitation?
   No, but close control of acid-base status is essential. Central venous blood gases provide clinically relevant information about acid-base status:

$$\text{Venous pH} + 0.05 = \text{arterial pH}$$
$$\text{Venous PCO}_2 - 5 \text{ mmHg} = \text{arterial PCO}_2$$

After you have adequate airway control and presumably are delivering 100% oxygen, you don't care what the arterial PO_2 is because you can do nothing about it. With a central line in place, frequent venous sampling is easy. To stick the femoral artery reliably and repeatedly during active CPR is incredibly difficult.

22. Which is preferred—colloid or crystalloid resuscitation fluid?
   Data support both sides. Colloid advocates claim that the solutions remain primarily in the intravascular space and thereby are more effective in elevating blood volume. Crystalloid advocates state that capillaries will leak albumin in the shock state. Many studies have shown that resuscitation with crystalloid is safe, especially with respect to pulmonary complications. Given its availability, low cost, and safety, crystalloid (lactated Ringer's solution) is the present choice for initial fluid resuscitation.

23. In a patient exhibiting asystole or fine fibrillation, what is your primary goal?
   To produce good, coarse fibrillation. It should be easy to cardiovert (shock) coarse fibrillation into a regular ventricular mechanism.

24. How do you convert fine fibrillation into coarse fibrillation?
   Normal acid-base status helps. By frequent monitoring of central venous blood gases (see question 21), you can give bicarbonate and control minute ventilation in a fashion that normalizes

pH and PCO_2, respectively. When acid-base status is okay, give 1 gm calcium gluconate and 1 mg (not microgram) of high-dose epinephrine. Repeat every 5 minutes.

25. Then what do you do?

As soon as you see good, coarse fibrillation on the EKG monitor, proceed with electrical cardioversion (see question 4).

26. What are the common causes of electromechanical dissociation (EMD)? How are they best treated?

EMD is defined as pulseless electrical activity, which is an orderly electrical rhythm in the absence of detectable blood pressure. In the setting of cardiac arrest, initial treatment consists of intravenous calcium chloride. Keep in mind the potentially correctable situations that commonly cause EMD: (1) tension pneumothorax (diagnosis: hyperresonant chest, decreased breath sounds), which is alleviated by placement of a large-bore needle into the pleural space on the side of the collapsed lung, and (2) pericardial tamponade (diagnosis: Beck's triad—distant heart sounds, distended neck veins/elevated central venous pressure, and hypotension), which is relieved by pericardiocentesis. EMD also is associated with hypovolemia (which already should have been corrected), ventricular rupture (traumatic or secondary to myocardial infarction), pulmonary embolism, and pump failure secondary to massive myocardial infarction.

27. List the drugs commonly used during resuscitation and the appropriate dosages.

1. **Oxygen:** to reverse hypoxia, always provide 100% oxygen; measurable pulmonary toxicity has not been detected in less than 36 hours.

2. **Sodium bicarbonate** ($NaHCO_3$): to reverse acidosis (hypoxia-induced anaerobic metabolism leads to acid accumulation; ventilatory failure leads to carbon dioxide retention [acidosis]). The initial dose is 1 mEq/kg. One ampule (50 ml) contains 50 mEq of sodium bicarbonate. Bicarbonate combines with hydrogen ions to form carbon dioxide and water; thus, adequate ventilation is required for bicarbonate therapy to be fully effective. Overzealous use of bicarbonate may result in hypokalemia (alkalosis shifts potassium ions intracellulary) and hypernatremia/hyperosmolality (each HCO_3^- is accompanied by a sodium ion).

3. **Epinephrine:** alpha- and beta-adrenergic agonist. Intravenous dosage is 5–10 ml of 1:10,000 solution. Because of the short duration of action, a repeat dose may be necessary after 5 minutes. Epinephrine is inactivated by alkali; do not mix with bicarbonate solutions. Although enhancing myocardial performance, epinephrine greatly increases myocardial oxygen demand. Ventilate!

4. **Calcium chloride or gluconate:** positive inotropic agent. Calcium ions bind to troponin (the cardiomyocyte-specific calcium regulatory protein that we use to diagnose an acute myocardial infarction), which enhances the formation of cross-bridges between muscle contractile filaments with resultant fiber shortening. Dose: calcium chloride (or gluconate), 500 mg IV push. Do not mix with bicarbonate because it will precipitate.

5. **Atropine:** parasympatholytic (vagolytic) agent that increases the discharge rate of the sinus (SA) node. Atropine is useful in treating sinus bradycardia associated with hemodynamic compromise. Dose of 0.5 mg IV is repeated at 5-minute intervals until a desirable rate is achieved (at least 60 beats/min). Increased heart rate increases myocardial oxygen demand; atropine should be used only if the bradycardia causes hemodynamic compromise (heart rate less than 60 beats/min).

6. **Lidocaine:** local anesthetic that suppresses ventricular arrhythmias (automatic and reentrant; see next chapter). An IV bolus of 1 mg/kg is followed by IV infusion at 2–4 mg/min. An additional IV bolus can be given at 10 minutes after initial dose if arrhythmias persist. Toxicity is limited to the central nervous systems and does not occur with a total dose less than 500 mg. Serious side effects include focal and grand mal seizures, which are treated with diazepam (5 mg IV).

7. **Bretylium tosylate:** a postganglionic adrenergic blocker with positive inotropic and antiarrhythmic effects that elevates ventricular fibrillation threshold (as does lidocaine). But because it is an alpha blocker, blood pressure drops. For ventricular tachycardia, infuse 500 mg over 8–10 minutes.

8. **Verapamil:** slow-channel calcium blocker used to block the AV node and to treat paroxysmal supraventricular tachycardia that causes hemodynamic compromise. Dose: 0.1 mg/kg. Dilute dose with 10 ml saline, and infuse 1 ml/min until the supraventricular tachycardia either breaks or blocks. Repeat dose after 30 minutes if not effective. The drug reduces systemic vascular resistance; therefore, blood pressure should be monitored closely during its use. A well-known property of verapamil is its direct depression of cardiac contractility, but *cardiac output* usually remains unchanged because of reflex sympathetic response.

9. **Adenosine:** a naturally occurring vasodilating hormone that is synthesized by vascular endothelial cells and dramatically slows AV nodal conduction. It is, therefore, useful in the therapy of supraventricular tachyarrhythmias. The dose is 6 mg injected in a rapid intravenous bolus (which may be repeated several times). The half-life of intravenous adenosine is only 12 seconds. Measurable systemic hypotension occurs in less than 2% of patients because adenosine is metabolized before it hits the systemic vessels.

BIBLIOGRAPHY

1. Lowenstein SR: Cardiopulmonary resuscitation in non-injured patients. In Wilmore DW, Cheung L, Harken AH, et al (eds): Scientific American Surgery, Vol. 1. New York, Scientific American, 1999.
2. Ballew KA: Cardiopulmonary resuscitation. BMJ 314:1462–1465, 1997.
3. Behringer W, Kittler H, Sterz F, et al: Cumulative epinephrine dose during cardiopulmonary resuscitation and neurologic outcome. Ann Intern Med 129:450–456, 1998.
4. Cummins RO, Hazinksi MF: The next chapter in the high-dose epinephrine story: Unfavorable neurologic outcomes? Ann Intern Med 129:501–502, 1998.
5. Frishman WH, Vahdat S, Bhatta S: Innovative pharmacologic approaches to cardiopulmonary resuscitation. J Clin Pharmacol 38:765–772, 1998.
6. Safar P, Bircher N, Pretto E Jr, et al: Reappraisal of mouth-to-mouth ventilation during bystander-initiated CPR. Circulation 98:608–610, 1998.

3. CARDIAC DYSRHYTHMIAS
Alden H. Harken, M.D.

1. Are cardiac dysrhythmias and cardiac arrhythmias the same?

Yes. Some purists will tell you that an arrhythmia can be only the absence of a cardiac rhythm. But these are the same purists who use the word *iatrogenic* to mean "caused by a doctor." The only things that can be truly iatrogenic are, of course, a physician's parents.

2. Are all cardiac dysrhythmias clinically important?

Most are not. Many of us have isolated premature ventricular contractions (PVCs) or depolarizations (PVDs) all of the time. And superbly conditioned athletes frequently exhibit resting heart rates in the thirties. A clinically important cardiac dysrhythmia is a rhythm that bothers the patient. As a rule, if the patient's ventricular rate is between 60 and 100 beats/min (regardless of mechanism), cardiac rhythm is not a problem.

3. What are your goals in the treatment of cardiac dysrhythmias?

Primary goal: to control ventricular rate between 60 and 100.
Secondary goal: to maintain sinus rhythm.

4. How important is sinus rhythm?

It depends on the patient's ventricular function. Induction of atrial fibrillation in a medical student volunteer causes no measurable hemodynamic effect. Your ventricular compliance is so good that you do not need an atrial "kick" to fill the ventricle completely. Conversely, the worse the patient's heart, the more you should try to maintain sinus rhythm. We once observed a patient with a 7% left ventricular ejection fraction who dropped his cardiac output by 40% when he spontaneously developed atrial fibrillation.

5. Do you need to be ankle-deep in EKG paper and personally acquainted with Drs. Mobitz, Lown, and Ganong to treat cardiac arrhythmias in the intensive care unit (ICU)?

No.

6. When you are called by the ICU nurse to see a patient with an "arrhythmia," what questions do you ask yourself?

1. *Does the patient really exhibit an arrhythmia?* Is the stuff that looks like ventricular fibrillation (VF) really just the patient brushing his teeth? Or is the rhythm strip that looks like asystole really just a loose lead? If the patient does exhibit an arrhythmia, ask yourself the following questions.

2. *Does the arrhythmia require intervention?* Isolated PVCs usually can be ignored safely. Similarly, a resting bradycardia in a triathlete is normal. This is the occasion to launch into your "two-second physical exam"—is the patient sweaty and confused or alert and happy?

3. *What is a two-second physical exam?* You look into the patient's eyes, hoping to determine whether he or she is perfusing his or her brain. If the patient looks back at you, you have some time. If the patient requires therapy, ask yourself the following questions.

4. *How soon is therapy required?* At this point the patient becomes (paradoxically) irrelevant. The most robust indicator dictating velocity of intervention is not how sick the patient is, but how frightened *you* are. The dean may have had his carotid arteries firmly ligated years ago. Conversely, to match the surgical residency of your choice, you need to be firing on a lot more cylinders than the dean. Thus, you must determine rapidly whether delay in therapy is likely to put the patient at risk. If the cardiac arrhythmia is likely to inflict psychopathologic (hypoxemic) consequences not only on the patient but also, by extension, on his or her extended (societal) family, *you* should be frightened. If you are frightened, you must ask yourself:

5. *What is the safest and most effective therapy?*

7. If the patient requires antiarrhythmic therapy, what is the safest and most effective strategy?

Although our cardiology colleagues try to complicate the issue, therapy for cardiac arrhythmias is startlingly simple—indeed, whole volumes about cardiac arrhythmias can be distilled into three comprehensible concepts:

1. If the patient is hemodynamically unstable (again, the sole determinant of instability is whether *you* are frightened), cardiovert with 360 joules.

2. If the patient has a wide-complex tachycardia, cardiovert with 360 joules.

3. If the patient has a narrow-complex tachycardia, infuse intravenously an AV nodal blocker. If at any time the patient becomes unstable, proceed with cardioversion.

8. In assessing a cardiac impulse, how do you distinguish supraventricular from ventricular origin?

Supraventricular origin. When an impulse originates above the AV node (supraventricular), it can access the ventricles only through the AV node. The AV node connects with the endocardial Purkinje system, which conducts impulses quite rapidly (2–3 meters/sec). Thus, a supraventricular impulse activates the ventricles quite rapidly (< 0.08 sec, 80 msec, or two little boxes on the EKG paper), producing a narrow-complex beat.

Ventricular origin. When an impulse originates directly from an ectopic site on the ventricle, it takes longer to access the high-speed Purkinje system. Thus, a ventricular impulse activates the entire ventricular mass slowly (> 0.08 sec, 80 msec, or two little boxes on the EKG paper), producing a wide-complex beat.

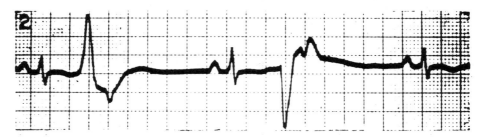

Wide complex beats are of ventricular origin. Narrow complex beats are of supraventricular origin.

9. Do all wide-complex beats derive from the ventricles?

No—but most do. An impulse of supraventricular origin that is conducted with aberrancy through the ventricle can take enough time to make it a wide-complex beat. In one study, 89% of 100 patients presenting to an emergency department with a wide-complex tachycardia eventually proved to exhibit ventricular tachycardia, whereas 11% were diagnosed with supraventricular tachycardia with aberrancy.

10. What do you do if you cannot tell whether a ventricular complex is wide or narrow?

Acutely and transiently (for 5 seconds) block the AV node by giving 6 mg of adenosine IV; if the ventricular complex persists, it is ventricular. if the ventricular complex stops, it was supraventricular.

11. To prevent lots of supraventricular impulses from getting to the ventricles, how do you block the AV node pharmacologically?

- In **seconds**: give 6 mg adenosine IV push.
- In **minutes**: draw up 10 mg verapamil (calcium channel blocker) in 10 ml saline and give 1 ml/min IV.
- In **hours**: put 0.5 mg digoxin in 100 ml Ringer's lactate and infuse by IV drip over 30 min.

12. Why give digoxin?

Digoxin is an effective AV nodal blocker, but it actually makes cardiomyocytes *more* excitable. By giving digoxin, you make supraventricular impulses *more* likely; but by blocking the AV node, you render these impulses *less* dangerous.

13. Why infuse digoxin over 30–60 minutes IV?

Studies indicate that a big pulse of digoxin (IV push) concentrates in the myocardium, making the myocytes hyperexcitable. Digoxin infused more slowly avoids this problem.

14. What are the steps in calling a dysrhythmia by name?

- **Bradycardia:** < 60 beats/min (bpm)
- **Tachycardia:** 100–250 bpm
- **Flutter:** atrial or ventricular rate between 250 and 400 bpm
- **Fibrillation:** atrial or ventricular rate above 400 bpm

15. *Extra credit:* **Correlate the EKG with cardiomyocyte membrane ion flux.**

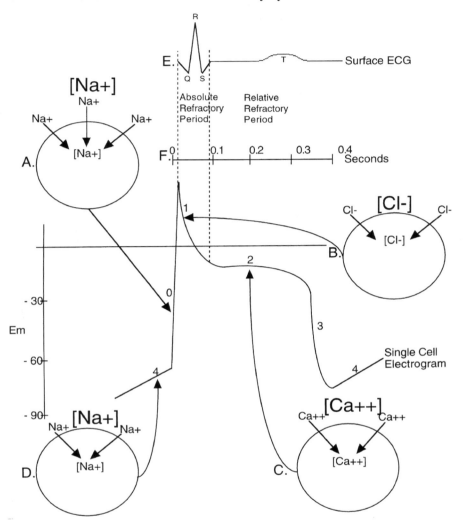

Typical action potential of a cardiac myocyte, the ionic shifts responsible for each phase, and correlation with the surface EKG. *A,* Phase 0 = rapid depolarization, characterized by rapid influx of sodium (Na$^+$) through the voltage-gated Na$^+$ channels. *B,* Phase 1 = brief repolarization, characterized by transient influx of chloride (Cl$^-$). *C,* Phase 2 = plateau phase, characterized by a rapid rise in calcium (Ca^{2+}) permeability through L-type Ca^{2+} channels. Phase 3 = repolarization with potassium (K$^+$) exiting the cell. *D,* Slow depolarization of pacemaker cells caused by slow influx of Na$^+$. (From Meldrum DR, Cleveland JC, Sheridan BC, et al: Cardiac surgical implications of calcium dyshomeostasis in the heart. Ann Thorac Surg 61:1273–1280, 1996, with permission.)

BIBLIOGRAPHY

Harken AH: Cardiac dysrhythmias. In Wilmore DW, Cheung L, Harken AH, et al (eds): Scientific American Surgery. New York, Scientific American, 1999.

4. SHOCK

Alden H. Harken, M.D.

1. What is shock?
Shock is: Not just low blood pressure
              Not just decreased peripheral perfusion
              Not just limited systemic oxygen delivery
Ultimately, shock is decreased tissue respiration. Shock is suboptimal consumption of oxygen and excretion of carbon dioxide at the cellular level.

2. Is shock related to cardiac output?
Of course. However, a healthy medical student can redistribute blood flow preferentially to vital organs.

3. Is organ perfusion democratic?
Absolutely not. Limited blood flow is always redirected toward the carotid and coronary arteries. Peripheral vasoconstriction steals blood initially from the mesentery, then skeletal muscle, then kidneys and liver.

4. Is this vascular autoregulatory capacity uniform in all patients?
No. With age and atherosclerosis, patients lose their ability to redistribute limited blood flow. Thus, a 20% decrease in cardiac output (or a fall in blood pressure to 90 mmHg) can be life-threatening to a Supreme Court justice, whereas it may be undetectable in a triathlete.

5. For diagnostic and therapeutic purposes, can shock be usefully classified?
Yes.
1. **Hypovolemic shock** mandates volume resuscitation.
2. **Cardiogenic shock** mandates cardiac stimulation (both pharmacologic and eventually mechanical).
3. **Peripheral vascular collapse shock** mandates pharmacologic manipulation of the peripheral vascular tone (and direct attention to the etiology of the vasodilation—typically sepsis).

6. Is it advisable to treat all shock in the same sequential fashion?
Ultimately, yes. Whether a cigar-chomping banker presents with a big GI bleed (hypovolemic shock) or crushing substernal chest pain (cardiogenic shock), the surgeon should take, in order, the following steps:
1. Optimize volume status; give volume until further increase in right-sided (central venous pressure) and left-sided (pulmonary capillary wedge pressure) preload confers no additional benefit for cardiac output or blood pressure. (This step is pure Starling's law—place the patient's heart at the top of the Starling curve.)
2. If cardiac output, blood pressure, and tissue perfusion remain inadequate despite adequate preload, the patient has a pump (cardiogenic shock) problem. Infuse cardiac inotropic drugs (beta agonist) to the point of toxicity (typically cardiac ectopy—lots of frightening, premature ventricular contractions. For pharmacologically refractory cardiogenic shock, insert an intraaortic balloon pump IABP).
3. If the patient exhibits a surprisingly high cardiac output and a paradoxically low blood pressure (such unusual loss of vascular autoregulatory control is associated typically—but not always—with sepsis), the surgeon may infuse a peripheral vasoconstrictor drug (alpha agonist).

7. What is the preferred access route for volume infusion?
Flow depends on catheter length and radius. Volume may be infused at twice the rate through a 5-cm, 14-gauge peripheral catheter as through a 20-cm, 16-gauge central line (see chapter 1). Assessment of central venous pressure (and left-sided filling pressure) may be necessary if the patient fails to respond to initial volume resuscitation.

8. Should one infuse crystalloid, colloid, or blood?
If the goal is only to improve preload and thus to repair cardiac output and blood pressure, crystalloid solution should be sufficient. It is controversial whether infused colloid remains in the vascular compartment. If the goal is to augment systemic oxygen delivery, red cells bind **much more** oxygen than plasma (see chapter 4).

9. When cardiac preload is adequate, what inotropic agents are useful?
The array of agents is mind-boggling. Pick several and get comfortable with them. Dobutamine, epinephrine, and norepinephrine are the chocolate, vanilla, and strawberry of the 32 flavors of cardiogenic drugs. These three drugs are all that the surgeon needs.

10. Is dopamine the same as dobutamine?
No. Dopamine stimulates renal dopaminergic receptors and may be quite useful in low doses (2 µg/kg/min) to counteract the renal arteriolar vasoconstriction that accompanies shock. Dopamine has no place as a primary cardiac inotropic agent.

11. Discuss the use of dobutamine, epinephrine, and norepinephrine.
Dobutamine is a beta-1 agonist (cardiac inotrope), but also has some beta-2 effects (peripheral vasodilation).
Start at: 5 µg/kg/min and increase to point of toxicity (cardiac ectopy).
Note: Infuse to desired effect (do not stick rigidly to a preconceived dose). Because dobutamine has some vasodilating effects, it may be difficult to infuse into typically hypotensive patients in shock.
Epinephrine is a combined beta- and alpha-adrenergic agonist, with the beta effects predominating at lower doses.
Start at: 0.05 µg/kg/min and increase to point of toxicity (cardiac ectopy).
Note: As with dobutamine, infuse to desired effect.
Norepinephrine is a combined alpha- and beta-adrenergic agonist, with the alpha effects predominating at all doses.
Start at: 0.5 µgkg/min and increase to point of toxicity (cardiac ectopy).
Note: Relatively pure peripheral vasoconstriction is uncommonly indicated and should be used only to modulate the peripheral vascular tone in peripheral vascular collapse shock.

12. When is an intraaortic balloon pump (IABP) indicated?
Mechanical circulatory support is indicated when the preload to both ventricles (CVP and PCWP) has been optimized and further cardiac stimulatory drugs are limited by frightening runs of premature ventricular contractions.

13. What does an IABP do?
Diastolic augmentation and systolic unloading.

14. What is diastolic augmentation?
A soft 40-ml balloon is inserted percutaneously through the common femoral artery into the descending thoracic aorta. The balloon is not occlusive, and it should not touch the walls of the aorta. When it is inflated, it is exactly like acutely transfusing 40 ml of blood into the aorta, thus

augmenting each left ventricular stroke volume by 40 ml. Balloon infusion is triggered off the QRS complex from a surface ECG (any lead). The balloon is always inflated during diastole to increase diastolic blood pressure and thus augment coronary blood flow (CBF). Eighty percent of CBF occurs during diastole.

15. What is systolic unloading?

Balloon deflation is an active (not a passive) process. Helium is abruptly sucked out of the balloon, leaving a 40-ml empty space in the aorta. The left ventricle can eject the first 40 ml of its stroke volume into this empty space—at dramatically reduced workload. An intraaortic balloon, therefore, increases coronary oxygen delivery (CBF) while decreasing cardiac oxygen consumption.

16. What are the contraindications to IABP?

Aortic insufficiency: diastolic augmentation distends and injures the left ventricle.
Atrial fibrillation: balloon inflation and deflation cannot be appropriately timed.

BIBLIOGRAPHY

Holcroft JW: Shock. In Wilmore DW, Cheung L, Harken AH, et al (eds): Scientific American Surgery. New York, Scientific American, 1999.

---

5. PULMONARY INSUFFICIENCY

Alden H. Harken, M.D.

---

1. What is pulmonary insufficiency?

The alveolar-capillary surface of the lung is the size of a singles tennis court. The purpose of the lung is to match alveolar ventilation (Va) to blood flow (Q). Mismatching leads to pulmonary insufficiency.

2. How is Va/Q mismatching characterized?

Shunt: decreased ventilation relative to regional blood flow
Dead space: decreased regional blood flow relative to ventilation

3. How much energy is expended in the work of breathing?

A healthy medical student expends about 3% of total oxygen consumption (energy utilization) on work of breathing. After injury, particularly a big burn, patients may increase fractional energy expenditure of breathing by as much as 20%.

4. What surgical incisions most significantly compromise a patient's vital capacity?

Intuitively, an extremity incision or injury influences vital capacity least, followed sequentially by a lower abdominal incision, median sternotomy, thoracotomy, and upper abdominal incision. An upper abdominal incision is worse than a thoracotomy.

5. Is a chest radiograph helpful in assessing respiratory failure?

Of course it is. But the radiograph must be interpreted carefully.

6. What should one look for on the chest radiograph of a patient with impending respiratory failure?
1. Are both lungs fully expanded?
2. Are there localized areas of infiltrate, atelectasis, or consolidation?
3. Are there generalized areas of infiltrate, atelectasis, or consolidation?
4. Are the endotracheal and other tubes in proper position?

7. Why is the local vs. generalized distinction important in assessing respiratory failure?
A local process may be assessed by aspiration or bronchoscopy to diagnose pneumonia or tumor. Generalized multilobar infiltrates are more likely to represent a diffuse alveolar-capillary leak syndrome such as ARDS.

8. What is ARDS?
Adult respiratory distress syndrome (ARDS) is a diffuse, multilobar capillary transudation of fluid into the pulmonary interstitium that dissociates the normal concordance of alveolar ventilation (Va) with lung perfusion (Q).

9. What governs fluid flux across pulmonary capillaries into the interstitium of the lung?
Starling initially described the balance between intravascular hydrostatic pressure (Pc), which tends to push fluid out of the capillaries, and colloid oncotic pressure (COP), which sucks fluid back in across the capillary endothelial barrier (K). Thus:

$$\text{Fluid flux} = K(Pc - COP)$$

10. What causes ARDS?
Anything that increases lung dysfunction by promoting wet lung:
1. **Heart failure** backs up pulmonary intravascular hydrostatic pressures (Pc), forcing fluid into the pulmonary interstitium.
2. **Malnutrition and liver failure** decrease plasma protein and thus COP. Fluid is not sucked back out of the lung (if the total protein and albumin are low).
3. **Sepsis** may break down the capillary endothelial barrier (K), thus permitting water and protein to leak into the lung.

11. What is high-pressure vs. low-pressure ARDS?
Purists appropriately note that lung congestion due to high intravascular hydrostatic pressure secondary to heart failure is really not primary respiratory distress syndrome. Thus, if the pulmonary capillary wedge pressure (PCWP) is greater than 18 mmHg, the diagnosis is high-pressure pulmonary edema (not ARDS).

12. What is a normal colloid osmotic pressure?
COP is normally 22 mmHg.

13. How is COP calculated?
Seventy-five percent of COP is normally created by serum albumin along with globulins and fibrinogen. Thus:

$$COP = 2.1 \text{ (total protein)}$$

If an osmotically active molecule such as hetastarch is infused, this calculation is fouled up.

14. What is low-pressure ARDS?
Low-pressure ARDS is a redundant term. To make the diagnosis of ARDS, the PCWP must be less than 18 mmHg. Better yet, pure ARDS exists only if the PCWP is more than 4 mmHg less than the COP.

15. How can the pulmonary capillaries leak if the COP exceeds the PCWP?

The current concept involves a septic expression of neutrophil CD11 and CD18 adhesion receptors, which stick to pulmonary vascular endothelial intercellular adhesion molecules (ICAM). Furthermore, septic stimuli provoke the adherent neutrophils to release intravascular proteases and oxygen radicals. Resultant endovascular damage breaks down the capillary endothelial barrier (K), permitting the lung leak—even at low hydrostatic pressure.

16. What is a Lasix sandwich?

Most surgeons, when their backs are against the wall, give 25 gm of albumin followed in 20 minutes by 20 mg Lasix IV. They reason that the albumin pulls fluid out of the water-logged lung and that the Lasix promotes diuresis to rid the patient of extra water. This therapeutic concept probably works only in patients who are not very sick. The sicker the patient, the faster the infused albumin leaks and equilibrates across the damaged endovascular endothelial barrier. Thus, little water is sucked out of the sick lung in preparation for diuresis.

17. What are the goals of the therapy for ARDS?

1. Reduce lung edema.
2. Reduce oxygen toxicity (inspired O_2 concentration < 60% is safe).
3. Limit lung barotrauma (avoid peak inspiratory pressure in excess of 40 cmH$_2$O).
4. Promote matching of ventilation (Va) and perfusion (Q).
5. Maintain systemic oxygen delivery (arterial oxygen content x cardiac output).

18. What governs the distribution of lung perfusion (Q)?

Mostly gravity. Thus, the dependent portions of the lung are always better perfused.

19. What is hypoxic pulmonary vasoconstriction (HPV)?

Most students believe that after dedicating the entire second year of medical school to pheochromocytoma and HPV, both entities may be safely forgotten. At least in the case of HPV, this is not true. A patient who has just undergone carotid endarterectomy illustrates the relevance of HPV. As the patient awakens from anesthesia, the blood pressure is 220/120 mmHg and arterial PO$_2$ with 100% oxygen is 500 mmHg. So that the patient will not blow the carotid anastomosis, the surgeon urgently infuses nitroprusside. In 20 minutes the blood pressure is 120/80, but PO$_2$ (still with 100% oxygen) has dropped to 125 mmHg!

Did the lab technician screw up the blood gas analysis? No—this is an example of the clinical significance of HPV, which directs pulmonary arteriolar delivery of deoxygenated blood toward ventilated alveoli and away from poorly ventilated lung regions. The patient was using HPV to attain a PO$_2$ of 500 mmHg. But all antihypertensive agents (such as nitroprusside) and most general anesthetics block HPV. Thus, the PO$_2$ increment from 125 to 500 mmHg is all due to HPV. HPV beautifully steered perfusion toward ventilated areas of the lung.

20. What governs the distribution of ventilation (Va) in lung?

A large pleural pressure gradient (more negative at the top of the lung by 20 cmH$_2$O) squeezes gas primarily out of the dependent lung during each exhaled breath. Thus, the regional compliance of dependent lung is much better than that of lung apex, which is still distended with gas at end of exhalation. Therefore, the usual approach is to perfuse and ventilate dependent lung preferentially.

21. How does ARDS compromise lung function?

The trachea is held open with cartilaginous rings, but terminal bronchioles are not. Wet lung collapses the terminal bronchioles, thus trapping distal alveolar gas. Persistent perfusion of these poorly ventilated regions is a shunt that results in hypoxia.

22. How long does it take for pulmonary arterial (deoxygenated) blood to equilibrate completely with trapped alveolar gas?

About three-fourths of a second. After that, no more oxygen is added and no more carbon dioxide is eliminated from the perfusing blood. Terminal bronchiolar closure producing trapped alveolar gas is bad.

23. What is the therapy for terminal airways closure and resultant shunt secondary to the wet lung of ARDS?

Positive end-expiratory pressure (PEEP) should hold open terminal bronchioles, thus promoting ventilation of previously trapped alveoli and minimizing the shunt.

24. When may the patient come off mechanical ventilation and be extubated safely?

The patient should be sufficiently alert to protect his airway, require an inspired oxygen concentration no greater than $FiO_2 = 0.4$, and be comfortable breathing on a T-piece (without mechanical ventilation) for 60 minutes at a respiratory rate less than 20 and a minute ventilation less than 10 L/min. The patient should be able to generate a negative inspiratory force (NIF) greater than -20 cmH_2O. Finally, after 1 hour on the T-piece oxygenation should provide a hemoglobin saturation greater than 85% without respiratory acidosis (see chapter 5).

25. What is nitric oxide (NO)?

Nitric oxide is synthesized in vascular endothelial cells both by constitutive nitric oxide synthase (cNOS) and inducible NOS (iNOS). Intuitively, inhaled NO should diffuse across ventilated alveoli to increase regional perfusion and improve matching of Va/Q.

26. Does inhaled NO work in ARDS?

Almost two dozen randomized controlled clinical trials have assessed the therapeutic efficacy of inhaled NO. Although systemic oxygenation and pulmonary hypertension improve transiently, ventilator time and ultimate survival are not influenced. Just say NO.

BIBLIOGRAPHY

1. Davidson TA, Caldwell ES, Curtis JR, et al: Reduced quality of life in survivors of acute respiratory distress syndrome compared with critically ill control patients. JAMA 281:354–360, 1999.
2. Ferreira E, Shalansky SJ: Nitric oxide for ARDS—what is the evidence? Pharmacotherapy 19:60–69, 1999.
3. Gust R, McCarthy TJ, Kozlowski J, et al: Response to inhaled nitric oxide in acute lung injury depends on distribution of pulmonary blood flow prior to its administration. Am J Respir Crit Care Med 159:563–570, 1999.
4. Marini JJ, Hotchkiss JR Jr: PEEP in the prone position: Reversing the perfusion imbalance. Crit Care Med 27:1–2, 1999.
5. Pesenti A, Fumagalli R: PEEP: Blood gas cosmetics or a therapy for ARDS? Crit Care Med 27:253–254, 1999.

6. ARTERIAL BLOOD GASES

Alden H. Harken, M.D.

1. Mr. O'Flaherty has just undergone an inguinal herniorrhaphy under local anesthesia. The recovery room nurse asks permission to sedate him. She says that he is confused and unruly and keeps trying to get out of bed. Is it safe to sedate Mr. O'Flaherty?

Absolutely not. A confused, agitated patient in the recovery room or surgical intensive care unit (SICU) **must** be recognized as acutely hypoxemic until proved otherwise.

2. Mr. O'Flaherty is moved to the SICU. At 2:00 AM the SICU calls to report that Mr. O'Flaherty has a PO$_2$ of 148 mmHg on face mask oxygen. Is it okay to roll over and go back to sleep?
Absolutely not. More information is needed.

3. You glance at the abandoned cup of coffee sitting on your well-worn copy of *Surgical Secrets*. What is the PO$_2$ of that cup of coffee?
148 mmHg.

4. How can Mr. O'Flaherty and the coffee have the same PO$_2$?
The abandoned coffee has presumably had time to equilibrate completely with atmospheric gas. At sea level the barometric pressure is 760 mmHg. To obtain the partial pressure of oxygen in the coffee, subtract water vapor pressure (47 mmHg) and multiply by the concentration of oxygen (20.8%) in the atmosphere. Thus:

$$PO_2 = (760 - 47) \times 20.8\% = 148 \text{ mmHg}$$

5. What is the difference between Mr. O'Flaherty's and the coffee's PO$_2$?
Nothing. Both represent the partial pressure of oxygen in fluid. A complete set of blood gases is necessary.

6. What is a complete set of blood gases?
PO$_2$
PCO$_2$
pH
Hemoglobin saturation
Hemoglobin concentration

7. If Mr. O'Flaherty and the coffee have the same PO$_2$, how would Mr. O'Flaherty do if he were exchange-transfused with coffee?
Badly.

8. Why?
Although the oxygen tensions are the same, the **amount** of oxygen in blood is vastly greater.

9. How does one quantitate the amount of oxygen in blood?
Arterial oxygen content (CaO$_2$) is quantitated as ml of oxygen /100 ml of blood. (**Watch out:** almost all other concentrations are traditionally provided per ml or per liter—**not** per 100 ml.) Because ml of oxygen is a volume in 100 ml of blood, these units are frequently abbreviated as vol. %.

10. Why is blood thicker than coffee (or wine)?
Because hemoglobin binds a huge amount of oxygen. Ten grams of fully saturated hemoglobin (hematocrit about 30%) binds 13.4 ml of oxygen, whereas 100 ml of plasma at a PO$_2$ of 100 mmHg contains only 0.3 ml of oxygen.

11. Does the position of the oxyhemoglobin dissociation curve make any difference?
• An increase in PCO$_2$.
• An increase in hydrogen ion concentrations (**not** pH).
• An increase in temperature.
All shift the oxyhemoglobin curve to the right; that is, oxygen is released more easily in the tissues. Within physiologic limits, however, Mae West probably said it best: "There is less to this than meets the eye."

12. If arterial oxygen content (CaO_2) or ultimately systemic oxygen delivery (cardiac output × CaO_2) is what the surgeon really wants to know, why does the nurse report Mr. O'Flaherty's PO_2 instead of his CaO_2 at 2:00 am?

No one knows.

13. What is the fastest and most practical method of increasing Mr. O'Flaherty's arterial oxygen content?

Transfusion of red blood cells. The patient's arterial oxygen content is increased by 25% with transfusion from a hemoglobin concentration of 8 to 10 gm%. The patient's arterial oxygen content is affected negligibly by an increase in arterial PO_2 from 100 to 200 mmHg (hemoglobin is fully saturated in both instances).

14. What is a transfusion trigger?

The hematocrit at which a patient is automatically transfused. This is **not** a useful concept. The NIH Consensus Conference, drawing data from Jehovah's Witnesses, patients with renal failure, and monkeys concluded that it is not necessary to transfuse a patient until the hematocrit reaches 21%. Traditional surgical dogma mandates a hematocrit above 30%. When the patient is in trouble, however, authorities in surgical critical care encourage transfusion to a hematocrit of 45% to optimize systemic oxygen delivery.

15. What governs respiratory drive?

PCO_2 and pH are inextricably intertwined by the Henderson-Hasselbach equation. By juggling this equation in the cerebrospinal fluid (CSF) of goats, it is clear that CSF hydrogen ion concentration (not PCO_2) controls respiratory drive. However, this distinction is not clinically important. What is important is that if a person becomes acidotic either with diabetic ketoacidosis or by running up a flight of stairs, minute ventilation ($\dot{V}_E$) is increased.

16. How tight is respiratory control? Or, if you hold your breath for 1 minute, how much do you want to breathe?

A lot.

17. After 60 seconds of apnea, what happens to $PaCO_2$?

It increases only from 40 to 47 mmHg. Thus, tiny changes in PCO_2 (and pH) translate into a huge respiratory stimulus. Normally, respiratory compensation for metabolic acidosis is very tight.

18. What is base excess?

Base excess is a poor man's indicator of the metabolic component of acid-base disorders. After correcting the PCO_2 to 40 mmHg, the base excess or base deficit is touted as an indirect measure of serum lactate. Although many parameters directing volume resuscitation in shock are more practical, expeditious, and direct (see chapter 3), base deficit has been advertised as helpful. The base excess or deficit is calculated from the Sigaard-Anderson nomogram in the blood gas laboratory. Normally, of course, there is no base excess of deficit. Acid-base status is "just right."

BIBLIOGRAPHY

1. Abrams JH, Cerra F, Holcroft JW: Cardiopulmonary monitoring. In Textbook of Surgery, vol 2. New York, Scientific American, 1998, p 3–26.
2. Bartlett RH: Critical Care Handbook, 13th ed. Ann Arbor, MI, University of Michigan Press, 1995.

7. FLUIDS AND ELECTROLYTES

Alden H. Harken, M.D.

1. What is hypertonic saline?

Normal saline is 0.9% sodium chloride. Hypertonic saline is 7.5% sodium chloride (8 times as concentrated as normal saline).

2. What is hypertonic saline good for?

Resuscitation. Infuse a little hypertonic saline, and it will pull extravascular water into the intravascular compartment, thus rapidly restoring volume.

3. Is hypertonic saline good for anything else?

Hypertonic saline also seems to pacify "primed" postinjury neutrophils, thus decreasing the risk of posttraumatic multiple organ failure.

4. How does one convert 1 mg of sodium into milliequivalents (mEq)?

Divide by the atomic weight of sodium. Thus, 1 gm (1,000 mg) of sodium divided by 23 equals 43.5 mEq.

5. How many mEq of sodium are in 1 teaspoon of salt?

One teaspoon of salt contains 2400 mg or 104 mEq of sodium.

6. How much does a 40-pound block of salt cost?

$3.40 at the feed store.

7. What is the electrolyte content of intravenous fluids?

Electrolyte Content of Intravenous Fluids

SOLUTION (mEq/L)	SODIUM	POTASSIUM	CHLORIDE	BICARBONATE/ LACTATE
Normal saline (0.9% NaCl)	154		154	
Ringer's lactate solution	130	4	109	28*
5% dextrose/½ normal saline	77		77	

* Lactate is immediately converted to bicarbonate.

8. How do these concentrations relate to body fluid and electrolyte compartments?

Electrolyte Concentrations in Body Fluids

COMPARTMENT (mEq/L)	SODIUM	POTASSIUM	CHLORIDE	BICARBONATE/ LACTATE
Plasma	142	4	103	27
Interstitial fluid	144	4	114	30
Intracellular fluid	10	150		10

9. What are the daily volumes (ml/24 hr) and electrolyte contents (mEq/L) of body secretions for a 70-kg medical student?

Daily Volumes and Electrolyte Contents of Body Secretions

	ml/24 hr	SODIUM	POTASSIUM	CHLORIDE	BICARBONATE
Saliva	+1500	10	25	10	30
Stomach	+1500	50	10	130	
Duodenum	+1000	140	5	80	
Ileum	+3000	140	5	104	30
Colon	−6000	60	30	40	
Pancreas	+ 500	140	5	75	100
Biliary	+ 500	140	5	100	30
Sweat*	+1000	50			
Gatorade		21		21	

* See question 7.

10. Are sweat glands responsive to aldosterone? Can they be trained?
Yes and yes. Thus, Archie Bunker's sweat contains 100 mEq/L sodium, whereas an Olympic marathon runner retains sodium (sweat sodium may be as low as 20–30 mEq/L).

11. Is Gatorade really just flavored athlete's sweat?
Yes.

12. What are the daily maintenance fluid and electrolyte requirements for a 70-kg medical student?
Total fluid volume   2500 ml
Sodium   70 mEq (1 mEq/kg)
Potassium   35 mEq (½ mEq/kg)

13. Does the routine postoperative patient require intravenous sodium or potassium supplementation? Routine serum electrolyte testing?
No and no.

14. Can a patient with a good heart and kidneys overcome all but the most woefully incompetent fluid and electrolyte management?
Yes.

15. Can one throw a healthy medical student into congestive heart failure by intravenous infusion of 100 ml of D_5/S per kg per hour?
No. One will simply be ankle-deep in urine.

16. What is subtraction alkalosis?
Vigorous nasogastric suction of a patient with a lot of gastric acid eliminates hydrochloric acid, leaving the patient alkalotic.

17. Which electrolyte is most useful in repairing a hypokalemic metabolic alkalosis?
Chloride.

18. What are the best indicators of a patient's volume status?
• Heart rate   • Urine output
• Blood pressure   • Big-toe temperature

19. Is a warm big toe indicative of a hemodynamically stable patient?

Most likely. The vascular autoregulatory ability of a young healthy patient is huge. The carotid and coronary circulations are maintained until the bitter end. Conversely, if the patient's big toe is warm and perfused, the patient is stable.

20. What is the minimal adequate postoperative urine output?

0.5 ml/kg/hr.

21. What is a typical postoperative urine sodium?

< 20 mEq/L.

22. Why?

Surgical stress prompts mineralocorticoid (aldosterone) secretions so that the normal kidney retains sodium.

23. What is paradoxical aciduria?

Postoperative patients, by virtue of nasogastric suction (loss of gastric acid), blood transfusions (the citrate in blood is converted to bicarbonate), and hyperventilation (decreased PCO_2) are typically alkalotic. Patients are also stressed, and their kidneys retain sodium and water. The renal tubules must exchange some other cations for the retained sodium. The kidney chooses to exchange potassium and hydrogen ions. Thus, even in the face of systemic alkalosis, the postoperative kidney absorbs sodium and excretes hydrogen ions, producing a paradoxical aciduria.

24. What is third-spacing?

Both hypotension and infection prime neutrophils (CD11 and CD18 receptor complexes), promoting adherence to vascular endothelial cells. Subsequent activation of adherent neutrophils spews out proteases and toxic superoxide radicals, blowing big holes in the vascular lining. Water and plasma albumin leak through the holes. The volume pulled out of the vascular space into the third space of the interstitial and hollow viscus (gut) creates relative hypovolemia and requires additional fluid replacement.

25. What is a Lasix sandwich?

Twenty-five percent albumin followed by 20 mg Lasix IV. If the patient is edematous, the intravenous albumin theoretically sucks water osmotically out of the interstitial third space. As the excessive water enters the vascular compartment, furosemide (Lasix) produces a healthy diuresis. In most intensive care patients, however, the infused albumin rapidly equilibrates across the damaged vascular endothelium. Thus, no additional water is pulled into the blood volume. Although surgeons often order Lasix sandwiches, they probably work only in healthy patients who do not need them.

BIBLIOGRAPHY

1. Burris D, Rhee P, Kaufmann C, et al: Controlled resuscitation for uncontrolled hemorrhagic shock. J Trauma 46:216–223, 1999.
2. O'Brenar D, Bruttig SP, Wade CE, Dubick MA: Hemodynamic and metabolic responses to repeated hemorrhage and resuscitation with hyperteonic saline dextran in conscious swine. Shock 10:223–228, 1998.
3. Ramsay JG: Cardiac management in the ICU. Chest 115:138S–144S, 1999.

8. NUTRITIONAL ASSESSMENT AND ENTERAL NUTRITION

Margaret M. McQuiggan, M.S., R.D., CSM, and Frederick A. Moore, M.D.

NUTRITIONAL ASSESSMENT

1. What does a nutritional assessment include?

1. The **medical and surgical history** is used to establish preexisting conditions, metabolic stress, and alterations in organ function that may influence nutritional support.

2. The **physical exam** focuses on muscle mass, adipose stores, skin integrity, and hydrational state.

3. **Laboratory data** should include the chemistry profile (sodium, potassium, carbon dioxide, chlorine, blood urea nitrogen, creatinine, glucose), complete blood count with differential, arterial blood gases (to assess acid-base status and carbon dioxide retention), albumin, transferrin, prealbumin, and urinary nitrogen.

4. The **drug profile** may reveal agents that affect the metabolism of nutrients (insulin, levothyroxine, corticosteroids) or alter energy expenditure (beta blockers, propofol).

5. **Anthropometric data** include height and weight and skinfold testing with calipers (once edema has resolved).

6. A **nutrition history** reveals information about the preexisting nutritional practices of the patient.

7. The **social history** explores economic data or substance abuse and may predict the potential for home care once the patient is discharged.

2. What are primary malnutrition and secondary malnutrition?

Primary malnutrition results when the patient consumes inadequate kilocalories, protein, vitamins, or minerals. It may be due to anorexia, poverty, or alcoholism. **Secondary malnutrition** may occur even when adequate food is infused or consumed. It may result from organ dysfunction (hypoalbuminemia with cirrhosis), malabsorption (Crohn's disease), immobility (muscle wasting), drug therapy (insulin resistance with corticosteroids), or inflammatory response (repriorization of hepatic synthesis of acute-phase instead of constitutive proteins).

3. What is the significance of serum proteins in nutritional assessment?

The most commonly cited and readily available proteins for nutritional assessment are albumin, transferrin, and prealbumin. Their half-lives are 21 days, 12 days, and 4 days, respectively. All three plummet shortly after injury or surgery. Then, as inflammation, infection, and stress resolve, the liver once again preferentially synthesizes these proteins as opposed to acute-phase proteins such as gammaglobulins and clotting factors. Adequate kilocalories and protein facilitate this process. Because of shorter half-lives, prealbumin and transferrin are the most useful indicators of nutritional status in the intensive care setting. Levels of both proteins, however, may be depleted in patients with hepatic failure. Prealbumin travels in the circulation bound to retinol binding protein (RBP) and vitamin A. Levels of prealbumin may be elevated in renal failure despite nutritional compromise because of decreased excretion of RBP.

4. What is the significance of urinary nitrogen in the surgical intensive care unit?

Total urinary nitrogen (TUN) is the most reliable indicator of nitrogen utilization and excretion. However, urinary urea nitrogen (UUN) is more readily available in most hospital laboratories. Although TUN and UUN are nearly equal in healthy ambulatory patients, critically ill patients exhibit a poor correlation. Optimal nutritional support should place a patient in +3 to +5 nitrogen balance. One may estimate the protein needs of the patient as follows:

[24-hr UUN gm + 2 gm N insensible losses + 5 gm] × 6.25 = required amount of protein (gm)

The total in brackets is multiplied by 6.25 to convert nitrogen grams to protein grams. Thus, if the lab reports a 24-hr UUN of 13 gm, add 2 gm N for insensible loss (skin, hair, feces) and 5 gm for optimal anabolism. The patient requires 20 gm N × 6.25 = 125 gm of protein to become anabolic.

5. How are protein requirements determined?

Protein need is based on the weight of the patient, current stress factors, extraordinary skin losses, and organ function. Although the daily protein requirement for healthy adults is only 0.8 gm protein/kg body weight, the following guidelines may be used in surgical patients:

Mild stress/injury	1.5 gm protein/kg
Moderate stress/injury	2.0 gm protein/kg
Severe stress/injury	2.5 gm protein/kg

6. Should protein be restricted in the surgical patient with hepatic or renal failure?

Protein should be restricted to 0.6 gm/kg in patients with **hepatic failure** and encephalopathy. However, only about 10% of patients with chronic liver disease are protein-sensitive; thus, other causes of encephalopathy, such as infection, constipation, and electrolyte disturbance, should be explored. If permissible, a more therapeutic postsurgical protein load (1.5 gm/kg) should be adopted.

In injured patients with **renal failure** one must balance the increased need for protein with the need for increased dialysis. One should provide the amount of protein required for healing and dialyze more frequently as necessary.

7. How are kilocalorie needs determined?

Kilocarlorie targets should be based on (1) standard predictive equations, (2) kcal/kg estimations, or (3) indirect calorimetry. The **Harris-Benedict equation** was developed in 1919 for use in ambulatory, healthy patients. Basal energy expenditure (BEE) is calculated using the following equations:

Female: BEE = 65.5 + 9.6 (kg) + 1.8 (cm) − 4.7 (age)
Male: BEE = 67 + 14 (kg) + 5 (cm) − 6.7 (age)

Subsequently, the above sums are multiplied by stress factors to determine total kilocalorie needs:

STRESS LEVEL	EXAMPLE	KCAL NEEDS
Mild stress	Closed fracture, pneumonia, or splenic laceration	BEE × 1.25
Moderate stress	Bowel resection, hepatorraphy, or thoracotomy	BEE × 1.5
Severe stress	Major bowel perforation with resection, major open wounds, intraabdominal abscess	BEE × 1.75

The accuracy of these elaborate calculations in stressed surgical patients has been challenged. A practical rule of thumb goal for total kcal/kg is as follows:

Underweight patients:	35 kcal/kg
Normal weight patients:	30 kcal/kg
Obese patients:	25 kcal/kg

8. What is indirect calorimetry?

It is a bedside test in which the patient's production of carbon dioxide and consumption of oxygen are measured for approximately 30 minutes:

$$MEE = [(3.796 \times VO_2) + (1.214 \times VCO_2)] \times 1440 \text{ min/day}$$

where MEE = measured energy expenditure (kcal/day), VO_2 = oxygen consumption (L/min), and VCO_2 = carbon dioxide exhaled (L/min). By measuring CO_2 produced and O_2 consumed, the cart reports the number of kilocalories that the patient is predicted to consume in 24 hours.

9. When is indirect calorimetry useful?

The test may be performed on the mechanically ventilated patient once he or she is relatively stable, with a fractional concentration of oxygen in inspired gas (FiO_2) < 60% and peak end-expiratory pressure (PEEP) < 10. Studies are helpful (1) when overfeeding (as in diabetes or chronic obstructive pulmonary disease) is undesirable; (2) when underfeeding (renal failure, large wounds) is especially detrimental; (3) in patients whose clinical factors (extensive burns) provoke energy expenditure that deviates from expected values; (4) when drugs are used that alter energy expenditure (paralytic agents, beta blockers), and (5) in patients who do not respond as expected to calculated regimens.

ENTERAL NUTRITION

10. When should enteral nutrition be considered?

Always—but especially when a patient is unlikely to meet > 70% of nutritional needs by mouth. Patients who have sustained major head injury (Glasgow Coma Scale score < 8), major torso trauma, trauma to the pelvis and long bones, or major chest trauma benefit from enteral nutrition. At least 85% of postoperative patients (even those undergoing gastrointestinal [GI] surgery) tolerate early enteral feeding (within 24 hours).

11. How do you access the GI tract for enteral feeding?

By blind placement of a nasogastric tube or duodenal placement of a nasoduodenal tube. More distal placement may be achieved endoscopically with a nasojejunal tube. Gastric decompression and nasojejunal feeds may be accomplished concurrently after percutaneous endoscopic gastrostomy/jejunostomy. Alternatively, a gastrostomy or feeding jejunostomy may be placed intraoperatively.

12. What types of enteral formulas are available?

Enteral feedings are soy-based, lactose-free products containing protein, carbohydrate, and fat. Most offer 1 kcal/ml and 50 gm protein per liter. Special modifications of the standard formulas include dietary fiber or "immune-enhancing" agents such as fish oil, arginine, glutamine, and nucleotides. Elemental formulas contain amino acids; di-, tri-, and quatrapeptides; dextrose; and minimal fat. Several concentrated formulas (2 kcal/ml) are available for use in patients with congestive heart failure, renal failure, and hepatic failure. In general, products that are disease-specific or contain nutrients in elemental form are much more expensive.

13. Are specialized formulas necessary for the critically ill patient with diabetes mellitus?

No. Formulas with reduced carbohydrate and increased fat are marketed as superior for maintaining glycemic control. The use of standard high-protein formulas in an isocaloric or hypocaloric fashion, combined with appropriate insulin therapy, may be the most effective treatment for insulin resistance in the stressed patient with type 2 diabetes.

14. What complications are related to enteral support?

Electrolyte abnormalities, hyperglycemia, GI intolerance, aspiration, and nasopharyngeal erosions.

15. Should enteral formulas be diluted for initial presentation?

No. Dilution usually delays the attainment of feeding goals. Furthermore, solution osmolarity is a relatively minor culprit in the incidence of diarrhea.

16. How should enteral feeding-related diarrhea be managed?

Mild-to-moderate diarrhea requires no treatment. Severe diarrhea requires feeding reduction, antidiarrheal agents, and smear/culture for *Clostridium difficile*. The medication profile should be evaluated for sorbitol-containing elixirs, laxatives, stool softeners, and prokinetic agents, Sanitation issues related to formula handling must be monitored. Success has been reported with lactobacillus (yogurt) in antibiotic-associated diarrhea.

17. Do enteral feedings contain enough water to meet all fluid needs?

Most 1-kcal/ml formulas (standard) contain 85% water by volume, whereas 2-kcal/ml formulas contain 70% water. Water is generally not an issue in the intensive care patient receiving multiple intravenous fluids and drugs. However, on the wards or in patients bound for home or post-care facilities, it is essential to write a water prescription with the tube feeding order. General guidelines for the total water needs of patients are as follows:

PATIENT	AGE (YR)	WATER NEEDS (ML/KG)
Young, active adult	18–25	40
Average adult	> 25–55	35
Adult	> 55–65	30
Elderly	> 65	25

Thus, if the total calculated need for fluid is 2400 ml for a 60-kg patient and the tube feeding provides 2000 ml of free water, an order should be written to deliver 200 ml of water to the patient twice daily.

18. How is enteral nutrition infused?

Enteral nutrition is infused continuously, in bolus form or cyclically. Continuous infusion is preferred in more critically ill patients requiring postpyloric feedings. Bolus feedings are used in more stable patients with gastric feedings. Cyclic feedings or nocturnal feedings benefit the patient who is on concurrent oral intake and in transition to full oral support.

19. Is enteral nutrition better than total parenteral nutrition (TPN)?

Yes. Substrates delivered enterally are better tolerated, are associated with fewer metabolic complications, and help to preserve normal gut mucosal integrity. A review of five studies contrasting TPN with no nutrition or early enteral nutrition concluded that TPN is associated with a greater incidence of septic morbidity.

CONTROVERSIES

20. How fat is fat? What is ideal body weight (IBW)?

Lean body mass is more metabolically active than adipose tissue. Multiple definitions of clinical obesity are available—e.g., > 120% IBW, > 130% IBW, body mass index (BMI) > 28, and body fat > 25% of body weight in men or > 30% in women. Measured weight is a poor indicator of relative adiposity. Self-reported weights or weights reported by family members are often erroneous. Fluid resuscitation and edema make visual assessment challenging and limit the usefulness of noninvasive technology, such as bioelectrical impedance, for measuring body composition. Although measured energy expenditure in kcal/kg of actual weight may approach that of normal-weight patients, feeding at the measured level may be associated with profound hyperglycemia, hypercapnea, and inability to clear triglycerides.

21. Should actual, ideal, or adjusted body weight be used in nutrition calculations for the obese patient?

Studies using an obesity-adjusted weight in kilocalorie calculations [IBW + 0.25 (actual-IBW)] report greater correlation with measured energy expenditure than when actual weight is used.

22. Which is more important—nitrogen or caloric balance?

Ultimately, maintaining positive nitrogen balance is more important than achieving positive kilocaloric balance.

23. Are postpyloric feedings superior to gastric feedings?

After major surgery or injury, the stomach exhibits decreased motility for several days. Early enteral feeding, with its known benefits, may not be accomplished through gastric feeding in the early stages of injury. Jejunostomy feedings are associated with higher kilocalorie intake, more timely return to anabolism, and a lower incidence of pneumonia than continuous gastric feeding.

24. Should one count all sources of kilocalories or merely the nonprotein kilocalories?

Once the amino group is removed from the protein molecule, the resulting carbon skeleton is used for energy production via the citric acid cycle. Thus, protein is a source of kilocalories.Since current nutrition practice may dictate the use of up to 2 gm protein per kg of body weight in the stressed trauma patient, failure to count the protein kilocalories results in a daily excess of 640 kilocalories for an 80-kg patient. Furthermore, both indirect calorimetry measurements and most standard prediction equations refer to total kilocalories—not nonprotein kilocalories.

25. When should immune-enhancing formulas be used?

Rarely. Immune-enhancing diets improve outcome and reduce septic morbidity in selected high-risk patients prone to intraabdominal sepsis after major torso trauma or major GI surgery and in some patients with gastric cancers. Because of the increased cost of immune-enhancing feedings, indications for their use should be considered carefully and length of use regulated.

BIBLIOGRAPHY

1. American Society of Parenteral and Enteral Nutrition: Guidelines for the use of parenteral and enteral nutrition in adult patients. J Parent Ent Nutr 17(Suppl 4):1SA–26SA, 1993.
2. Cutts ME, Dowdy RP, Ellersieck MR, Edes TE: Predicting energy needs in ventilator dependent critically ill patients: Effect of adjusting weight for edema or adiposity. Am J Clin Nutr 66:1250–1256, 1997.
3. Hunter DC, Jaksic T, Lewis D, et al: Resting energy expenditure in the critically ill: Estimation versus measurement. Br J Surg 75:875–878, 1988.
4. Konstantinides FN, Konstantinides NN, Li JC, et al: Urinary urea nitrogen: Too sensitive for calculating nitrogen balance studies in surgical clinical nutrition. J Parent Ent Nutr 15:189–193, 1991.
5. McClave SA, Snider HL: Understanding the metabolic response to critical illness: Factors that cause patients to deviate from the expected pattern of hypermetabolism. N Horiz 2:139–146, 1994.
6. McMahon M, Rizza RA: Nutrition support in hospitalized patients with diabetes mellitus. Mayo Clin Proc 71:587–594, 1996.
7. McQuiggan MM, Marvin RG, McKinley BA, Moore FA: Enteral feeding following major torso trauma: From theory to practice. N Horiz 7:131–140, 1999.
8. Montecalvo MA, Steger KA, Farber HW, et al: Nutritional outcome and pneumonia in critical care patients randomized to gastric versus jejunal tube feedings. Crit Care Med 20:1377–1387, 1992.
9. Moore FA, Feliciano DV, Andrassy R, et al: Enteral feeding reduces postoperative septic complications: A meta analysis. Ann Surg 216:62–71, 1992.

9. PARENTERAL NUTRITION

Margaret M. McQuiggan, M.S., R.D., CSM, and Frederick A. Moore, M.D.

1. What is parenteral nutrition?

Parenteral nutrition is the provision of amino acids (4 kcal/gm), dextrose (3.4 kcal/gm), fat (lipid 20% in a solution that delivers 2 kcal/ml), vitamins, minerals, trace elements, fluid, and sometimes insulin through an intravenous infusion. Acid-base status may be influenced by the amount of chloride and acetate used in providing sodium and potassium. The concentrations of calcium and phosphorus are limited to avoid precipitation of a calcium phosphate salt.

2. What are the indications for total parenteral nutrition (TPN)?

TPN should be used when the gastrointestinal tract is totally nonfunctional, as in major bowel resection, "short gut," high-volume enterocutaneous fistulas, ileus, and severe intractable diarrhea.

3. What types of access are available for the delivery of parenteral nutrition?

Central parenteral solutions are highly concentrated with osmolarities up to 3000 mOsm/L. They should be delivered into a large-lumen vein (e.g., subclavian) or, less commonly, a femoral vein. If a multiple-port catheter is used, a "virgin port" should be reserved exclusively for nutrient infusion. When long-term parenteral nutrition is planned in the postacute setting, a long-term access device may be used, such as a Hickman or Broviac catheter. This approach may not be necessary, however, when the central venous catheter is placed under sterile conditions and the patient and family are taught meticulous care.

4. What is peripheral parenteral nutrition (PPN)?

PPN may be used when parenteral nutrition is required for less than 10 days and central line placement is contraindicated. Solutions must have a low osmolarity (< 800 mOsm/L) to prevent thrombosis at the entry site. The inclusion of fat emulsion, which has a near-isotonic osmolarity, helps to decrease the overall osmolarity while increasing total kilocalories. Because of the dilute nature of the solution, a large volume is required to provide ample nutrition to the patient. Thus, PPN may not be desirable in fluid-restricted patients (e.g., those with congestive heart failure).

5. What is intradialytic parenteral nutrition (IDPN)?

Occasionally, limited quantities of parenteral nutrition may be infused during standard hemodialysis. This strategy, which affords the opportunity to provide nutrition while simultaneously removing volume and urea, may be useful in a limited subset of hemodialysis patients who are malnourished and cannot achieve adequate nutrition support orally or enterally.

6. When should concentrated amino acid and dextrose solutions be used?

The concentration of amino acids in standard solutions is generally 8.5% (8.5 gm/100 ml) or 10%. Concentrated solutions contain 15%. Dextrose is maximally concentrated at 70%, although 50% dextrose (D50%) is used more commonly in standard TPN solutions. Maximally concentrated TPN may be desirable in patients with congestive heart failure, acute renal failure, or hepatic failure.

7. Should iron be included in parenteral nutrition?

Iron deficiency is rarely an acute problem in the intensive care unit. Patients receive 250 mg elemental iron per unit of blood transfusion. In longer-term TPN, iron supplementation may become necessary. Ideally it should be provided by the enteral route because of the high anaphylactic potential of intravenous and intramuscular iron.

8. What complications are associated with parenteral nutrition?

Fluid and electrolyte imbalance, altered glucose metabolism, increased values on liver function tests, hepatic steatosis (fatty liver), and gut atrophy are associated with TPN. Hemothorax or pneumothorax may occur during central line placement. Although rare, air emboli or extravascular placement of central lines have been reported.

9. What factors play a role in catheter-related sepsis (CRS)?

Preventive measures can be divided into three categories: (1) catheter insertion, (2) catheter maintenance, and (3) catheter removal. During insertion the skin should be prepared with chlorhexadine rather than alcohol or povidone iodine and maximal sterile barriers should be used. Although it is commonly thought that multiple-lumen catheters have a higher rate of CRS than single-lumen catheters, randomized studies using rigorous central venous catheter protocols demonstrate comparable rates of CRS. Catheter care includes (1) scheduled dressing and tubing change every 72 hours, (2) antibiotic ointment (of questionable merit but commonly used), and (3) use of gauze, which is superior to transparent occlusive dressings. Finally, removing the catheter at set intervals effectively reduces CRS, but the benefits must be weighed against the risks of mechanical complications associated with placement of a new catheter at a different site. Guidewire changes are an effective method for early diagnosis of local catheter colonization or infection.

10. Why do parenterally fed patients often develop hyperglycemia?

Increased stress (catecholamines), the inflammatory response, limited mobility, concurrent steroid therapy, and excessive kilocalorie intake are contributing factors. Glucose infusion rates should not exceed 5 mg/kg/minute. Maintaining the blood glucose at < 150 mg/dl during parenteral nutrition is recommended to increase immunocompetence, maintain hydrational status, and enhance wound healing.

11. How should hyperglycemia be managed?

Regular insulin may be required in the initial TPN solution in patients with baseline hyperglycemia, insulin resistance, or insulinopenia. Supplemental insulin needs should be evaluated daily before reordering TPN. Neutral protamine Hagedorn (NPH) insulin is geared toward patients who consume meals at regular intervals and thus is not appropriate with continuous intravenous feedings.

12. Why are intravenous fat emulsions used? When are they contraindicated?

Theoretically, fat emulsions are used to prevent essential fatty acid deficiency. In reality, this condition is rare, takes several weeks to develop, and requires only 3–4% of kilocalories as linoleic acid (or 10% of kilocalories as a standard fat emulsion). Fat emulsions also are used to provide additional kilocalories once glucose infusion has reached 5 mg/kg/min. Practically speaking, lipids are packaged in 100-ml, 250-ml, and 500-ml units.

Fat emulsions should be avoided with hyperlipidemia-induced pancreatitis (a small percentage of the total cases of pancreatitis) and significantly elevated serum triglycerides (e.g., > 500 mg/dl). When delivered in total-nutrient admixtures (3-in-1 solutions), lipid emulsions are stable for 24 hours. When they are infused as a sole nutrient, hang times should not exceed 12 hours because of the potential for bacterial growth.

13. What is refeeding syndrome?

Refeeding syndrome occurs when a patient is moderately-to-severely malnourished and has limited substrate reserves. It is characteristic of patients with chronic alcoholism, anorexia nervosa, or chronic starvation. When presented with a large nutrient load, the patient rapidly develops clinically significant drops in serum potassium, phosphorus, calcium, and magnesium due to compartment shifts of these elements. Hyperglycemia is commonly due to blunted basal insulin secretion.

14. How is refeeding syndrome best managed?

Ample quantities of potassium, phosphorus, calcium, and magnesium should be provided with the initial parenteral mixtures. The initial kilocalorie provision should be reduced by 25% of goal by reducing dextrose kilocalories. Serial blood glucose determinations (3–4 daily) and serum potassium, phosphorus, calcium, and magnesium should be evaluated daily for 5 days after initiating feeding.

15. How should parenteral nutrition be monitored?

Parenteral nutrition should be monitored daily with a chemistry profile (sodium, potassium, chloride, carbon diozide, glucose), magnesium, phosphorus, and calcium during the first several days of initial therapy in the critical care setting. Accucheck blood glucose determinations are needed every 6 hours. As the fluid and electrolyte balance stabilizes, frequency may be reduced to once weekly. Home TPN therapy may require as little as once-monthly monitoring. The adequacy of the regimen may be assessed by evidence of proper wound healing, maintenance of body cell mass, and timely repletion of constitutive protein (albumin, transferrin) levels. Overfeeding may be evidenced by insulin resistance, hypertriglyceridemia, increased values on liver function tests, and hypercapnea.

16. What infusion schedules are used for TPN?

TPN most often is delivered by continuous infusion. In more ambulatory patients and those on home therapy, a cyclic or nighttime infusion schedule may be adopted, as along as adequate hydration can be maintained. This approach dictates a 12–18-hour infusion period.

17. How should TPN be discontinued?

When TPN is no longer needed, the infusion rate should be reduced by one-half for 2 hours, halved again for 2 hours, and then discontinued. This "ramp down" prevents reactive hypoglycemia.

18. What is the cost of parenteral nutrition?

The cost of parenteral solutions may vary widely, depending on the constituents. The cost of TPN solution components and preparation is 10 times that of a standard enteral feeding. Most third-party payers do not provide more reimbursement for parenteral than for enteral therapy in the hospital setting.

CONTROVERSIES

19. Does preoperative TPN improve surgical outcome?

It is well documented that malnourished patients are at an increased risk for septic complications, problems with wound healing, longer hospital stays, and increased mortality. However, results of recent studies evaluating preoperative TPN and outcome are variable. Recent trials suggest that TPN, in fact, may increase postoperative septic complications. For mildly or moderately malnourished patients, the risks of preoperative TPN appear to outweigh the benefits. However, a small subgroup of severely malnourished patients appear to benefit from 10 days of preoperative TPN.

20. Should TPN solutions contain the same percentage of fat kilocalories recommended in the diet of healthy Americans (i.e., 30% of kilocalories)?

The American Heart Association (AHA) recommendation for 30% of total kilocalories as fat is geared toward prevention of cardiovascular disease in healthy people and was not intended for intravenous feeding in critically ill patients. Furthermore, the AHA suggests that fat kilocalories should be divided equally among saturated, monounsaturated, and polyunsaturated fat, including omega-3 series fatty acids. Lipid formulations currently available in the United States are made from either soybean oil or a mixture of soybean and safflower oil; thus, they are predominantly polyunsaturated (omega-6) fat. Glucose kilocalories are the most cost-effective kilocalories, followed, in order, by standard amino acid kilocalories and lipid calories. Lipid infusions exceeding 1 gm/kg of body weight are associated with decreased immunocompetence and compromised oxygenation in critically ill patients. Some of these dilemmas may be resolved once mixed lipids, structured lipids, and fish oil become available in the United States.

21. Do stress or hepatic failure formulas containing increased levels of branched-chain amino acids enhance clinical outcomes?

Specialty amino acid formulas designed to meet specific organ-failure requirements include "stress" formulas with high levels of branched-chain amino acids (BCAAs) and low levels of aromatic amino acids (AAAs). Renal specialty formulas high in essential amino acids (EAAs) were developed to maximize protein provision during acute renal failure in the absence of dialysis. The specialty formulas generally deliver isonitrogenous loads at 20 times the cost of standard amino acids. Studies comparing BCAAs with standard solutions in stressed patients have shown improvements in nitrogen retention, visceral protein levels, and immune function but failed to show reduced morbidity and mortality rates. The use of specific organ-failure formulas (hepatic and renal) does not improve nutritional status or outcome.

22. Should all patients with pancreatitis be supported with parenteral nutrition?

TPN has been a standard of care to provide nutrients while "resting" the pancreas. However, recent studies indicate that enteral feedings into the jejunum are feasible. Compared with TPN, jejunal feeding does not increase pancreatic stimulation and is associated with reduced septic complications because of modulation of the inflammatory and sepsis response. Early enteral support is well tolerated and is a cost-effective alternative to parenteral nutrition. The type of formula and level of the gastrointestinal tract into which nutrients are infused determine the degree of pancreatic exocrine stimulation.

23. Does parenteral glutamine enhance outcome in patients with bone marrow transplant (BMT)?

Glutamine, the most prevalent amino acid in muscle and plasma, decreases after surgery, injury, or stress. Thus, it is considered a conditionally essential amino acid. Glutamine is a metabolic substrate for rapidly replicating cells, is thought to maintain the integrity and function of the intestinal barrier, and protects against free radical damage by maintaining glutathione levels. Glutamine is not included in the standard amino acid solutions because of limited solubility and stability; its dipeptide form, which is bound to alanine or glycine, is more stable and soluble. Although oral glutamine does decrease the severity and duration of oropharyngeal mucositis in patients with autologous BMT, parenteral glutamine improves nitrogen balance, lowers clinical signs of infection, decreases length of hospital stay and hospital costs, and supports lymphocyte recovery after BMT.

BIBLIOGRAPHY

1. ASPEN guidelines for the use of parenteral and enteral nutrition in adult patients. J Parent Ent Nutr 17(Suppl 4):1SA–26SA, 1993.
2. Gottschlich MM: Selection of optimal lipid sources in enteral and parenteral nutrition. Nutr Clin Pract 7:152–165, 1992.
3. Havala T, Shronts E: Managing the complications associated with refeeding. Nutr Clin Pract 5:23–29, 1990.
4. MacBurney M, Young LS, Ziegler TR, Wilmore DW: A cost evaluation of glutamine-supplemented parenteral nutrition in adult bone marrow transplant patients. J Am Diet Assoc 11:1263–1266, 1994.
5. McClave SA, Snider H, Owens N, Sexton LK: Clinical nutrition in pancreatitis. Dig Dis Sci 42:2035–2044, 1997.
6. McMahon M, Manji N, Driscoll DF, Bistrian BR: Parenteral nutrition in patients with diabetes mellitus: Theoretical and practical considerations. J Parent Ent Nutr 13:545–553, 1989.
7. Nakad A, Piessevaux H, Marot JC, et al: Is early enteral nutrition in acute pancreatitis dangerous? About 20 patients fed by an endoscopically-placed nasogastrojejunal tube. Pancreas 17:187–193, 1998.
8. Veterans Affair Total Parenteral Cooperative Study Group: Perioperative total parenteral nutrition in surgical patients. N Engl J Med 325:525–532, 1991.
9. Wolfson M, Foulks CJ: Intradialytic parenteral nutrition: A useful therapy? Nutr Clin Pract 11:5–11, 1996.

10. POSTOPERATIVE FEVER

Alden H. Harken, M.D.

1. What is a fever?

Normal core temperature varies between 36°C and 38°C. Because we hibernate a little at night, we are cool (36°C) just before rising in the morning; after revving our engines all day, we are hot at night (up to 38°C). A fever is a pathologic state reflecting a systemic inflammatory process. The core temperature is above 38°C but rarely above 40°C.

2. What is malignant hyperthermia?

Malignant hyperthermia is a rare, life-threatening response to inhaled anesthetics or some muscle relaxants. Core temperature rises above 40°C. Abnormal calcium metabolism in skeletal muscle produces heat, acidosis, hypokalemia, muscle rigidity, coagulopathy, and circulatory collapse.

3. How is malignant hyperthermia treated?

- Stop the anesthetic.
- Give sodium bicarbonate (2 mEq/kg IV).
- Give dantrolene (calcium channel blocker at 2.5 mg/kg IV).
- Continue dantrolene (1 mg/kg every 6 hr for 48 hr).
- Cool patient with alcohol sponges and ice.

4. What causes fever?

Macrophages are activated by bacteria and endotoxin. Activated macrophages release interleukin-1, tumor necrosis factor, and interferon, which reset the hypothalamic thermoregulatory center.

5. Can fever be treated?

Yes. Aspirin, acetaminophen, and ibuprofen are cyclooxygenase inhibitors that block the formation of prostaglandins (PGE_2) in the hypothalamus and effectively treat fever.

6. Should fever be treated?

Treatment of fever is controversial. No evidence suggests that suppression of fever improves patient outcome. Patients are more comfortable, however, and the surgeon receives fewer calls from the nurses.

7. Should fever be investigated?

Absolutely. Fever indicates that something (frequently treatable) is going on. The threshold for inquiry depends on the patient. A transplant patient with a temperature of 38°C requires scrutiny, whereas a healthy medical student with an identical temperature of 38°C 24 hours after an appendectomy can be cheerfully ignored.

8. What is a fever work-up?

- Order blood cultures, urine Gram stain and culture, and sputum Gram stain and culture.
- Look at the surgical incisions.
- Look at old and current IV sites for evidence of septic thrombophlebitis.
- If breath sounds are worrisome, order a chest radiograph.

9. What is the most common cause of fever during the early postoperative period (1–3 days)?

The traditional answer is atelectasis. A total pneumothorax, however, does not cause fever. Why does a little atelectasis cause fever, whereas a lot of atelectasis (pneumothorax) does not? The most likely explanation is that sterile atelectasis (and early postoperative lung collapse is typically not infected) has nothing to do with fever.

10. Do surgical incisions compromise spontaneous breathing patterns?

Absolutely. Vital capacity has been measured in a large group of patients 24 hours after various surgical procedures. An upper abdominal incision is the worst, followed by lower abdomen incision and then (counterintuitively) by thoracotomy, median sternotomy, and extremity incision.

11. Should atelectasis be treated with incentive spirometry?

Yes—but not to avoid fever.

12. What is a wound infection?

By definition, a wound infection contains more than 10^5 organisms per gram of tissue.

13. Are certain wounds prone to infection?

Each milliliter of human saliva contains up to 10^8 aerobic and anaerobic, gram-positive and gram-negative bacteria. Thus, all human bite wounds must be considered as contaminated. Surprisingly, animal bite wounds are typically less contaminated. (It is safer to kiss your dog than your fiancé[e]).

14. Do incisions become infected early after surgery?

The incision must be examined in a patient with a fever (39°C) less than 12 hours after surgery. Look for a foul-smelling, serous discharge in a particularly painful wound (all incisions hurt) with or without crepitus. Gram stain of the serous discharge for gram-positive rods confirms or excludes the diagnosis of clostridial infection.

15. What is the therapy for clostridial gas gangrene?

- The wound should be opened immediately, with fluid resuscitation of the patient. The mainstay of therapy is aggressive surgical debridement of necrotic tissue (skin, muscle, fascia). Make a big hole, and do not worry about closing it.
- Give penicillin, 12 million U/day IV for 1 week.
- Hyperbaric oxygen is not convincingly helpful.

16. Are nonclostridial necrotizing wound infections a cause of concern?

Hemolytic streptococcal gangrene, idiopathic scrotal gangrene, and gram-negative synergistic necrotizing cellulitis are distinct entities but have been lumped into the single category of necrotizing fasciitis. All require the same initial approach:
1. Fluid and electrolyte resuscitation.
2. Broad-spectrum antibiotics ("triples").
3. Aggressive surgical debridement of all necrotic tissue.

17. What are triple antibiotics?

Triple antibiotics are a shotgun approach to potentially life-threatening infections when the patient is seriously ill and the surgeon is seriously concerned:
1. Gram-positive coverage (e.g., ampicillin)
2. Gram-negative coverage (e.g., gentamicin)
3. Anaerobic coverage (e.g., flagyl)

To avoid overgrowth of yeast and resistant bacteria, one should focus on the culprit bacteria as soon as the cultures come back.

18. What types of surgical procedures predispose to wound infections?
Gastrointestinal procedures, especially when the colon is opened.

19. When do wound infections typically occur?
Twelve hours to 7 days postoperatively.

20. How is a wound infection treated?
The wound should be opened and completely drained.

21. Is it necessary to irrigate an infected wound?
Tap water irrigation decreases the bacterial load and promotes healing. Alcohol is toxic to tissues. Sodium hydrochlorite (Dakin's solution) and hydrogen peroxide kill fibroblasts and slow epithelialization. As a rule of thumb, put nothing into a wound that you would not put in your eye.

22. When do urinary tract infections occur?
The longer the urethral (Foley) catheter is in place, the more likely the infection. Urologic instrumentation at the time of surgery may accelerate the process considerably. Bugs crawl up the outside of the urethral catheter, and by 5–7 days after surgery most patients harbor infected urine.

23. How is a urinary tract infection (UTI) diagnosed?
Urine culture with more than 10^5 bacteria/ml defines a UTI. White cells on urinalysis are highly suspicious.

24. What are the most common late causes of postoperative fever?
Septic thrombophlebitis (from an IV line) and occult (usually intraabdominal) abscesses tend to present even 2 weeks or more after surgery.

BIBLIOGRAPHY

1. Mabika M, Laburn H: The role of tumor necrosis factor-alpha (TNF-alpha) in fever and the acute phase reaction in rabbits. Pflügers Arch 438:218–223, 1999.
2. Roth J, Martin D, Storr B, Zeisberger E: Neutralization of pyrogen-induced tumor necrosis factor by its type I soluble receptor in guinea-pigs: Effects on fever and interleukin-6 release. J Physiol 509:267–275, 1998.

11. OXYGEN MONITORING AND ASSESSMENT

James B. Haenel, RRT, and Patrick J. Offner, M.D., M.P.H.

1. How does a pulse oximeter work?
Light-absorption characteristics differ for the four most common circulating species of hemoglobin in adults:
- Reduced hemoglobin (RHb)
- Oxygenated hemoglobin (O_2Hb)
- Methemoglobin (Met Hb)
- Carboxyhemoglobin (CO Hb)

Current pulse oximeters transmit two wavelengths of light, red (680 nm) and infrared (940 nm), which best differentiate O_2Hb from RHb. Using optical plethysmography, the pulse oximeter measures hemoglobin saturation only during arterial pulsation.

2. What is the accuracy of pulse oximetry?

The device is highly accurate over a hemoglobin range of 70–95%.

3. How accurate are clinicians in determining arterial desaturation by "visual oximetry"?

Not very good. Pulse oximetry should be regarded as the fifth vital sign.

4. How does the pulse oximeter respond to an abnormal species of hemoglobin?

In carbon monoxide or cyanide poisoning, the oximeter interprets an abnormal hemoglobin as a combination of O_2Hb and RHb, which results in an erroneously high saturation. Underestimation of arterial hemoglobin saturation occurs with methemoglobinemia.

5. Can any other environmental or clinical conditions result in inaccurate pulse oximetry values?

Reliability depends on a strong arterial pulse plus good light transmission. Therefore, inaccuracy results with hypotension (mean arterial pressure < 50 mmHg), hypothermia (< 35°C), vascular disease (poor peripheral perfusion), and vasopressor therapy (vasoconstriction). In addition, bright lights, intravenous dyes, nail polish, and excessive motion produce an artifact in signal transmission.

6. What is the relationship between oxyhemoglobin saturation (SaO_2) and partial pressure of oxygen (PaO_2)?

Proper use of pulse oximetry requires recall of the oxyhemoglobin dissociation curve. A rightward shift (decreased hemoglobin affinity for oxygen) facilitates oxygen unloading at the tissue level. Increasing temperature, increasing $PaCO_2$, increasing 2,3-DPG, and increasing hydrogen ion concentration—all "increases"—shift the curve to the right. When the PaO_2 exceeds 100 mmHg, however, the curve is virtually flat. Consequently, a large drop in PaO_2 may occur with no discernible change in SaO_2.

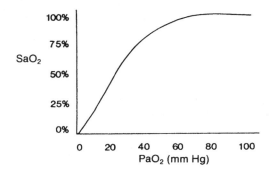

Oxyhemoglobin dissociation curve.

7. What are the indications for continuous pulse oximetry?

Pulse oximetry should be considered standard monitoring in critical care units. Pulse oximetry is uniquely valuable during patient transport, weaning from the ventilator, and following major ventilator changes. In addition, critically ill patients who are outside the ICU (emergency department or radiology suite) should be monitored by pulse oximetry.

8. How does a continuous mixed venous oximeter work?

Mixed venous oximetry uses reflective spectrophotometry. Narrow wavebands of light are transmitted via a fiberoptic bundle to the blood flowing past the tip of the catheter and are reflected by a separate fiberoptic bundle to a photodetector that determines relative absorption of the specific wavelength. A microprocessor then calculates mixed venous hemoglobin saturation (SvO_2).

9. What is the normal value for mixed venous O_2 saturation?

The normal oxygen tension in mixed venous blood (PvO_2) is 40 mmHg. Under standard conditions this value is equivalent to an SvO_2 of 75%, which is on the steep portion of the oxyhemoglobin dissociation curve. Therefore, three-fourths of the oxygen (see chapter 5) delivered out the aorta (DO_2) actually returns to the right heart.

10. Using a pulmonary artery catheter, how can oxygen delivery and consumption be determined?

The Fick equation shows the relationship between systemic oxygen delivery (DO_2) and oxygen consumption (VO_2):

$$VO_2 = CO \times (CaO_2 - CvO_2)$$

where CaO2 is arterial oxygen content, CvO_2 is mixed venous oxygen content, and CO is cardiac output. Oxygen delivery is determined by the following equation:

$$DO_2 = CaO_2 \times CO$$

where CaO_2 is (1.36 × [hemoglobin concentration] × [arterial oxygen saturation]) + PaO_2 × 0.003) and CvO_2 is (1.36 × [hemoglobin concentration] × [venous oxygen saturation]) + PaO_2 × 0.003).

11. Describe the four primary causes of a sudden fall in SvO_2.

A stable, normal SvO_2 ensures a balance of DO_2 and VO_2, whereas a sudden fall in SvO_2 provides an early warning of (1) low CO, (2) arterial oxygen desaturation, (3) drop in hemoglobin, or (4) increased VO_2.

12. Why does SvO_2 rise during general anesthesia? Why does it rise with septic shock?

General anesthesia suppresses metabolic demands; thus, VO_2 decreases and SvO_2 rises. During sepsis large peripheral shunts, high cardiac output, and poor oxygen extraction contribute to an elevated SvO_2.

13. What are the advantages of continuous monitoring of venous oxygen saturation?

SvO_2 provides prompt feedback about therapeutic interventions and disease progression. But SvO_2 trends are more important than absolute values. The catheter tip is easily gummed up with tissue proteins; the catheter should be recalibrated every 12–24 hours.

14. Are there any disadvantages to computer-generated hemodynamic profiling?

Yes—even when it is wrong, we tend to believe it. Hemodynamic profiling is a constellation of parameters: cardiac output, PaO_2, SvO_2, urine output, serum lactate level, and big-toe temperature.

15. What is dual oximetry?

Dual oximetry consists of simultaneous monitoring of arterial (SaO_2) and mixed venous (SvO_2) hemoglobin saturation to provide real-time, continuous information about pulmonary function, oxygen transport, and oxygen consumption. Dual oximetry is particularly useful for real-time assessment during a best trial of positive end-expiratory pressure (PEEP).

16. What is transcutaneous oxygen monitoring (TCM)?

TCM is a method of continuously recording skin PO_2 ($P_{tc}O_2$), which is not necessarily equal to arterial PO_2. In 1975 Van Duzee observed that the lipid component of the stratum corneum melts as skin temperature increases and gas diffusion increases by as much as 1,000-fold. The $P_{tc}O_2$ electrode, therefore, is designed to heat the skin to 44–45°C. The elevated temperature also increases dermal blood flow and "arterializes" the capillary blood. The interpretation of pulse oximetry and TCM are the same, however.

17. If the skin beneath the sensor is arterialized, why is the $Pa_{tc}O_2$ not equal to the PaO_2?

Four factors contribute to the difference between $P_{tc}O_2$ and PaO_2: (1) the rightward shift of the oxygen-hemoglobin dissociation curve with heating, (2) variations in the skin O_2 permeability, (3) metabolic consumption of oxygen by the dermal tissue, and (4) cutaneous blood flow. Because factors 1 and 3 tend to cancel each other, the relationship between $P_{tc}O_2$ and PaO_2 is effectively linear and depends only on O_2 permeability and skin blood flow.

18. What is an oxygen debt?

An oxygen debt is the net cumulative difference between oxygen consumption measured at baseline and during any pathologic state. In other words, an oxygen debt is the amount of oxygen needed by the cells to compensate for the mismatch between oxygen delivery and oxygen demand.

19. How should a hypoxic event be managed?

Once a hypoxic event has been identified, supplemental oxygen is applied. The first maneuver for intubated patients is to hand-ventilate with an ambu bag. A ruptured endotracheal tube cuff is self-evident, whereas difficult bagging implies airway obstruction, bronchospasm, or tension pneumothorax. Inability to pass a suction catheter confirms endotracheal tube obstruction. if the obstruction is not reversible by changing head position or by cuff deflation, the endotracheal tube must be replaced immediately. If there is difficulty with bagging and no evidence of airway obstruction, a quick chest examination excludes a tension pneumothorax. The mechanical ventilator and breathing circuit are inspected. Arterial blood gases are measured to confirm hypoxia and rule out hypoventilation.

Additional work-up generally includes portable chest radiograph and review of recent medications, interventions (e.g., suctioning, position changes, nursing care), and changes in clinical status. Most acute hypoxic events in the intensive care unit are due to easily identified and reversible mechanical problems, such as disconnects from oxygen delivery systems or mucus plugging that requires suctioning.

ICU HYPOXIC EVENTS

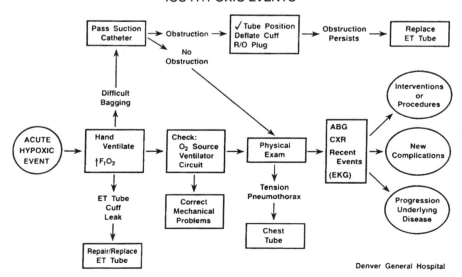

Denver General Hospital

EXTRA-CREDIT QUESTIONS

20. Four hours after your patient undergoes an exploratory laparotomy following a motor vehicle accident, the nurse reports that the patient's vital signs, urine output, and oxygen transport numbers are normal. Can the patient still be in trouble?

The Advanced Trauma Life Support Program defines shock as an abnormality of the circulatory system that results in inadequate organ perfusion and tissue oxygenation. This definition is easy to understand with uncompensated shock. However, critically injured patients rarely make the transition from uncompensated shock to normal physiology without some evidence of continued suboptimal tissue perfusion. This altered physiologic state may exist in up to 85% of patients who exhibit normal blood pressure, heart rate, and urine output. Assessing the sufficiency of blood flow to vital organs based on normal oxygen transport indices offers little information about the adequacy of flow distribution and whether cellular O_2 utilization is appropriate. To correct fully an oxygen debt in a high-risk patient, oxygen transport variables should be maximized with simultaneous monitoring of indirect biochemical indices of perfusion, such as lactate, base deficit, and gastric mucosal pHi.

21. Do supranormal oxygen transport indices (DO_2, VO_2, cardiac index) serve as useful resuscitation end points?

Yes, but this issue is controversial. The supranormal oxygen delivery goals most often reported are a cardiac index of 4.5 L/min/m², oxygen delivery index > 600 ml/min/m², and oxygen consumption index > 170 ml/min/m². Based on clinical experience, most young, otherwise healthy patients achieve these objectives with little extra assistance. Conversely, cardiovascular disease may place the older patient at higher risk, and supranormal oxygen transport goals may increase mortality. The purpose of pushing resuscitation is to reverse or "pay back" the accumulated oxygen debt. Although the final answer about the efficacy of supranormal resuscitation is unknown, the message is clear. The patient must be rewarmed, mechanical ventilation must be optimized, adequate sedation and pain control must be provided, and the patient must be appropriately volume-resuscitated.

22. Are there any organ-specific indicators of the adequacy of blood flow?

Electrocardiography and urine output can be used to assess cardiac and renal perfusion, respectively. Cerebral perfusion is probably adequate if the patient can recall "how many dudes jumped me." Gastric tonometry is a method of assessing the adequacy of the splanchnic circulation. Splanchnic hypoperfusion occurs early in the course of shock (see chapter 3) and may precede changes in systemic hemodynamic indices, oxygen transport variables, and acid-base balance.

23. How is gastric tonometry performed?

The gastric tonometer consists of a CO_2-permeable balloon secured to the distal end of a nasogastric tube. CO_2 in the adjacent gastric mucosa is allowed to equilibrate with the saline-filled balloon. After 60 minutes of equilibration, the saline is aspirated as a measure of the gastric mucosal PCO_2, and arterial blood gases are obtained for bicarbonate concentration [HCO_3^-]. Gastric intramucosal pH is then calculated from the Henderson-Hasselbach equation:

$$pHi = 6.1 + \log_{10} \frac{\text{arterial [HCO}_3^-]}{\text{saline PCO}_2 \times 0.03}$$

Normal pHi is approximately 7.38 (range: 7.35–7.41). Survival benefits in critically ill patients have been demonstrated if admission pHi can be corrected and maintained at values greater then 7.32 within the initial 24 hours.

BIBLIOGRAPHY

1. Bongard FS, Leighton TA: Continuous dual oximetry in surgical critical care. Ann Surg 216:60–68, 1992.
2. Comroe JH, Botello S: Unreliability of cyanosis in recognition of arterial anoxemia. Am J Surg 214:1, 1947.
3. Elliott DC: An evaluation of the end points of resuscitation. J Am Coll Surg 187:536–547, 1998.
4. Ivatury RR, Simon RJ, Islam S, et al: A prospective randomized study of end points of resuscitation after major trauma: Global oxygen transport indices versus organ-specific gastric mucosal pH. J Am Coll Surg 183:145–154, 1996.
5. Marino PI: The ICU Book, 2nd ed. Baltimore, Williams & Wilkins, 1998.
6. Moore FA, Haenel JB, Moore EE, Whitehill TA: Incommensurate oxygen consumption in response to maximal oxygen availability predicts postinjury multiple organ failure. J Trauma 33:58–67, 1992.
7. Neff TA: Routine oximetry: A fifth vital sign? Chest 94:227, 1988.
8. Porter JM, Ivatury RR: In search of the optimal end points of resuscitation in trauma patients: A review. J Trauma 44:908–914, 1998.

12. CENTRAL VENOUS AND PULMONARY ARTERY PRESSURE MONITORING

Thomas A. Whitehill, M.D., Glenn J.R. Whitman, M.D., and Alden H. Harken, M.D.

1. What is central venous pressure (CVP)?

Central venous or right atrial pressure is the pressure that pushes blood into the right ventricle during the period of diastolic filling. The higher the CVP, the more the blood will flow into the right ventricle. Starling's law indicates that with increasing end-diastolic volume (to a point), more blood will be ejected during systole; thus, increased CVP usually leads to an increased stroke volume. Normally, the right ventricle can fill adequately with an astonishingly low CVP (3–5 mmHg).

2. What are the indications for placement of a CVP monitoring catheter?

Facilitation of fluid administration and management, emergency insertion of a transvenous pacemaker, lack of adequate peripheral veins, and administration of long-term hypertonic solutions (total parenteral nutrition) or antibiotics.

3. How do you measure CVP?

A catheter must be placed in the superior vena cava (SVC) or right atrium. Because of the negligible pressure drop between the SVC and the right atrium, either one of these locations is acceptable; all intrathoracic veins have nearly the same pressure. The catheter can be threaded into the intrathoracic position from either an antecubital vain cutdown site or a percutaneous central subclavian/internal jugular approach. Either fluid column manometric or electronic transducer systems can be used to interpret the resultant pressure wave.

4. What are the contraindications to percutaneous subclavian or internal jugular venous catheterization?

Bleeding and pneumothorax. During percutaneous subclavian vein or jugular venous access the risk of bleeding is low—but not zero. In a patient who has abnormal clotting studies (for whatever reasons), who is anticoagulated, or who has a platelet count less than 20,000, it is typically safer to place a CVP line by peripheral cutdown. Similarly, a patient with hyperinflated lungs, chronic obstructive pulmonary disease, and some respiratory distress may not tolerate a pneumothorax very well. Of interest, inadvertent arterial puncture is tolerated fairly well unless the patient is coagulopathic.

5. How do you place a CVP or Swan-Ganz catheter by percutaneous subclavian vein puncture?

1. Place the patient the mild head-down (Trendelenburg) position.

2. Using sterile technique, insert an 18-gauge "finder" needle on a 10-ml syringe in the mid-clavicular line, pointing the suprasternal notch. Hug the undersurface of the clavicle. Apply gentle suction with the syringe. When you hit the vein, dark (nonpulsatile) blood easily flows back into the syringe.

3. Insert a soft, flexible wire down the 18-gauge needle.

4. Remove the needle, leaving the flexible wire stylet in place.

5. Slide a plastic sheath over the guidewire stylet. Remove the wire.

6. A plastic (or Swan-Ganz) catheter should pass easily down inside the introducer sheath.

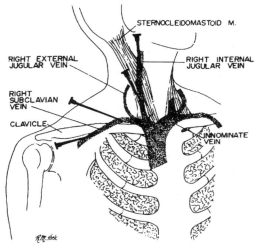

Catheter placement by percutaneous subclavian vein puncture.

6. How do you confirm position of the central venous or pulmonary (Swan-Ganz) catheter?

Chest radiograph.

7. Why would anyone want to place a pulmonary artery (Swan-Ganz) catheter?

To measure (1) pressure (left ventricular filling pressure), (2) flow (cardiac output), and (3) saturation (systemic oxygen extraction).

8. What are the assumptions inherent in pulmonary artery pressure monitoring?

1. Pulmonary artery diastolic pressure equals pulmonary capillary wedge pressure.

2. Pulmonary capillary wedge pressure equals pulmonary venous pressure.

3. Pulmonary venous pressure equals left atrial pressure.

4. Left atrial pressure equals left ventricular end-diastolic pressure.

5. Left ventricular end-diastolic pressure reflects left ventricular end-diastolic volume.

6. Left ventricular end-diastolic volume relates to stroke volume.

7. Stroke volume times heart rate equals cardiac output.

9. Is that a lot of assumptions?

Yes.

10. As you insert a Swan-Ganz catheter, what do the pressure waveforms look like?

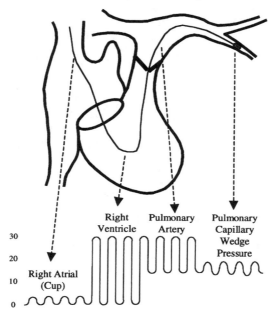

Pressure waveforms after insertion of a Swan-Ganz catheter.

11. How is cardiac output measured by thermodilution?

Inject 10 ml of cold (10°C) saline into the proximal port of a Swan-Ganz catheter. A temperature probe at the distal catheter tip integrates the bolus of cold blood as it flows by and electronically converts this signal into blood flow (L/min). Because cardiac output changes during the respiratory cycle, injection should be synchronized with end-expiration (functional residual capacity [FRC]) to standardize variability. Even so, expect a variation of ± 15%.

12. When is a thermodilution measurement of cardiac output inaccurate?

A left-to-right shunt adds shunted blood to the cold saline bolus, giving a falsely elevated measurement of cardiac output. Similarly, tricuspid regurgitation generates an abnormal curve with a falsely elevated reading. The higher the cardiac output, the less accurate the computation.

13. How do you determine the systemic (peripheral) vascular resistance?

$$SVR = \frac{\overline{BP} - \overline{CVP} \times 80}{CO}$$

where SVR = systemic vascular resistance (dynes/sec/cm^{-5}), BP = mean arterial blood pressure (mmHg), CVP = central venous pressure (mmHg), and CO = cardiac output (L/min). Normal SVR is 800–1200 dynes/sec/cm^{-5}.

14. How are right- or left-sided filling pressures used to evaluate shock?

Management of the patient in shock requires knowledge of arterial pressure as well as right arterial pressure, pulmonary artery pressure, pulmonary capillary wedge pressure (PCWP), and cardiac output. Prompt characterization of the hemodynamic pattern allows an etiologic diagnosis and points the way to therapy.

Hypovolemic shock. Right and left filling pressures are low, as is cardiac output. Peripheral vascular resistance is high. (In patients with heart disease, CVP is frequently a poor reflection of left ventricular filling). The diagnosis is confirmed when volume repletion with rising filling pressure is associated with increased cardiac output, normalization of system pressure, and decreased peripheral vascular resistance.

Cardiogenic shock. Shock despite adequate right (CVP) and left (PCWP) heart filling pressures means that volume status is okay; the problem is the pump (heart). Cardiac output is low. If SVR is high, infuse dobutamine, 5 µg/kg/min, to stimulate the heart and reduce SVR. If SVR is low, infuse epinephrine, 0.05 µg/kg/min, to stimulate the heart and increase SVR.

Septic shock. The hallmarks of septic shock are normal or low-normal filling pressure, supranormal cardiac output, and low peripheral vascular resistance (< 600 dynes/sec/cm^{-5}). Treatment requires fluid resuscitation and systemic vasoconstriction while the underlying cause (e.g., abdominal abscess) is treated.

15. What is an oximetric Swan-Ganz catheter?

A catheter with a fiberoptic monitor at its distal tip that continuously measures HbO_2 saturation [$SO_2(\%)$]. When properly positioned, the distal catheter tip is in the pulmonary artery, and O_2 saturation reflects that of mixed venous blood (SvO_2).

16. What is the significance of mixed venous oxygen saturation? What is the difference between PaO_2, O_2 saturation, and oxygen content?

Please see Chapter 5.

1. **Arterial oxygen content (C_aO_2)**

O_2 dissolved in blood + O_2 combined with hemoglobin

O_2 dissolved = $0.003 \times PO_2$

O_2 combined with hemoglobin = $1.38 \times Hgb \times SaO_2$

For example, if Hgb = 12 gm %, PO_2 = 60 torr, and SaO_2 = 90%, C_aO_2 = (0.003×60) = $(1.38 \times 12 \times 0.90)$ = 15.08 ml O_2/100 ml/blood or 15.08 vol %. As is usually the case, dissolved O2 makes up only a small percentage of C_aO_2 (in this example, 1%). Therefore, its contribution to C_aO_2 is omitted in further discussion.

2. **A-VO$_2$ difference.** Understanding how to determine the oxygen content of blood permits determination of the difference in arterial vs. mixed venous O_2 content, or the A-VO$_2$ difference. When the pulmonary artery or mixed venous HbO_2 saturation (SvO_2) is known, the computation is straightforward:

A-VO$_2$ difference $(C_aO_2 - C_vO_2)$ = Hb 1.38 · SaO_2 – Hb 1.38 · SvO_2

= Hb 1.38 $(SaO_2 - SvO_2)$

In the typical situation, Hb = 15 (mg)%, SaO_2 = 96%, and SvO_2 = 75%. Thus, the A-VO$_2$ difference = 15 · 1.38 · $(SaO_2 - SvO_2)$

= 15 · 1.38 · (97 – 75)

= 20.7 (0.21)

= 4.35 vol%

In other words, every 100 ml of blood that travels around the body gives up 4.35 ml of O_2. The normal range for the A-VO$_2$ difference is 3–5 vol%.

3. **Fick principle.** In a steady-state situation, the body uses O_2 at the rate of 125 ml/min/m^2. Therefore, one can roughly determine the minute O_2 consumption. By measuring the A-VO$_2$ difference, one can determine the contribution of each 100 ml of blood that travels around the body to the total minute O_2 consumption (VO_2). Thus, in a man with a body surface area of 2 m^2, minute O_2 consumption (VO_2) = 250 ml. If the measured A-VO$_2$ difference = 4.35 ml, as in the example above, one may conclude that every 100 ml of blood contributes 4.35 ml to the VO_2 of 250 ml. Thus, 4.75 L of blood must travel around the patient's body each minute to meet the O_2 requirement. By assuming VO_2 and measuring the A-VO$_2$ difference, one can estimate cardiac output:

$$CO = \frac{VO_2}{\text{A-VO}_2 \text{ difference}} \times 10$$

17. What is the meaning of mixed venous oxygen saturation (SVO₂)?

If your head is not already swimming with assumptions, let's make some more:

1. Assume that the patient's total body oxygen consumption (VO₂) is stable (as it probably is over short periods).

2. Assume that the patient's arterial oxygen content (C$_a$O₂) is stable (as it probably is over short periods).

As cardiac output increases (delivering more oxygen to meet fixed demand), the patient extracts less oxygen peripherally and mixed venous O_2 will rise. Conversely, as cardiac output decreases (delivering less oxygen peripherally to meet fixed demand), tissue oxygen extraction must increase, driving mixed oxygen saturation down. Thus, we assume (over short periods) that the only parameter that influences mixed venous oxygen saturation (SvO₂) is cardiac output. Again, over short periods these assumptions are not bad:

Green zone SvO₂ (happy patient)   = 75% or above
Yellow zone SvO₂ (trouble)   = 55% or above
Red zone SvO₂ (impending doom) = 55% or below

18. When is the oximetric Swan-Ganz catheter inaccurate or misleading?

When the catheter has been in place for prolonged periods (24–72 hr), the fiberoptic tip may become covered with gunk. The transmitted light intensity then diminishes, and the readings become inaccurate. The new oximetric Swan-Ganz catheters have a light-intensity measurement that alerts the clinician when the device is covered with fibrin. A drop in hematocrit also may lower the SvO₂. This phenomenon is real—it is not an artifact (because O_2 delivery really decreases). If the A-VO₂ difference is 5 vol% and the Hbg is 15 gm%, the SvO₂ = 75%. However, if the Hbg is 7.5, the SvO₂ = 50%. The SvO₂ can change on the basis of Hbg alone, with no change in cardiac output.

BIBLIOGRAPHY

1. Swan HJC, Ganz W: Complications of flow-directed balloon-tipped catheters. Ann Intern Med 91:494, 1979.
2. Swan HJC, Ganz W: Use of balloon flotation catheters in critically ill patients. Surg Clin North Am 55:501, 1975.
3. Woods M, Scott RN, Harken AH: Practical considerations in the use of a pulmonary artery catheter. Surgery 79:469–475, 1976.

13. SURGICAL WOUND INFECTION

Steven L. Peterson, D.V.M, M.D.

1. How are surgical wound infections defined and classified?

Surgical wound infections or, more appropriately, **surgical site infections** (SSIs), occur within 30 days of surgery unless a foreign body is left in situ. In the case of implanted foreign material, 1 year must elapse before surgery can be excluded as causative. SSIs are subdivided based on depth of tissue involvement into three clinically relevant categories:

1. Superficial incisional SSIs
2. Deep incisional SSIs (involving fascia and muscle)
3. Organ space SSIs (any anatomic structure opened or manipulated during the operative procedure)

2. What are the classic signs of superficial, deep incisional, and organ space SSIs?
Superficial and deep incisional SSIs
- Calor (heat)   • Tumor (swelling)
- Rubor (redness)   • Dolor (pain)

Organ space SSIs should be suspected in the presence of systemic signs and symptoms, such as fever, ileus, and/or shock. Definitive diagnosis may require imaging studies.

3. Can you predict the potential for development of an SSI based on the type of wound?

Yes. Based on degree of gross contamination, wounds may be stratified into one of four categories: clean, clean-contaminated, contaminated, and dirty-infected. **Clean wounds** are atraumatic wounds in which no inflammation is encountered, no breaks in sterile technique occur, and no hollow viscus is entered. **Clean-contaminated wounds** are identical except that a hollow viscus is entered. **Contaminated wounds** are caused by trauma from a clean source or by minor spillage of infected materials. **Dirty-infected wounds** are caused by trauma from a contaminated source or gross spillage of infected material into an incision. Reported infection rates for each category are 2.1%, 3.3%, 6.4%, and 7.1%, respectively.

4. What factors other than wound class help to predict the probability of wound infection?

Physical status as classified by the American Society of Anesthesiologists, results of intraoperative cultures, and duration of preoperative hospital stay are significant predictors of postoperative SSIs. Adequacy of regional blood supply is also important, as evidenced by the low infection rate in facial wounds.

5. What factors can the surgeon control to decrease SSIs?

Limiting the duration of surgery, obliterating dead space, meticulous hemostasis, minimizing placement of foreign material (to include excessive suture), and gentle tissue handling help to decrease postoperative infection. Appropriate use of electrocautery for hemostasis does not increase wound infection rates.

6. Does prophylaxis with systemic antibiotics decrease the probability of infection?

The use of antibiotics in contaminated and dirty-infected wounds is clearly indicated and represents therapy rather than prophylaxis. In clean-contaminated wounds consensus supports their routine use as prophylaxis. The use of prophylactic antibiotics in clean wounds was initially advocated only in cases in which prosthetic material was implanted. The general attitude was that any benefit from the use of prophylactic antibiotics in clean surgery was outweighed by potential untoward side effects from spurious use. Strictly speaking, however, all operations leave some foreign material (i.e., suture), and even a single suture may cause suppuration with a bacterial inoculum that by itself does not result in infection. In addition, a large multicenter, prospective, randomized study of antibiotic prophylaxis in clean surgery has shown the apparent value of prophylaxis in reducing SSIs.

7. If antibiotics are used, when should they be administered?

Maximal benefit is obtained when tissue concentrations are therapeutic at the time of contamination. Efficacy, therefore, is enhanced when prophylactic antibiotics are administered immediately before surgical incision; late administration is similar to no administration. Multiple-dose regimens have no proven benefit over single-dose regimens. Indiscriminate antibiotic selection outside recommended hospital protocols may actually increase the incidence of SSIs.

8. Does all that pulsatile lavage used in the operating room really do any good?

Yes. High-pressure pulsatile lavage has been extensively evaluated in soft tissue contamination and has been shown to be seven times more effective in reducing bacterial load than bulb syringe lavage. The inherent elastic recoil of the soft tissues allows particulate matter to escape between pulses of fluid. The optimal pressure and pulse frequency appear to be 50–70 pounds/square inch and 800 pulses/minute, respectively.

9. With antibiotics and high-pressure lavage, can primary closure be used more frequently for obviously dirty or contaminated wounds?

Despite these adjuvant therapies, primary closure remains a difficult surgical decision requiring experience and good judgment. Primary closure is always tempting because of the decreased morbidity and improved cosmesis. However, if infection develops, the consequences are serious and the wound must be reopened. Factors that affect the decision include degree of contamination, amount of necrotic tissue or dead space left in the wound, adequacy of blood supply, efficacy of drains, interval since injury, and presence of foreign material. In general, it is safer to leave a questionable wound open and allow it to heal secondarily or to use delayed primary closure 3–5 days later. Delayed primary closure is a compromise that often differentiates the experienced surgeon from the enthusiastic amateur.

10. List commonly reported infection rates for specific operations.

Cholecystectomy	3%	Inguinal herniorrhaphy	2%
Appendectomy	5%	Thoracotomy	6%
Colectomy	12%		

11. When infections occurs, what are the most commonly involved organisms?

Because staphylococci are the most common skin organism, they are also the most common etiologic agent in SSIs. Certain organisms, however, are more commonly associated with SSIs in specific wound sites. If the gut was violated, enterobacteriaceae and anaerobes are common; biliary tract and esophageal incisions yield these organisms plus enterococci. Other areas, such as the urinary tract or vagina, contain organisms such as group D streptococci, *Pseudomonas* sp, and *Proteus* sp.

12. How are wound infections temporally related to surgery?

The typical wound infection occurs 5–7 days postoperatively; however, peracute infections may occur. Clostridial infections associated with massive amounts of devitalized tissue in an enclosed space are the classic example of the peracute SSI.

13. What is the first line of therapy in SSIs?

Drainage, which often is established by reopening the wound or, in the case of deep space infections, by computed tomography- or ultrasound-guided techniques. Antibiotic therapy is also used to control associated cellulitis and generalized sepsis.

14. What may happen with untreated superficial or deep incisional SSIs?

Locally the wound breaks down, and the infection dissects through tissue planes and continues to advance. If the infection progresses rapidly, necrotizing fasciitis may develop. Finally, the strength layers of the wound closure break open (dehisce).

15. What is wound dehiscence? Evisceration?

Wound dehiscence is the partial or total disruption of any or all layers of the operative wound. **Evisceration** is rupture of all layers of the abdominal wall and extrusion of the abdominal viscera.

16. What factors predispose to dehiscence?

Age greater than 60 years, obesity and increased intraabdominal pressure, malnutrition, renal or hepatic insufficiency, diabetes mellitus, use of corticosteroids or cytotoxic drugs, and radiation have been implicated in wound dehiscence. Infection also plays an important role; an infective agent is identified in over one-half of wounds that undergo dehiscence. Despite these excuses, the single most important factor in wound dehiscence is the adequacy of closure. Fascial edges should not be devitalized. The linea alba sutures ideally should be placed neither too laterally nor too medially. Excessively lateral placement may incorporate the variable blood supply of the rectus abdominis muscle and compromise fascial circulation. Excessively medial placement misses the point of maximal strength at the transition zone between the linea alba and rectus abdominis sheath. In addition, sutures should be tied correctly without excessive tension, and suture material of adequate tensile strength should be chosen.

17. When does wound dehiscence occur?

Wound dehiscence may occur at any time after surgery; however, it is most common between the fifth and tenth postoperative days when wound strength is at a minimum.

18. What are the signs and symptoms of wound dehiscence?

Normally a ridge of palpable thickening (healing ridge) extends about 0.5 cm on each side of the incision within 1 week. Absence of this ridge may be a strong predictor of impending wound breakdown. More commonly, leakage of serosanguinous fluid from the wound is the first sign. In some instances, sudden evisceration may be the first indication of abdominal wound dehiscence. The patient also may describe a sensation of tearing or popping associated with coughing or retching.

19. Describe the proper management of wound dehiscence.

If the dehiscence is not associated with infection, elective reclosure may be the appropriate therapeutic course. However, if the condition of the patient or wound makes reclosure unacceptable, the wound should be allowed to heal by second intention. An unstable scar or incisional hernia may be dealt with at a later, safer time. Dehiscence of a laparotomy wound with evisceration represents a surgical emergency with a reported mortality rate of 10–20%. Initial treatment in this instance consists of appropriate resuscitation while protecting the eviscerated organs with moist towels; the next step is prompt surgical closure. Exposed bowel and/or omentum should be lavaged thoroughly and returned to the abdomen; the abdominal wall should be closed; and the skin wound should be packed open.

BIBLIOGRAPHY

1. Bhandari M, Adili A, Lachowski RJ: High pressure pulsatile lavage of contaminated human tibiae. An in vitro study. J Orthop Trauma 12:478–484, 1998.
2. Classen DC, Evans RS, Pestotnik SL, et al: The timing of prophylactic administration of antibiotics and the risk of surgical-wound infection. N Engl J Med 326:281–286, 1992.
3. Emmerson M: A microbiologist's view of factors contributing to infection. New Horizons 6(Suppl 2):S3–S10, 1998.
4. McDonald M, Grabsch E, Marshall C, Frobes A: Single- versus multiple-dose antimicrobial prophylaxis for major surgery: A systematic review. Aust N Z J Surg 68:388–396, 1998.
5. Platt R, Zaleznik DF, Hopkins CC, et al: Perioperative antibiotic prophylaxis for herniorrhaphy and breast surgery. N Engl J Med 322:153–160, 1990.
6. Platt R, Zucker JR, Zaleznik DF, et al: Prophylaxis against wound infection following herniorrhaphy and breast surgery. J Infect Dis 166:556–560, 1992.
7. Velasco E, Thuler LC, Martins CA, et al: Risk index for prediction of surgical site infection after oncology operations. Am J Infect Control 26:217–223, 1998.

14. ACUTE ABDOMEN

Alden H. Harken, M.D.

1. What is the surgeon's responsibility when confronted by a patient with an acute abdomen?

(1) To identify how sick the patient is and (2) to determine whether the patient needs to go directly to the operating room, should be admitted for resuscitation or observation, or can safely be sent home.

2. Which is the most dangerous course?

To send the patient home.

3. Is it important to make the diagnosis in the emergency department?

No. Frequently time spent confirming a diagnosis in the emergency department is lost to in-hospital resuscitation and/or treatment in the operating room. The only patient who needs a relatively firm diagnosis is a patient who is to be sent home.

4. If the essential goal is not to make the diagnosis, what should the surgeon do?

1. Resuscitate the patient. Most patients do not eat or drink when they are getting sick. Thus, most patients are depleted of at least several liters of fluid. Depletion is worse in patients with diarrhea or vomiting.

2. Start a big IV line.

3. Replace lost electrolytes (see chapter 6).

4. Insert a Foley catheter (this approach does not hurt the patient, and it is a real crowd-pleaser).

5. Examine the patient.

5. Are symptoms and signs uniquely misleading in any groups of patients?

Yes. Watch out for the following groups:
- The very young, who cannot talk.
- Diabetics, because of visceral neuropathy.
- The very old, in whom, much as in diabetics, abdominal innervation is dulled.
- Patients taking steroids, which depress inflammation and mask everything.
- Patients with immunosuppression (a heart transplant patient may act cheerful even with dead or gangrenous bowel).

6. What history is needed?

1. **The patient's age.** Neonates present with intussusception; young women present with ectopic pregnancy, pelvic inflammatory disease, and appendicitis; the elderly present with colon cancer, diverticulitis, and appendicitis.

2. **Associated problems.** Previous hospitalizations, prior abdominal surgery, medications, heart and lung disease? An extensive gynecologic history is valuable; however, it is probably safer to assume that all women between 12 and 40 years old are pregnant.

3. **Location of abdominal pain.** *Right upper quadrant:* gallbladder or biliary disease, duodenal ulcer. *Right flank:* pyelonephritis, hepatitis. *Midepigastrium:* duodenal or gastric ulcer, pancreatitis, gastritis. *Left upper quadrant:* ruptured spleen, subdiaphragmatic abscess. *Right lower quadrant:* appendicitis (see chapter 37), ectopic pregnancy, incarcerated hernia, rectus hematoma. *Left lower quadrant:* diverticulitis, incarcerated hernia, rectus hematoma. *Note:* Cancer, unless it obstructs (colon cancer), and bleeding (diverticulosis) typically do not hurt.

4. **Duration of pain.** The pain of a perforated duodenal ulcer or perforated sigmoid diverticulum is sudden, whereas the pain of pyelonephritis is gradual and persistent. The pain of intestinal obstruction is intermittent and crampy. *Note:* Although the surgeon is rotating through a GI service, the patient may not know this and may present with urologic, gynecologic, or vascular pathology.

PHYSICAL EXAMINATION

7. Are vital signs important?

Yes. They are vital. If both heart rate and blood pressure are on the wrong side of 100 (heart rate > 100, systolic blood pressure < 100), watch out! Tachypnea (respiratory rate > 16) reflects either pain or systemic acidosis. Fever may develop late, particularly in the immunosuppressed patient who may be afebrile in the face of florid peritonitis.

8. What is rebound?

The peritoneum is well innervated and exquisitely sensitive. It is not necessary to hurt the patient to elicit peritoneal signs. Depress the abdomen gently and release. If the patient winces, the peritoneum is inflamed (rebound tenderness).

9. What is mittelschmerz?

Mittelschmerz is pain in the middle of the menstrual cycle. Ovulation is frequently associated with intraperitoneal bleeding. Blood irritates the sensitive peritoneum and hurts.

10. What do bowel sounds mean?

If something hurts (like a sprained ankle), the patient tends not to use it. Thus, inflamed bowel is quiet. Bowel contents squeezed through a partial obstruction produce high-pitched tinkles. Bowel sounds are notoriously unreliable, however.

11. What is the significance of abdominal distention?

Distention may derive from either intra- or extraenteric gas or fluid (worst of all, blood). Abdominal distention is always significant and bad.

12. Is abdominal palpation important?

Yes. But remember, the patient is (or should be) the surgeon's friend. There is no need to cause pain. Palpation guides the surgeon to the anatomic zone of most tenderness (usually the diseased area). It is best to start palpation in an area that does not hurt. Rectal (test stool for blood) and pelvic examinations further localize pathology.

13. What is Kehr's sign?

The diaphragm and the back of the left shoulder enjoy parallel innervation. Thus, concurrent left upper quadrant and left shoulder pain indicate diaphragmatic irritation from a ruptured spleen or subdiaphragmatic abscess.

14. What is a psoas sign?

Irritation of the retroperitoneal psoas muscle by an inflamed retrocecal appendix causes pain on flexion of the right hip or extension of the thigh.

LABORATORY STUDIES

15. How is a complete blood count helpful?

1. **Hematocrit.** If the hematocrit is high (> 45%), the patient is most likely very dry and/or may have chronic obstructive lung disease. If it is low (< 30%), the patient probably has a more chronic blood disease.

2. **White blood cell count.** It takes time (hours) for inflammation to release cytokines and elevate the white cell count. A normal white blood cell count is entirely consistent with significant abdominal trouble.

16. Is urinalysis necessary?

Absolutely. White cells in the urine may redirect attention to the diagnosis of pyelonephritis or cystitis. Hematuria points to renal or ureteral stones. Because an inflamed appendix may lie directly on the right ureter, both red and white blood cells may be found in the urine of patients with appendicitis.

17. What is a "three-way of the abdomen"?

1. **Upright chest radiograph.** Look for free air under the diaphragm (perforated viscus) and pneumonia or pneumothorax.

2. **Upright abdomen.** Look for free air under the diaphragm and air-fluid levels (intestinal obstruction). Remember to look for sigmoid or rectal air (partial obstruction).

3. **Supine abdomen.** This radiograph tells nothing.

Most ureteral stones can be visualized. Only 10% of gallstones are radiopaque, and appendiceal fecaliths are rarely noted. **Honors:** Air in the biliary system indicates a biliary-enteric fistula. In association with intestinal air-fluid levels, the diagnosis is gallstone ileus.

18. What is a sentinel loop?

Except in children (who swallow everything, including air), small bowel gas is always pathologic. A single loop of small bowel gas adjacent to an inflamed organ (e.g., the pancreas) may point to the disease.

19. Is ultrasound valuable?

Yes—if the working diagnosis is cholecystitis, gallstones, ectopic pregnancy, or ovarian cyst.

20. Is abdominal computed tomography (CT) scanning valuable?

Yes—if the working diagnosis is an intraabdominal abscess (sigmoid diverticulitis), pancreatitis, retroperitoneal bleeding (leaking abdominal aortic aneurysm; this patient should have gone straight to the operating room), or intrahepatic or splenic pathology.

21. What is a double-contrast CT scan?

The bowel is delineated with barium or gastrografin. The blood vessels are delineated with an iodinated vascular dye. Thus, the CT scan precisely displays the abdominal contents relative to vascular and intestinal landmarks. Contrast CT imaging of pancreatitis is valuable to assess zones of perfusion and/or necrosis.

SURGICAL TREATMENT

22. If the patient is sick (and not getting better), what should be done?

After fluid resuscitation, the patient's abdomen should be explored. An exploratory laparotomy has been touted as the logical conclusion of a complete physical examination.

23. Is a negative laparotomy harmful?

Yes. But patients can uncomfortably survive a negative laparotomy, whereas missed bowel infarction (or even appendicitis) can be life-threatening.

24. What is the most challenging problem in all of medicine?

An acute abdomen.

BIBLIOGRAPHY

1. Abernathy CM, Hamm RM: Surgical Scripts. Philadelphia, Hanley & Belfus, 1994.
2. Graber MA, Ely JW, Clarke S, et al: Informed consent and the general surgeons' attitudes toward the use of pain medication in the acute abdomen. Am J Emerg Med 17:113–116, 1999.
3. Gordon LA: Gordon's Guide to the Surgical Morbidity and Mortality Conference. Philadelphia, Hanley & Belfus, 1994.
4. Mindelzun RE, Jeffrey RB: The acute abdomen: Current CT imaging techniques. Semin Ultrasound CT MR 20:63–67, 1999.
5. Richardson NG, Jones PM: Informed consent in patients with acute abdominal pain. Br J Surg 86:426, 1999.
6. Saeian K, Reddy KR: Diagnostic laparoscopy: An update. Endoscopy 31:103–109, 1999.

15. SURGICAL SEPSIS: PREVENTION AND MANAGEMENT

Glenn W. Geelhoed, M.D., M.P.H., FACS

MICROBIAL CONTAMINATION AND INFECTION

1. Modern antibiotic developments have controlled many, if not most, of the problems of surgical infection—right?

Quite wrong! In seriously ill surgical patients in intensive care settings, the problems of sepsis have increased and remain among the principal causes of death in patients with multiple organ failure and impairments of host defense. Antibiotic treatment may change the biographical sketch of the flora associated with patients' deaths but cannot overcome the multiple causes of failing host resistance to infection that accompany barrier breeches to microbial invasion and the inflammatory and immunologic responses to the "usual suspects."

2. What kinds of barrier breech allow microbial invasion that may set up surgical infection?

The skin and mucosal linings of the body maintain a barrier between the multifloral outside world and the sterile interior milieu of tissues and organs (even when the outside world is a tube of heavily populated flora through the middle of usually sterile body cavities, such as the gastrointestinal [GI] tract). It is easy to see the barrier breech when a knife penetrates the skin, carrying exterior flora beneath the skin, or when that knife perforates and spills the contaminated contents of the gut into the abdomen. It is less obvious when the breech is caused by a low-flow state or when inadequate nutrition or toxins impair mucosal immunoglobulins, making the "bug-body barrier" permeable. These polymicrobial communities of organisms may begin to invade through the breech in such barriers, particularly if there are further failures in the third line of defense in humoral and cellular resistance.

3. What is the difference between contamination and infection?

The presence of microorganisms does not an infection make!

Resident communities of flora on body surfaces do little harm, and gut flora are downright beneficial when contained in the gut. It is even possible for bacteria to be transiently present outside their usual commensal residences without constituting an infection in the normally intact host. For example, in vigorously brushing your teeth this morning, gram-negative bacteria of various kinds that are resident in the oral cavity were introduced into your blood stream but probably were quickly eliminated by normal defense mechanisms—unless they met lowered host resistance or seeded a prosthetic heart valve.

4. How can the enormous load of bacteria in the lower GI tract be beneficial?

Bugs can be beautiful. These are the same bacteria that have lived with and in humans symbiotically for millennia. They synthesize vitamin K—something we literally cannot do without—or crowd out pathogenic organisms by their overwhelming numbers. They also help to metabolize bile salts and play a role in detoxifying some environmental hazards. You are familiar with other forms of plumbing known as septic systems?

5. Whenever intraabdominal bowel spillage is encountered, it is mandatory to culture the fecal contamination and obtain sensitivities of all identified organisms—right?

Have you already forgotten the difference between contamination and infection? What edifying information will cultures of fecal spillage into the peritoneum give you? Do you think that the contaminant, just because of its change in position with reference to the bowel wall, is likely to be sterile? When would you like the laboratory to quit? Will you be content to hear a report of *Escherichia coli* and bacteroides—two of the more than 800 species that even the most compulsive laboratory can hardly be competent to identify, given the exposure to air and time lapse until processing on different media? How will information from a sampling error of mixed, community-acquired contaminants change your therapy? If, for instance, no anaerobes are identified from the fecal specimen, will you be so confident that they are not present as to exclude these species from coverage?

The lesson to be learned is that culture of community-acquired **contaminants** is expensive, incomplete, and unedifying; the culture of invading microbes in **infections**, particularly hospital-acquired microbes that persist after treatment, may give critical information and is a more appropriate use of microbiologic resources.

6. What are preps, such as bowel preps?

Preps are decontamination procedures, designed to reduce resident flora before an elective invasive procedure. Preps may take the form of a simple process such as the alcohol swab smeared over the skin before the quick prick of the subcutaneous injection, or may involve preparation of a larger area of the skin surface for the surgical field of incision (see question 7).

A bowel prep is similarly designed to reduce the resident flora in the gut and may do so by (1) mechanical catharsis (i.e., purge); (2) osmotic or volume dilution with large volumes of saline, other electrolyte solutions, or mannitol; or (3) oral administration of nonabsorbed antibiotics. Of these methods, the most important is clearly mechanical catharsis because it purges huge amounts of flora, which may account for up to two-thirds the dry weight of colon contents. One of the most cogent reasons for the choice of certain oral antibiotics in bowel preps (see question 9) is their vigorous cathartic action.

7. How do we sterilize the skin or mucosal cavities of a patient to prepare a sterile field for operative incision?

I can think of one way, hardly recommended, by which patients can be "sterilized"; like instruments and drapes, they can be placed in an autoclave. But short of this absurd example, *the skin is never sterile*. Decontamination processes are never perfect, particularly in so complex a tissue with crevices and accessory skin structures in which bacteria reside. Resting gloved hands on a "sterile field" does not include the skin or mucosal surfaces.

At best we simply *reduce* the flora to the low-level inoculum that can be handled by most intact host defense systems—as in the example of brushing your teeth—but living tissue surfaces are never "sterile." A method that kills all microbial organisms from such surfaces also would devitalize mammalian cells and render them more susceptible to lower-level microbial inocula.

8. What means can be used to reduce surface resident flora without further injuring skin or mucosa?

1. **Volume lavage** (for mnemonic value only, dilution is the solution to pollution)
2. **De-fatting**, which solubilizes the sebaceous oils that may trap flora
3. **Microbicidal killing** with a bacteriostatic agent

To an amazing extent, one cheap, simple fluid may serve as diluent, fat solvent, and antimicrobial—alcohol. Alcohol is nearly ideal as as prepping solution, with the minor disadvantages that it is dehydrating and minimally flammable. Because it vaporizes and disappears, flora may spread from interstices, outside the field, or even via aerosolized fallout onto the field, thus requiring the addition of extended-duration bacteriostasis to the alcohol prep.

Iodine also kills bacteria, but with a greater hazard to sensitive mammalian cells (it oxidizes the cell walls of small plants). A lower initial concentration of iodine and a longer duration of action can be achieved by incorporation of an iodophor, a substance in nearly universal use in preps. The application of moisture- and vapor-permeable "incise drapes" or desiccation-preventing "ring drapes" may further retard repopulation of flora over the prepped (but still not sterile) field.

9. What are "pipe cleaner" antibiotics?

Pipe cleaners are orally administered antibiotic regimens that reduce the flora in the GI tract, from which they are not well absorbed. They are an almost ideal component of bowel preps because they are potent cathartic agents and accomplish the vast majority of their "pipe cleaning" by mechanical purgative action. The most popular pipe cleaners include a neomycin/erythromycin base.

10. What is selective gut decontamination? How does it work?

It doesn't work. This method used pipe cleaners in patients at high risk for the development of sepsis from multiple organ failure with the theoretic aim of reducing the risk involved in barrier breech of the GI tract and inoculation with gut flora. Good experimental evidence indicated that this method should reduce the high mortality rate in seriously ill patients at high risk of surgical sepsis. After prolonged clinical trials, however, it failed to demonstrate a benefit in patient survival. The likely reason is that the laboratory studies were done in intact animal models with functioning host defense systems, whereas failures of defense beyond the barrier breech may explain why selective gut decontamination failed to benefit seriously ill patients. Furthermore, flora repopulated the purged gut over time, but with virulent forms of microbes selected by their resistance to the broad-spectrum antibiotics. The method still has some utility in patients undergoing procedures such as high-dose chemotherapy or bone marrow transplantation and, in some patients isolated in "life islands" (e.g., patients with immunodeficiency diseases or burns).

ANTIBIOTICS

11. Are antibiotics the classic wonder drugs?

Yes, they are wonderful. You wonder if they are going to work; if they are going to cause more harm than good; and if the next generation will be unaffordable as well as toxic.

Skepticism is healthy in regard to any procedure or agent in heath care, but especially in regard to antibiotics, which are embraced almost universally as agents that both prevent and cure infections. The primacy of the host defense in this vital process and the potential interference by the very drugs given credit for infection control are overlooked. We must look critically at the limited role that antibiotics should play in health care and restrain their overuse, which generates even more harm than unnecessary expense.

12. What is meant by generations of antibiotics, as in third-generation cephalosporins?

The earliest antibiotics were bacteriostatic, largely through interference in protein synthesis, so that they might keep a microorganism from reproducing even if they did not kill it. The difference between **infestation** (presence of living microbes in the host) and **infection** (replication and spread of microorganisms in the host) may be useful in understanding how earlier drugs possibly controlled infection but were less capable of eliminating organisms in any brief period of therapy.

Penicillin changed all that. It may be the first antibiotic with a legitimate claim to the title "wonder drug" because it has the microbicidal capability of eradicating sensitive organisms. Penicillin was the first generation of the beta-lactam antibiotics, joined by the congener first-generation cephalosporins (e.g., cefazolin). They shared beta-lactam structure and had good gram-positive coverage with less range in any effect over gram-negative microbes.

The second-generation beta-lactam antibiotics (e.g., cefoxitin) covered new classes of microbes beyond gram-positive aerobes, such as many of the *Bacteroides* species, but had little effect on gram-negative aerobic microbes. Because the third-generation cephalosporins covered some of the latter microbes, they were touted as single-agent therapy for all principal-risk flora.

As with penicillin, the original wonder drug, the wonderment waned with failures of the new agents because of rapidly induced antimicrobial resistance. The most easily measured and calculated difference in the generations is cost: wholesale values are about $2.00/gm for the first generation, $5.00/gm for the second, and $30.00/gm for the third. Despite this bracket creep in cost, the higher generations lose some of their potency against the original gram-positive organisms for which the first-generation agents were truly wonderful. Therefore, it takes two grams of moxalactam to be half as good as one gram of cefazolin for gram-positive coverage. It does not take a pharmacoeconomist to ask, "What have I got in return for this 60-fold surcharge?"

13. What is the role of third-generation cephalosporins in surgical prophylaxis?

None. No more wondering here! If the principal-risk flora are gram-positive, the first generation is better; if the anaerobic risk is sizable, the second generation is better. And either class is cheaper by far and seems to have generated less resistance than the the the third-generation cephalosporins, which are unconscionably expensive for use in prophylaxis and rarely as effective as other single-agent therapy for established surgical infection. Specific indications, of course, might use or exclude these agents, such as pediatric meningitis, hospital-acquired pneumonia, or other specific infections outside the indications of surgical predominance.

14. How do enzyme inhibitors combined with antibiotics enhance their antimicrobial spectrum?

Microorganisms have defense mechanisms of their own, and the strains that have the capacity to make antibiotic-degrading enzymes achieve an unnatural selection advantage with the widespread use of antibiotics. This is what happened to penicillin. Penicillinases emerged. But clever pharmaceutical manufacturers closed that loophole for bacterial ingenuity in degrading penicillin by strategic placement of a methyl group to ruin the survival fitness of penicillinase producers. Methicillin was the result, but the persistence of the microbes means that we now have a plague of methicillin-resistant *Staphylococcus aureus* (MRSA). Besides, microbes outnumber pharmaceutical manufacturers and have a shorter turnaround time than the approval process of the Food and Drug Administration (FDA). Microbes will always be ahead of us in ingenuity if only because of their numbers.

Newer strategies by the bacteria included the production of beta-lactamases. The response of the pharmaceutical industry was a group of inhibitors of beta-lactamase, such as clavulonic acid or sulbactam. The combination of a beta-lactamase inhibitor with a modified penicillin such as ampicillin should have enhanced activity against bacteria that produce beta-lactamase, provided that they were ampicillin-sensitive in the first place. Higher doses of the original agent for a shorter time may accomplish the same effect, often at lower cost, because the combined drugs were developed much more recently and are under patent protection.

15. What are the most expensive kinds of antibiotic therapy?

1. Drugs that are given when they are not needed.
2. Drugs that are badly needed but do not work.
3. Drugs that cause more harm than good because of host toxicity, whatever their antibiotic potential.

16. Can oral antibiotics be given in place of intravenous antibiotics in seriously ill surgical patients?

Yes—if only they could take them! The kind of patient we are talking about almost invariably can take nothing by mouth (NPO), often is unconscious, and is as likely as not to be on a ventilator. In addition, the gut has been put out of commission by nasogastric suction tubes, laparotomy, and ileus, and primary intraabdominal problems often associated with the need for the antibiotics, such as intraabdominal sepsis and pancreatitis. Usually such patients are on complete gut rest and are likely to be on parenteral nutrition as well.

The attempt to use some form of gut-delivered antibiotic is based on the favorable pharmacokinetics and spectrum of quinolones, which can be started intravenously and switched as soon as possible to the oral form when feeding has resumed. Nearly all such patients begin on some form of intravenous antibiotic program, and the start-up of the antibiotic regimen is more important than the form to which patients are tapered before treatment is discontinued.

PROPHYLAXIS

17. Should systemic antibiotic prophylaxis be used in elective colon resection?

Yes—beyond any statistical shadow of a doubt. At least two dozen clinical trials have been carried out using placebo controls against a variety of antibiotics, principally those active against at least the anaerobic-predominant flora, and nearly all have shown a reduction in infectious complications in the antibiotic group. Never again should this point need repeating, and no patient should be placed at risk when systemic antibiotic prophylaxis has been established as the standard of care. No new clinical trials against placebo in this group of patients with known risk can be performed ethically, given the confirmed risk reduction.

Other risk groups besides patients undergoing colon resection have been standardized by trials in large patient populations and have shown similar risk reduction, such as cesarean section after membrane rupture. The benefit of prophylaxis has been demonstrated. In other groups of patients that cannot be standardized because of unusual contamination factors or unique factors of host resistance impairment, guidelines for rational prophylaxis should follow similar principles.

18. Are two prophylactic doses better than one in preventing infection? Are three doses better still?

Only one dose of prophylactic antibiotic can be proved, beyond statistical or clinical doubt, to be efficacious—the dose in systemic circulation at the time of the inoculum. Whether the dose needs to be repeated one or more times during the 24 hours after the inoculum depends on the blood levels of the drug, which are largely a function of protein binding and clearance rate. We also know for sure that 10 days of the same prophylactic drug that is efficacious if given immediately before the inoculum results in a higher risk of infection than no antibiotic at all.

19. What factors determine the timing of antibiotic administration under the criteria of prophylaxis?

The one immutable principle has been set out above—the most important element in timing of prophylaxis is that the drug be **circulating** before the inoculum. When should it stop? When the reduction in infection risk is no longer provable and before continued use will defeat the prophylactic purpose (as explained above). To summarize with an arbitrary rule of thumb: *there is no justification for prophylactic antibiotic 24 hours after the inoculum of an invasive procedure.*

What does this rule imply? Should we not continue prophylaxis for weeks to cover the presence of a prosthetic hip joint? Presumably, the prosthetic hip will be in the patient for many years—but surely you do not argue that the antibiotic should continue on a daily basis as long as the hip is in place! What is "prophylaxed" is not the prosthetic hip, but the procedure of implantation. And it is not only implantation that poses a risk to the patient with a prosthesis—so does hemorrhoidectomy done years later, for which prophylaxis is made mandatory by the presence of the hip prosthesis.

The prosthetic or rheumatic heart valve is a risk, but the indication for the use of prophylactic antibiotics is an invasive procedure—the root canal is an example in which the inoculum is unavoidable. *Operations are covered by prophylactic antibiotics; the conditions that are risk factors during the operation are not.*

20. To be safe, why not administer prophylactic antibiotics to all patients undergoing any kind of operation?

Wait a minute. Can you give me the indication for a prophylactic antibiotic in a patient undergoing a clean elective surgical procedure that implants no prosthesis, such as hernia repair?

"Sure," one of my brighter students once responded, "the patient who has a serious impairment in host response, such as acute granulocytic leukemia in blast crisis."

To which I responded: "Why on earth are you fixing his hernia? That is a clean error (hopefully not a clean kill) in surgical judgment that has nothing to do with antibiotics at all. A patient with that degree of host impairment does not undergo an elective surgical procedure."

Rule of thumb: *If you can give me the indication for a prophylactic antibiotic to cover a clean elective nonprosthetic operation for a patient, you have just given me the contraindication for the operation.*

MANAGEMENT OF SURGICAL INFECTIONS

21. What is the drug of choice for the treatment of an abscess?

Bard-Parker (drain the abscess). Abscesses have no circulation of blood within them to deliver an antibiotic. The antibiotic, even if injected directly into the abscess, would be worthless, because the abscess has a soup of dead microorganisms and white cells. Even if the organisms were barely alive, they would not be reproducing and incorporating the antibiotic. The drug most likely would not work at all at the pH and pKa conditions of the abscess environment—and you still want to treat this localized pus with a systemic drug? (You will do better sending a letter to the North Pole for Santa Claus or a letter to the tooth fairy or current resident.)

If there is an indication for an antibiotic, it would be in the circulation around the compressed inflammatory edge of the abscess and the cellulitis (at the vascularized peel of the orange) and uncontaminated tissue planes through which the necessary drainage must be carried out. A *focal* infection is managed by a *local* treatment, which is both *necessary* in all abscesses and *sufficient* treatment in many. Adjunctive systemic antibiotics occasionally are indicated for protection of the tissues through which drainage is carried out. If it helps to make this fundamental surgical principle clear, here is the rule of thumb for management of abscesses: *Where there is pus, let there be steel.* Perhaps one of the most gratifying procedures in all of medicine is the drainage of pus with immediate relief of local and systemic symptoms (e.g., a perirectal abscess).

22. Which abscess treatment is the important one in determining the outcome of a patient with intraabdominal sepsis?

It is the drainage of the *last* abscess that counts. There should be little applause for drainage of a pelvic abscess in the patient who retains a subphrenic abscess. The patient responds dramatically when the *last* pus is drained.

This has been an area of significant advance in managing surgical infections, because noninvasive scanning capability has facilitated the finding of multiple pockets of pus. Furthermore, such modalities as the computed tomography (CT) scan not only *find* but also percutaneously *direct the fixing* of the last abscess. What might have been an indication for an exploratory return trip to the operating room only a decade before (i.e., a failing patient on appropriate therapy should trigger the first response, "Where's the pus?") is now a good indication for a CT scan to find and drain the focal infection.

23. What is the preferred method of drainage of an intraabdominal abscess—by needle or by knife?

Which can be done most expeditiously? The patient with intraabdominal sepsis is very ill, and the earliest, safe drainage is the procedure of choice. There may be advantages to the less invasive CT scanning, which can be repeated and has less morbidity if the results are negative. Surgery, on the other hand, can fix associated conditions that may have caused the abscess, such as the devitalized loop of bowel or the leak in the anastomosis that can be exteriorized. Each method is likely to find multiple collections, and each can leave external drains for lavage and continuing drainage. Whether by needle or by knife, urgency and adequacy of local treatment of focal infection determine which methods takes precedence.

24. What is the role of gallium scintiscanning in early finding of abscesses in the abdomen?
Zip (I mean zippo). Ordering a gallium scan is a temporizing means of self-deception that some progress is being made in finding out what is wrong with the patient. In fact, it merely postpones decisions about intervention in critical illness for several days, often to a point beyond salvage. Gallium scanning involves bowel prepping, a vigorous white cell response from an active bone marrow, and false positives at the sites of tubes and incisions. It is a time-consuming and unreliable test that is the obverse of the principles of *early* and *definitive* management. Do not order a gallium scan for any patient you like or to satisfy a consultant that "something is being done for this patient."

BIBLIOGRAPHY

1. Bartlett JG: Intra-abdominal sepsis. Med Clin North Am 79:599–617, 1995.
2. Bilik R, Burnweit C, Shandling B: Is abdominal cavity culture of any value in appendicitis? Am J Surg 175:267–270, 1998.
3. Christou NV, Turgeon P, Wassef R, et al: Management of intra-abdominal infections. The case for intra-operative cultures and comprehensive broad-spectrum antibiotic coverage. The Canadian Intra-abdominal Infection Study Group. Arch Surg 131:1193–1201, 1996.
4. Ciftci AO, Tanyei FC, Buyukpamukcu N, Hicsonmea A: Comparative trial of four antibiotic combinations for perforated appendicitis in children. Eur J Surg 163:591–596, 1997.
5. Falagas ME, Barefoot L, Griffith J, et al: Risk factors leading to clinical failure in the treatment of intra-abdominal or skin/soft tissue infections. Eur J Clin Microbiol Infect Dis 15:913–921, 1996.
6. Geelhoed GW: Preoperative skin preparation: Evaluation of efficacy, timing, convenience, and cost. Infect Surg 648–669, 1985.
7. Geelhoed GW: Cultures of the peritoneal cavity. Postgrad Gen Surg 3:164–166, 1991.
8. Geelhoed GW: New approaches to serious infections in the surgical patient. Clin Ther 12B:2–8, 1990.
9. Graninger W, Zedwitz-Liebenstein K, Laferi H, Burgmann H: Quinolones in gastrointestinal infections. Chemotherapy 42(Suppl 1): 43–45, 1996.
10. Simon GL, Geelhoed GW: Diagnosis of intra-abdominal abscesses. Am Surg 51:431–436, 1985.
11. Solomkin JS, Dellinger EP, Bohnen JM, Rostein OD: The role of oral antimicrobials for the management of intra-abdominal infections. New Horizons 6(Suppl 2):S46–S52, 1998.
12. Walker AP, Nichols RL, Wilson RF, et al: Efficacy of a beta-lactamase inhibitor combination for serious intraabdominal infections. Ann Surg 217:115–121, 1993.
13. Wilson SE, Faulkner K: Impact of anatomical site on bacteriological and clinical outcome in the management of intra-abdominal infections. Am Surg 64:402–417, 1998.
14. Wittmann DH, Schein M: Let us shorten antibiotic prophylaxis and therapy in surgery. Am Surg 172(6A): 25S–32S, 1996.
15. Wittmann DH, Schein M, Condon RE: Management of secondary peritonitis. Ann Surg 224:10–18, 1996.

II. Trauma

16. INITIAL ASSESSMENT

Douglas Y. Tamura, M.D., and Walter L. Biffl, M.D.

1. What are the three major components of initial assessment in trauma?
Primary survey, resuscitation, and secondary survey.

2. What are the ABCDEs of the primary survey?
Airway maintenance with cervical spine control
Breathing and ventilation
Circulation with control of hemorrhage
Disability: neurologic status
Exposure of the entire patient
Resuscitation is performed simultaneously. Additional early interventions include **F**oley catheterization and **G**astric tube placement. The primary survey must be repeated frequently in the emergency department.

3. What is the most common cause of upper airway obstruction in trauma patients?
The tongue, followed by blood, loose teeth or dentures, and vomit.

4. What initial maneuvers are used to restore an open airway?
The chin lift and jaw thrust physically displace the mandible and tongue anteriorly to open the airway; manual clearance of debris and suctioning of the oropharynx optimize patency. Nasopharyngeal and oropharyngeal airways are useful adjuncts in maintaining an open airway in obtunded patients. All of these maneuvers must be accomplished with the patient's head still taped to the backboard (before clearing the cervical spine).

5. What are the indications for a definitive airway? What types are available?
The indications for a definitive airway include apnea, inability to maintain an airway, need to protect an airway, need for hyperventilation, inability to maintain oxygenation, hemodynamic instability, and need for sedation/muscle relaxation. The three types of definitive airway are orotracheal intubation, nasotracheal intubation, and surgical airway (cricothyroidotomy or tracheostomy).

6. What are the indications and contraindications to a surgical airway?
Extensive maxillofacial trauma, which precludes airway access via the oral or nasal route, is the principal indication for a surgical airway. Furthermore, nasotracheal intubation cannot be performed in apneic patients, and morbid obesity or cervical swelling may limit the feasibility of orotracheal access. Contraindications to cricothyroidotomy include direct laryngeal trauma, tracheal disruption, and age less than 12 years. Tracheostomy and percutaneous transtracheal ventilation are the alternatives.

7. What does "clearing the C-spine" mean?
Before manipulating the patient's head, injury to the cervical spine (C-spine) must be excluded. Alert patients without other "significant painful injuries" may be moved without radiographs if they have no cervical tenderness by direct palpation. Patients with symptoms or a major

injury require a minimum of three views (lateral, anteroposterior, and odontoid) to image the C-spine. Visualization of C7–T1 is mandatory and may require supine oblique or "swimmer's" views (the patient's arm is placed above the head with the x-ray focused at the axilla). In high-risk patients with symptoms, bilateral supine oblique views or computed tomography scan of the neck may be required. Upright lateral or delayed flexion/extension films to rule out ligamentous injury may be obtained in symptomatic patients with five normal views. In patients with equivocal images or in whom physical examination is not possible, a cervical spine collar should be left in place.

8. Does a Philadelphia collar adequately stabilize the cervical spine?
No. The Philadelphia collar allows approximately 30% of normal flexion and extension, over 40% of rotation, and 66% of lateral motion. Immobilization must also include sandbags taped to a backboard.

9. What nonairway conditions pose an immediate threat to ventilation?
Tension pneumothorax, most commonly seen after blunt chest trauma, is treated by tube thoracostomy (36-French tube in the midaxillary line). An **open pneumothorax** may compromise ventilation if the chest wall defect is greater than two-thirds the diameter of the trachea. The defect should be sealed with petroleum gauze or cellophane wrap taped on three sides to allow egress of air or, better yet, taped on four sides with concomitant chest tube placement. **Hemothorax** should be drained with a large-bore thoracostomy tube and watched for continued bleeding that may require thoracotomy. Impaired ventilation associated with a **flail chest** is usually due to underlying pulmonary contusion, not to rib fractures.

10. What are the preferred sites for emergent venous access?
Peripheral venous access usually of the upper extremity (i.e., antecubital vein), with a large-bore catheter is preferred. Saphenous vein cutdown provides an alternative access site when percutaneous access is unobtainable. Central venous access is indicated primarily to monitor central venous pressure. It is useful in hemodynamically unstable patients and patients with chronic cardiopulmonary disease. Good flow rates can be achieved with 8.5-Fr catheters. In young children (< 6 yr old), interosseous catheter placed in the distal femur or proximal tibia provides a viable alternative.

11. What are five rapidly assessed elements to determine hemodynamic instability?
1. Diminished level of consciousness   4. Oliguria/anuria
2. Pale, cool skin   5. Low blood pressure
3. Diminished pulses
Peripheral pulses are useful in grossly estimating blood pressure. A palpable radial pulse indicates a systolic blood pressure ≥ 80 mmHg, a femoral pulse indicates a systolic blood pressure ≥ 70 mmHg, and a carotid pulse indicates a systolic blood pressure ≥ 60 mmHg.

12. What is the most common cause of shock in multiply injured patients? What fluids should be used for initial resuscitation?
Acute blood loss resulting in hypovolemia is the most common cause of postinjury shock. The mainstay of fluid resuscitation is rapid crystalloid infusion. Colloid solutions are costly and have not proved advantageous. Hypertonic saline solutions remain controversial. Blood should be administered to optimize oxygen-carrying capacity when crystalloid infusion exceeds 50 ml/kg. Type O-negative blood is acceptable because it can be obtained 10 minutes before type-specific, non-crossmatched blood and 20 minutes before crossmatched blood.

13. What are the most common causes of cardiogenic shock after injury? How are they recognized and treated?
Tension pneumothorax impairs venous return to the heart. The physical signs are ipsilateral hyperresonance and diminished breath sounds and contralateral tracheal deviation. Empirical

tube thoracostomy is indicated (do not wait for a chest radiograph). Traumatic **pericardial tamponade** is caused by the accumulation of blood (as little as 100 ml) or air in the pericardial sac. The classic Beck's triad (arterial hypotension, central venous hypertension, and muffled heart sounds), however, is lacking in most patients. Pericardiocentesis frequently stabilizes the patient and confirms the diagnosis for transport to the operating room for definitive treatment. **Myocardial contusion** is manifested primarily by dysrhythmias and occasionally by pump failure.

14. What are the indications for thoracotomy in the emergency department?
Cardiac arrest or profound hypotension (< 60 mmHg) due to suspected pericardial tamponade or uncontrolled intrathoracic bleeding that is refractory to initial resuscitative measures. Thoracotomy allows access to decompress the pericardium, to control intrathoracic hemorrhage, to institute open cardiac massage, and to cross-clamp the descending aorta to improve coronary and cerebral perfusion and decrease subdiaphragmatic hemorrhage. Emergency department thoracotomy for blunt trauma has a low yield, particularly in patients devoid of vital signs after blunt trauma (< 1% survival rate).

15. What are the three main components of the Glasgow coma scale?
1. Best eye-opening response is scored from 1–4.
2. Best verbal response is scored from 1–5.
3. Best motor response is scored from 1–6.

Points from each component are added up. An overall score below 8 represents a comatose state, whereas a score of 15 represents normal consciousness. The mnemonic **AVPU** is a simple method to assess neurologic status during the primary survey:
A **a**lert
V response to **v**ocal stimuli
P response to **p**ainful stimuli
U **u**nresponsiveness

16. During the primary survey what other actions should be conducted?
While the ABCs are being assessed and treated, large-bore IV access should be obtained for fluid resuscitation. The patient should be monitored with blood pressure cuff, pulse oximetry, and electrocardiography. Oxygen supplementation should be supplied either by face mask or nasal cannula. Foley catheter should be placed in major to assess urine output. Naso- or orogastric tubes are placed if stomach distention is suspected, aspiration is a risk, or deep peritoneal lavage is anticipated. Radiographs should be obtained of the C-spine, chest, and pelvis.

17. What are the main components of the secondary survey?
The secondary survey is divided into the patient's history and a detailed physical exam.

18. What is an AMPLE medical history?
Allergies, **m**edications, **p**ast medical history, **l**ast meal, and **e**vents related to the injury.

19. What are the most commonly overlooked injuries?
Fractures, most notably cervical spine injuries.

CONTROVERSIES

20. What is the role of the pneumatic antishock garment?
Also known as military antishock trousers (MAST), the pneumatic antishock garment was once believed to autotransfuse blood from extremities to the central circulation. The MAST garment now appears to increase total peripheral resistance and may be detrimental with major thoracoabdominal injuries. Currently it is used primarily to stabilize and control refractory pelvic venous hemorrhage, but the penalty of soft tissue ischemia is problematic.

21. In a patient in shock with an obvious head injury, grossly positive peritoneal aspirate, and suggestion of a thoracic aortic injury on chest radiograph, what are the priorities after initial resuscitation?

An exploratory laparotomy is indicated based on hemodynamic instability in the face of a grossly positive peritoneal tap. The patient should have a computed tomographic scan of the head and chest immediately thereafter. Intraoperative intracranial pressure monitoring may be both diagnostic and therapeutic.

BIBLIOGRAPHY

1. American College of Surgeons, Committee on Trauma: Advanced Trauma Life Support Course, 6th ed. Chicago, American College of Surgeons, 1997.
2. Biffl WL, Moore EE, Harken AH: Emergency department thoracotomy. In Mattox KL, Feliciano DV, Moore EE (eds): Trauma, 4th ed. Norwalk, CT, Appleton & Lange, 1999.
3. Gould SA, Moore EE, Hoyt DB, et al: The first randomized trial of human polymerized hemoglobin as a blood substitute in acute trauma and emergent surgery. J Am Coll Surg 187:113, 1998.
4. Krantz BE: Initial assessment. In Feliciano DV, Moore EE, Mattox KL (eds): Trauma, 3rd ed. Norwalk, CT, Appleton & Lange, 1996, pp 123–139.
5. Mattox KL, Moore EE, Mateer J, et al: Hypertonic saline-dextran solution in the prehospital treatment of post-traumatic hypotension: The USA multicenter trial. Ann Surg 213:482, 1991.

17. POSTTRAUMATIC HEMORRHAGIC SHOCK

Garret Zallen, MD, and Ernest E. Moore, MD

1. What is hemorrhagic shock?

The loss of intravascular volume due to hemorrhage. Attempts at rapid control of hemorrhage and blood transfusions have decreased the mortality rate, but it remains unacceptably high.

2. What is irreversible hemorrhagic shock?

In the 1940s C.J. Wiggers demonstrated that hemorrhagic shock produced effects that were not reversible by simply replacing the lost blood. Animals subjected to severe hemorrhage exhibited a mortality rate of 80% at 24 hours despite the return of shed blood. This "irreversible shock" was due to a continuing loss of intravascular fluid through leaking endothelial cells and isotonic swelling of skeletal muscle. Wiggers demonstrated that this loss could be overcome with additional infusions of isotonic salt solutions.

3. How is hemorrhagic shock classified?

Class 1 hemorrhage: blood volume loss up to 15%, minimal symptoms, occasionally mild tachycardia.

Class 2 hemorrhage: blood volume loss 15–30% (750–1500 ml in a 70-kg man), tachycardia, tachypnea, and decreased pulse pressure.

Class 3 hemorrhage: blood volume loss 30–40% (approximately 2000 ml in an adult), marked tachycardia, tachypnea, decreased mental status, hypotension, decreased urinary output.

Class 4 hemorrhage: blood volume loss greater than 40%, immediately life-threatening, marked tachycardia, significantly depressed systolic blood pressure to nonpalpable pulses, no urinary output, cold, pale skin.

4. What is the normal blood volume?

Blood volume is normally 7% of body weight in an adult or approximately 70 ml/kg. In a child the blood volume is slightly higher at 9% of body weight or 90 ml/kg.

5. What mechanisms lead to hypotension?

Nearly 70% of blood volume resides in the venous system and represents the reservoir that provides the preload to the heart. Depletion of venous volume leads to decreased cardiac filling. According to Starling's law, the more the heart muscle is stretched, the greater the contractility; hence decreased cardiac filling leads to decreased contractility, decreased stroke volume, and decreased cardiac output. In addition, persistent hemorrhagic shock leads to membrane depolarization in skeletal muscle, which permits increased movement of water from the extracellular compartment to the intracellular compartment. This shift further exacerbates the deficit in circulating blood volume.

6. How does the body compensate for decreased circulating volume?

A fall in great vessel pressure leads to excitation of the sympathetic nervous system and subsequent release of endogenous catecholamines. This response, coupled with inhibition of the medullovagal center (Marey's reflex), leads to tachycardia, increased strength of cardiac contraction, and vasoconstriction. There is a differential response in various vascular beds to vasoconstriction (this process is not democratic); the skin, mesenteric, and renal circulations exhibit the greatest degrees of vasoconstriction. Decreased renal blood flow leads to release of renin, which augments the conversion of angiotensin I to angiotensin II. Angiotensin II is a potent vasoconstrictor that also stimulates the release of aldosterone and antidiuretic hormone, leading to increased reabsorption of salt and water by the renal tubules, which in turn augments vascular volume.

7. Does this response change with age?

Unfortunately, yes. Old age is not for wimps. As a rule you can increase cardiac output by increasing your heart rate up to 200 beats per minute (bpm) minus your age (maximal heart rate = 220 – age). At the other end of the age spectrum, infants have a relatively fixed stroke volume and can increase cardiac output only by an increase in heart rate.

8. What are the cellular manifestations of hemorrhagic shock?

Inadequately perfused and oxygenated cells are unable to perform normal aerobic metabolism. This inability results in the production of lactic acid, creating a gap metabolic acidosis. The production of adenosine triphosphate (ATP) is decreased, and the cell can no longer maintain membrane polarization. The first evidence of this process is swelling of the endoplasmic reticulum, followed by mitochondrial damage, lysozyme rupture, and entry of sodium and water into the cell. The loss of water into the cells exacerbates the extracellular and intravascular volume deficit.

9. What are the clinical manifestations of hemorrhagic shock?

Rapid pulse and low blood pressure. Invasive monitoring reveals decreases in urine output, central venous pressure, pulmonary capillary wedge pressure, cardiac output, and mixed venous oxygen saturation.

10. Does a normal hematocrit exclude hemorrhagic shock?

No. The concentration of red blood cells does not fall until either exogenous fluids are given or interstitial fluid shifts into the circulating volume. The second process usually occurs over 24 hours without fluid resuscitation.

11. How does hemorrhagic shock differ from other types of shock?

Cardiac compressive shock (tamponade or tension pneumothorax) is manifested by increased central venous pressure and equalization of right and left heart pressures. Neurogenic shock may look similar to hemorrhagic shock since the cause is decreased circulating volume secondary to venous pooling and loss of arterial tone below the spinal cord injury. Septic shock may occur in victims of trauma who are delayed in presentation; it is characterized initially by fever; warm, pink skin; and increased cardiac output.

12. What is tachycardia?

Tachycardia is defined as > 160 bpm in infants, > 140 bpm in preschool children, and > 100 bpm in adults. Be wary if the patient is taking medications that can affect heart rates, such as beta blockers.

13. Where can blood loss hide?

As opposed to obvious blood loss from external injuries, the abdominal and chest cavities, the retroperitoneum (following pelvic fracture), and thighs can hold sufficient blood to cause fatal hemorrhagic shock.

14. What is the initial management of hypovolemic shock?

Stop the bleeding, and give volume. Start large-bore (14- or 16-gauge) peripheral intravenous lines. Poiseuille's law states that fluid resistance is proportional to the fourth power of the radius of the catheter. If peripheral veins are not accessible, large-bore central venous lines (femoral, subclavian, or jugular) should be placed. In an infant or child interosseous catheters placed into the tibia can be surprisingly effective.

15. How much and what type of fluid should be administered for initial resuscitation?

Adults should receive a rapid bolus of 1–2 liters of warm Ringer's lactate; infants and small children should receive 20 ml/kg.

16. Is there a role for colloid resuscitation?

The debate over resuscitation with crystalloid vs. colloid (albumin or dextran solutions) continues. A meta-analysis of multiple prospective clinical studies indicates a decrease in mortality in trauma patients resuscitated with crystalloid solutions as opposed to colloid solution. Perhaps surprisingly, these studies found no difference in lung edema, transfusion requirement, or length of stay with crystalloid resuscitation.

17. When is blood transfusion indicated during initial resuscitation?

If the clinical setting is really frightening, give blood. The patient should be transfused with uncrossed, O negative packed red blood cells (O positive can be used for males who have not received previous blood transfusions; females should always receive O negative blood to prevent sensitization that may complicate future pregnancies).

18. What are the physiologic complications of blood transfusions?

The most common complication is hypothermia caused by administration of cold banked blood. This problem can be eliminated by running banked blood through a rapid warming system. Replacement of lost blood with only packed red blood cells and crystalloid may lead to dilution of coagulation factors and require the concomitant administration of fresh frozen plasma. Banked blood contains calcium scavengers such as citrate (give 250 mg calcium gluconate after transfusing each 4 units of blood). Evidence is accruing that older units of blood may contain lipid breakdown products that are proinflammatory and promote neutrophil-mediated tissue injury with subsequent multiple organ failure. Finally, there is the risk of transmitting hepatitis B and C, HIV, and HTLV.

19. What are the alternatives to banked blood?

Blood autotransfusion from tube thoracostomy is commercially available. Blood is collected, filtered, anticoagulated (citrate), and reinfused. Intraoperative devices for the collection and reinfusion of blood are occasionally used, but the number of units that can be retransfused is limited. Currently no blood substitution products are commercially available, but several are in the process of approval by the Food and Drug Administration. These substitutes consist of various kinds of purified hemoglobin (without red cells) that has been purified and cross-linked to delay renal excretion. They function like native hemoglobin, but their circulating half-life is short.

Blood substitutes require no cross-matching, are free from infectious agents, and have much longer unrefrigerated shelf life.

20. How does hemorrhagic shock lead to multiple organ dysfunction?

Severe hemorrhagic shock begins an inflammatory cascade that cannot be reversed in some patients despite adequate resuscitation. During the Vietnam War patients in hemorrhagic shock were rapidly treated but later succumbed to pulmonary failure or adult respiratory distress syndrome (ARDS). Patients with ARDS can be mechanically ventilated but later die from a combination of liver, renal, cardiac and bone marrow failure or multiple organ failure (MOF). MOF remains the leading cause of late postinjury mortality. In addition to the cellular derangement in ATP synthesis, shock causes the release of platelet-activating factor, interleukin-8, and arachidonic acid metabolites that activate neutrophils to adhere to endothelial cells and release cytotoxic mediators, causing organ damage. The mesenteric circulation is a hotbed of proinflammatory agent synthesis (the gut is the motor for MOF). In addition to directly activating neutrophils, the mesenteric circulation appears to release agents into the mesenteric lymph that cause neutrophil activation and lung injury.

BIBLIOGRAPHY

1. American College of Surgeons: Advanced Trauma Life Support, 6th ed. Chicago, American College of Surgeons, 1997.
2. Choi P, Yip G, Quinonez L, Cook D: Crystalloids vs. colloids in fluid resuscitation: A systematic review. Crit Care Med 27:200, 1999.
3. Consensus conference: Perioperative red blood cell transfusion. JAMA 260:2700, 1988.
4. Feliciano D, Moore E, Mattox K: Trauma, 3rd ed. Stamford, CT, Appleton & Lange, 1996.
5. Gould SA, Moore EE, Hoyt DB, et al: The first randomized trial of human polymerized hemoglobin as a blood substitute in acute trauma and emergent surgery. J Am Coll Surg 187:113–120; discussion, 120–122, 1998.
6. Holcroft J: Shock. In Wilmore D, Cheing L, Harken A, et al (eds): Scientific American Surgery. New York, Scientific American, 1999.
7. Moore FA, Moore EE: Evolving concepts in the pathogenesis of postinjury multiple organ failure. Surg Clin North Am 75:257, 1995.
8. Zallen G, Moore EE, Johnson JL, et al: Posthemorrhagic shock mesenteric lymph primes circulating neutrophils and provokes lung injury. J Surg Res 83(2):83–88, 1999.

18. TRAUMATIC BRAIN INJURY

J. Paul Elliott, M.D., and Kerry Brega, M.D.

1. Is traumatic brain injury (TBI) a common problem?

Yes. One in 12 deaths in the United States is due to injury. One-third of traumatic deaths are associated with TBI. Of deaths resulting from motor vehicle accidents, 60% are due to brain injury. Even more common is minor TBI, which accounts for 70–80% of admissions for head trauma.

2. What is a concussion?

Concussion denotes the relatively common occurrence of transient loss of neurologic function without macroscopic brain abnormality. The Glasgow Coma Scale (GCS) score is used to categorize brain injuries as follows: mild, 14–15; moderate, 9–13; and severe, ≤ 8.

3. How is the GCS score derived?

The GCS is a means of identifying change in neurologic status. Its principal strengths are ease of use and reproducibility among observers. It is a 15-point scale; 15 is the best score and 3 is the worst. The score is derived from the addition of the three individual components: best eye-opening response (1–4 points), best verbal response (1–5 points), and best motor response (1–6 points). The GCS, however, is insensitive to pupillary response and focality. A patient with a perfect score of 15 may have hemiparesis and a life-threatening lesion.

4. When should a neurosurgeon be consulted?

A neurosurgeon should be consulted for patients with loss of consciousness and subsequent neurologic abnormality or abnormality on computed tomography (CT) scan. Such patients usually but not always have a GCS score ≤ 13.

5. How does one initially assess the brain-injured patient?

Just like any trauma patient. The first steps are assessment of the ABCs (airway, breathing, circulation) and aggressive physiologic resuscitation. The neurologic examination is critical. The initial exam includes (1) level of consciousness, (2) pupillary exam, and (3) motor exam. Repetition of the neurologic exam is also critical. If deterioration is missed and appropriate treatment is not quickly initiated, irreversible brain injury may result. Finally, watch for concurrent cervical spine injury.

6. What takes priority in a hypotensive patient with TBI?

Hypotension in patients with head injury frequently accompanies other injuries. Do *not* assume that hypotension is due to the brain injury alone. Hypotension due to brain injury is a terminal event.

7. What is the significance of anisocoria in an injured patient?

Anisocoria (unequal pupils) is a true neurologic emergency. Commonly a mass lesion (e.g., subdural or epidural hematoma, contusion, or diffuse swelling of one hemisphere) leads to uncal herniation and stretching of the ipsilateral third nerve. Time is critical. Give mannitol, get a CT scan, and proceed with surgical decompression (if possible).

8. What if the larger pupil is reactive?

If the larger pupil is reactive, the third cranial nerve is functioning. Think of Horner's syndrome (miosis, ptosis, and anhydrosis) on the other side. This syndrome may be due to injury to the sympathetic nerves traveling with the carotid artery in the neck. Consider evaluation (angiography) for a carotid dissection.

9. Are terms such as semicomatose nonsense?

Yes. Patients are either alert (like medical students and surgeons), lethargic (like internists, in whom arousal is maintained by verbal interaction), obtunded (like hospital administrators, who require constant mechanical stimulation to maintain arousal), or comatose (like most deans, in whom neither verbal nor mechanical stimulation elicits arousal). Change in level of consciousness is often the first sign of increasing intracranial pressure (ICP); it is also the most poorly documented part of the neurologic exam. Document all findings!

10. How is motor response tested?

Ascertain the ability to follow commands by asking the patient to hold up fingers and move his or her arms and legs. If the patient does not follow commands (he or she may be a dean), test response to painful central stimulus. Localization of painful stimulus is confirmed by the patient's hand reaching toward a sternal rub. But the patient may be in even bigger trouble if in response to pain he or she exhibits flexor posturing (decorticate), extensor posturing (decerebrate), or no response. Flexor posturing indicates a high brainstem injury, and extensor posturing is associated with low brainstem dysfunction. The patient with no motor response may have a cervical spine injury.

11. What is the significance of periorbital ecchymosis (raccoon eyes) and ecchymosis over the mastoid (Battle's sign)?

In the absence of direct trauma to the eyes or mastoid regions, periorbital ecchymosis and ecchymosis over the mastoid are reliable signs of basilar skull fractures. Ten percent of patients with basilar skull fractures have cerebrospinal fluid (CSF) leaks, including rhinorrhea or otorrhea. Persistent CSF leaks are associated with meningitis.

12. Should scalp lacerations be explored in the emergency department?

Yes—but gently. You want to know whether there is an underlying fracture. A laceration over a linear nondisplaced fracture can be cleaned and closed. If CSF or brain tissue is evident in the wound or if a depressed fracture is identified, surgical intervention is required to debride the wound and to close any dural tears. If you are worried, get a head CT.

13. Which patients need CT scans of the head?

If you are worried, get a head CT. The CT scan is used partly as a triage tool with minor brain injuries and can be cost-effective compared with admission to the intensive care unit for observation. Conversely, patients with focality on exam do not proceed to the operating room without a CT scan.

14. What are the common traumatic surgical lesions?

If the ventricles are large (ventriculomegaly), a ventriculostomy can drain excessive CSF. Epidural hematomas (from arterial bleeding), subdural hematomas (from venous bleeding), and intraparenchymal hematomas with significant mass effect should be surgically evacuated. A depressed skull fracture or foreign body (like a bullet) also requires a trip to the operating room.

15. When is ICP monitoring indicated?

When the neurologic exam becomes insensitive (when the patient is unconscious) to changes in ICP.

16. Describe the initial treatment of patients with a suspected increase in ICP.

The brain, like every other organ, must have adequate blood flow and oxygen delivery. The ABCs come first. Systolic blood pressures < 90 mmHg and partial pressure of oxygen in arterial blood (PaO_2) < 60 are significantly correlated with poor outcomes in patients with TBI.

17. Should all patients with elevated ICP be hyperventilated?

Decreasing the partial pressure of carbon dioxide (pCO_2) is the most rapidly effective treatment for elevated ICP. The goal is usually a pCO_2 of 30 mmHg. Any patient with depressed level of consciousness and inability to protect the airway should be intubated. Before a CT scan is obtained, patients thought to have a mass lesion by neurologic exam should be hyperventilated.

18. In hemodynamically stable patients, how do you decrease ICP?

Mannitol, 1 gm/kg, as an intravenous bolus.

19. What is the endpoint of diuresis?

Serum sodium of 150 mEq/L and serum osmolarity of 320 mOsm are the upper limits of diuresis. Blood volume should be maintained with colloids to help form an osmotic gradient between the extravascular and the intravascular spaces. Anticipate intravascular hypovolemia, and treat with colloids and blood products as necessary.

20. What is the significance of cerebral perfusion pressure?

Cerebral perfusion pressure (CPP) is the difference between mean arterial pressure (MAP) and ICP:

$$CPP = MAP - ICP$$

CPP is important. Neurologic outcome is best in patients with CPPs in the 70s. Some patients require treatment with pressors to maintain the CCP—if CPP is lower than 60 mmHg, you are creating a dean.

21. Why should all children with TBI be undressed and thoroughly examined?
One-half of children suffering nonaccidental trauma (child abuse) have TBI.

22. Should posttraumatic seizures be treated prophylactically?
Patients with brain parenchymal abnormalities on CT following head injury benefit from 1 week of antiseizure prophylaxis. Early seizures can increase the metabolic demand of the injured brain and adversely affect ICP (and IQ). Ten percent of patients who have seizures within the first 7 days of injury also have late seizures. Prevention of early seizures, however, does not reduce the incidence of late seizures.

23. Which coagulopathy is associated with severe brain injury?
Disseminated intravascular coagulation (DIC). The presumed mechanism is massive release of thromboplastin from the injured brain into the circulation. The serum levels of fibrin degradation products roughly correlate with the extent of brain parenchymal injury. All severely brain-injured patients should be evaluated with prothrombin time (PT), partial thromboplastin time (PTT), platelet counts, and fibrinogen levels.

24. What other medical complications may result from severe head injury?
Diabetes insipidus (DI) due to the inadequate secretion of antidiuretic hormone is caused by injury to the pituitary or hypothalamic tracts. The kidney is unable to decrease free water loss. Usually the urine output is > 200 ml/hr, and the urine specific gravity is < 1.003. The serum sodium may rise precipitously if DI is not treated promptly. The treatment of choice in trauma is intravenous infusion of synthetic vasopressin (pitressin), which has a 20-minute half-life and can be titrated to produce the appropriate urine output. Because most trauma-induced DI is self-limited, 1-deamino-8-D-arginine vasopressin (DDAVP), which has a 12-hour half-life, is not necessary.

25. If a patient is awake with significant neurologic symptoms but no abnormality on CT scan, what are the likely explanations?
A spinal cord injury or carotid or vertebral artery dissection.

26. Are gunshot wounds that cross the midline of the brain uniformly fatal?
No (although such a wound killed Lincoln). The tract that the bullet takes is important, but so is the energy that it imparts to the brain.

27. What is the significance of concussion?
In most studies of minor TBI, > 50% of patients have complaints of headache, fatigue, dizziness, irritability, and alterations of cognition and short-term memory. It is important to alert the patient to the likelihood of developing such symptoms. The neurobehavioral problems significantly affect patients' lives. The symptoms usually resolve within 6 months after injury.

28. Can patients with minor brain injuries be discharged from the emergency department?
Patients with minor TBIs whose exam (including short-term memory) returns to normal and who have a normal head CT scan can be discharged to home, assuming that they are accompanied by a responsible person.

29. Is brain injury permanent? Is the outcome always poor?
No. Brain injury occurs in two phases. The primary injury occurs at the moment of impact. Secondary injury, however, is both preventable and treatable. Examples include hypoxia, hypotension, elevated ICP, and decreased perfusion to the brain due to ischemia, brain swelling, and expanding mass lesions. Rapid surgical management and avoidance of secondary injury improve outcome. Although previously it was believed that the brain was not capable of repair, it is now clear that neuronal repair and reorganization occur after injury.

BIBLIOGRAPHY

1. Biegler ED: Neuroimaging in pediatric traumatic head injury: Diagnostic considerations and relationships to neurobehavioral outcome. J Head Trauma Rehabil 14:406–423, 1999.
2. Bullock R, et al: Guidelines for the Management of Severe Head Injury. New York, Brain Trauma Foundation, 1995.
3. Narayan RK, Wilberger JE, Povlishock JT: Neurotrauma. New York, McGraw-Hill, 1996.
4. Reinert MM, Bullock R: Clinical trials in head injury. Neurol Res 21:330–338, 1999.
5. Vigue B, Ract C, Benayed M, et al: Early SvO$_2$ monitoring in patients with severe brain trauma. Intens Care Med 25:445–451, 1999.
6. Wu JJ, Hsu CC, Liao SY, Wong YK: Surgical outcome of traumatic intracranial hematoma at a regional hospital in Taiwan. J Trauma 47:39–43, 1999.
7. Yamamoto M, Marmarou CR, Stiefel MF, et al: Neuroprotective effect of hypothermia on neuronal injury in diffuse traumatic brain injury coupled with hypoxia and hypotension. J Neurotrauma 16:487–500, 1999.

19. SPINAL CORD INJURIES

Kerry Brega, M.D., and J. Paul Elliott, M.D.

1. What other injuries are commonly associated with cervical spine injury?

Forces associated with significant head and brain injury may be transmitted through the cervical spine. Fifty percent of patients with spinal cord injuries have associated head injuries. Approximately 15% of patients with one spine injury have a second injury elsewhere in the spine.

2. What does this association imply?

All victims with evidence of craniofacial trauma should be treated with a rigid cervical collar. The thoracic and lumbar spine should be immobilized on a board, and the patient should be log-rolled only.

3. Describe the evaluation of patients with potential spine injuries.

First, be sure that the patient is adequately immobilized. Second, do a neurologic exam, including all four extremities; test strength, sensation (light touch/proprioception and pain/temperature), and reflexes. Be sure to document the results.

4. How can the spinal cord be evaluated in patients with associated head injury?

All patients should have a rectal exam to evaluate tone. A patulous anus is a good indication of spinal cord or cauda equina injury. Flaccid motor tone and absent reflexes should raise suspicion of spinal cord injury. Such findings are extremely unusual with brain injury. Priapism is common with spinal cord injury but never caused by head injury.

5. How is the level of the spinal cord injury defined?

The level does not refer to the level of the injury to the spinal column (vertebrae, discs, and ligaments) but to the most caudal level in the cord with intact function. For example, if a patient has normal function of the deltoids (C5) and little or no function of the biceps (C6) or below, the patient has a C5 motor level injury. Right and left sides should be documented separately.

6. Can a patient have a spinal cord injury and normal plain radiographs?

Yes—with purely ligamentous injuries between vertebrae. Spinal cord injury without radiographic abnormality (SCIWORA) is common in children; 30% of children with spinal cord injuries have no radiographic abnormality. SCIWORA is less common in adults (about 5% of spinal cord injuries). In patients with preexisting cervical stenosis, either congenital or degenerative, hyperextension or flexion may result in cord injury without spinal column disruption.

7. What is an adequate radiologic evaluation?
Minimal views include cross-table lateral, anteroposterior, and open-mouth odontoid views. The relationship between C7 and the top of T1 must be visualized. Mild traction on the shoulders with the lateral film or swimmer's views help in patients with large shoulders. If this area cannot be seen on plain films, a lateral tomogram or computed tomography (CT) scan may be needed. Oblique views are helpful in viewing the pedicles and facet joints. Patients with evident or possible fractures should have CT scans to define the injury in greater detail.

8. Are magnetic resonance imaging (MRI) scans ever needed in the acute evaluation of cervical spine trauma?
Yes. If plain radiographs and CT scans do not adequately explain the extent of injury noted on the neurologic exam, MRI should be used to evaluate the cervical spine for herniated discs and ligamentous injuries and to visualize damaged areas within the spinal cord.

9. Describe the proper way to read a lateral cervical spine film.
Make a habit of doing a thorough systematic review in the same way with every film. First look at the prevertebral soft tissue space, which may be the only radiographic abnormality in as many as 40% of C1 and C2 fractures. The space anterior to C3 should not exceed one-third of the body of C3. At the C6 level the entire body of C6 generally fits into the prevertebral soft tissue space. Check the alignment of the anterior, then posterior edges of the vertebral bodies. Be sure that the intervertebral disc spaces are of relatively equal height. Check the spinous processes for alignment and abnormal splaying. Finally, evaluate each vertebra for fracture.

10. What about the anteroposterior (AP) film?
Carefully inspect the alignment of the midline spinous processes. Abrupt angulations suggest unilateral facet dislocation. Fractures of the bodies may be more obvious in the AP view.

11. Fractures of C1 and C2 are best visualized with which view?
The odontoid view. Look for overhang of the lateral mass of C1 off the lateral edges of C2, which should not be greater than 2 mm on either side. Abnormal overhang is seen in **Jefferson's fractures** (burst fractures of the C1 ring). The three types of odontoid fractures should be apparent: type I occurs in the body of the odontoid, type II at the junction of the odontoid and the body of C2, and type III through the body of C2 below the odontoid.

12. What is hangman's fracture?
Bilateral fractures through the pedicles or pars interarticularis of C2 that are caused by a severe hyperextension injury, usually due to high-speed motor vehicle accidents. Think about the mechanism of injury: the C2–C3 disc space may be disrupted anteriorly. In judicial hangings the fatal injury is the spinal cord stretch caused by the drop in combination with the C2 fracture. Most patients with hangman's fracture present neurologically intact.

13. Define deficits in complete transverse myelopathy, anterior cord syndrome, central cord syndrome, and Brown-Séquard syndrome.
Complete transverse myelopathy may result from transection, stretch, or contusion of the cord. All function below the level of the lesion—motor, sensory, and reflexive—is lost. Complete transverse myelopathy may be accompanied by spinal shock and/or neurogenic shock. Approximately 50% of spinal cord injuries are complete.

Anterior cord syndrome results from loss of the anterior two-thirds of the spinal cord (the distribution of the anterior spinal artery), which carries motor, pain, and temperature tracts. Light touch and proprioception are intact because the posterior columns are preserved.

Central cord syndrome results from injury to the central area of the spinal cord. Often it is found in patients with preexisting cervical stenosis due to spondylotic changes. Characteristically, motor deficits are more severe in the upper extremities than in the lower extremities. Motor function usually is affected more than sensory function.

Brown-Séquard syndrome characteristically is seen in penetrating injuries but also may be seen in blunt injury, especially with unilateral, traumatically herniated discs. The syndrome results from injury to one-half of the spinal cord. Clinically, motor, position, and vibration sense are affected on the side ipsilateral to the injury; these tracts cross in the brainstem. Pain and temperature sensation are abolished contralateral to the lesion; these tracts cross in the cord at or near the level of innervation.

14. What is spinal shock?

Absence of all spinal cord function below the level of the lesion results in flaccid motor tone and areflexia. Neurogenic shock refers to the hypotension that may result from cervical or upper thoracic complete spinal cord lesions. The hypotension is due to the lack of sympathetic vasomotor innervation below the lesion and is characterized by bradycardia from unbalanced vagal input to the heart. Fluid resuscitation and pressors with both alpha and beta stimulation work best. Strictly alpha stimulation may result in profound bradycardia or asystole. Usually the spinal shock resolves and vasomotor tone returns over the first few days.

15. What is the role of methylprednisolone in the treatment of acute cord injury?

The results of the Second National Acute Spinal Cord Injury Study (NASCIS II) suggest that high-dose methylprednisolone results in a statistically significant improvement in outcome. The dose is a 30-mg/kg load, followed by 5.4 mg/kg/hr for 23 hours. The NASCIS III trial reported that patients dosed between 3 and 8 hours after injury had improved outcomes when treated 48 hours rather than 24 hours with the methylprednisolone. In patients dosed within 3 hours of injury no further gains were documented by treating beyond 24 hours. This regimen should be followed in any patient suspected of having a spinal cord injury. Penetrating trauma was not evaluated in the study.

16. Do patients with spinal cord injuries ever undergo acute surgery?

Yes. Patients with deterioration in the neurologic exam may undergo urgent spinal cord decompression. Deterioration may be due to herniated disc material, epidural hemorrhage, or cord swelling in a narrowed canal, causing cord compression and worsening symptoms.

17. How is the bony injury treated?

The two most important factors in planning treatment of the spine injury are alignment and stability:

1. **Bad alignment: traction.** If good alignment is obtained, halo with or without operative fixation is recommended. If good alignment is not obtained, open reduction and fixation are generally required.

2. **Good alignment but unstable** (significant ligamentous disruption): halo with or without operative fixation.

3. **Good alignment and stable:** usually treated in a rigid collar.

18. What is the outcome in patients with spinal cord injury?

With complete lesions (no motor or sensory function below the lesion) the chances of recovery are poor; 2% of patients recover ambulation. The prognosis is markedly better for patients with incomplete lesions—75% recover. Appropriate treatment of bony injuries helps to prevent pain and late neurologic deterioration.

19. What other significant injury may present as a high thoracic cord lesion?

Thoracic aortic dissection may present as a T4 region cord injury. T4 is a watershed zone in the cord between the vertebral arterial distribution and the aortic radicular arteries.

BIBLIOGRAPHY

1. Bracken MB, Shepard MJ, Collins WF, et al: A randomized controlled trial of methylprednisolone or naloxone in the treatment of acute spinal-cord injury. N Engl J Med 322:1405–1411, 1990.
2. Bracken MB, Shepard MJ, Holford TR, et al: Administration of methylprednisolone for 24 or 48 hours or tirilazad mesylate for 48 hours in the treatment of acute spinal cord injury. Results of the Third National Acute Spinal Cord Injury randomized controlled trial. JAMA 277:1597–1604, 1997.
3. Bracken MB, Shepard MJ, Holford TR, et al: Methylprednisolone or tirilazad mesylate administration after acute spinal cord injury: 1 year follow up. Results of the Third National Acute Spinal Cord Injury randomized controlled trial. J Neurosurg 89:699–706, 1998.
4. Copper PR: Head Injury: Epidemiology of Head Injury. Baltimore, Williams & Wilkins, 1993.
5. Mangaiardi JR: Neurologic injuries. Top Emerg Med 11:1–84, 1990.
6. Pang D: Disorders of the Pediatric Spine. New York, Raven Press, 1995, pp 509–516.
7. Narayan RK, Wilberger JE Jr, Povlishock JT: Neurotrauma. New York, McGraw-Hill, 1996.

20. PENETRATING NECK TRAUMA

Walter L. Biffl, M.D., and Ernest E. Moore, M.D.

1. Why are penetrating neck wounds unique?

Although comprising only a small percentage of body surface area, the neck contains a heavy concentration of vital structures.

2. What constitutes a penetrating neck wound?

Violation of the platysma muscle defines a penetrating neck wound. This investing fascial layer of the neck is superficial to vital structures. If the platysma is not penetrated, the wound is managed as a simple laceration.

3. What are anterior and posterior neck injuries?

The anterior cervical triangle is bounded by the lower border of the mandible and the anterior borders of the sternocleidomastoid muscles. The posterior cervical triangle is formed by the posterior border of the sternocleidomastoid muscle, the middle one-third of the clavicle, and the anterior border of the trapezius muscle. Wounds entering in the anterior triangle should arouse suspicion of vascular and tracheoesophageal injuries.

4. What are the boundaries of the three zones of the neck?

Zone I extends from the sternal notch to the cricoid cartilage; zone II from the cricoid cartilage to the angle of the mandible; and zone III comprises the area cephalad to the angle of the mandible. These zones have distinct management implications.

5. Which side of the neck is more likely to be injured?

The left side of the neck is more likely to be injured, because most assailants are right-handed.

6. Do gunshot wounds and knife wounds cause the same relative injuries?

Gunshot wounds generally tend to inflict more tissue damage:

STRUCTURE	GUNSHOT WOUNDS	STAB WOUNDS
Artery	20%	5%
Vein	15%	10%
Airway	10%	5%
Digestive	20%	<5%

7. What are the priorities in the management of penetrating neck trauma?

Airway patency and control of hemorrhage. The ABCs (airway, breathing , and circulation) are the first priority in every trauma patient. Patients who are neurologically intact should be intubated orally. Patients who present with a neurologic deficit require simultaneous protection of the cervical spine and airway; orotracheal intubation is still preferred, although cricothyrotomy may be necessary with an extensive neck wound. Although the patient may present with a patent airway, early elective airway control is uniquely valuable in patients with expanding cervical hematomas. While hemorrhage is being controlled, intravenous access is secured with two large-bore peripheral lines. Central venous access may be diagnostic (high despite concurrent hypotension), suggesting the possibility of pericardial tamponade.

8. How should deep cervical bleeding be controlled at the accident scene and in the emergency department?

Direct pressure is nearly always successful, even for major arterial lesions. Do not blindly place clamps, because the risk of injury to vital structures is high. Occasionally, a patient with zone I vascular injury (base of the neck) requires an emergency department thoracotomy for proximal arterial (great vessel) control.

9. What specific historical details and physical signs are important?

The type of weapon used, blood loss before arrival at the emergency department, and hemodynamic status. Shock or substantial blood loss at the scene, ongoing hemorrhage, expanding hematoma, hemoptysis, hematemesis, neurologic deficits, dysphagia, dysphonia, hoarseness, stridor, and crepitus mandate an early trip to the operating room.

10. How often do patients with crepitus have a significant injury?

One-third of patients with crepitus have an injury of the pharynx, esophagus, larynx, or trachea. In two-thirds of such patients, however, the air has been introduced through the wound entrance site and there is no significant underlying injury.

11. What is selective management of penetrating neck trauma?

Do not explore all penetrating neck wounds. Up to 50% of penetrating neck wounds are not associated with significant injury. Alert and asymptomatic patients are either evaluated with a combination of diagnostic studies or observed expectantly with frequent serial physical examinations. Wounds that cannot be reliably observed are promptly explored in the operating room—explore all drunks.

12. What are the advantages of selective management?

The morbidity and cost of unnecessary neck surgery are avoided; however, the savings may be nullified by extensive diagnostic testing.

13. Should arteriography be performed on all patients?

Preoperative arteriograms are generally performed in hemodynamically stable patients with zone I injuries. Their value is to identify injuries to major vessels in the thoracic outlet that may require a thoracic operative approach. Wounds in zone III are best treated by angioembolization.

14. What is the value of other diagnostic studies, such as esophagography, esophagoscopy, laryngoscopy, bronchoscopy, and computed tomography scans?

Patients undergoing neck exploration generally do not require additional studies. A questionable injury may be demonstrated by intraoperative endoscopy, or insufflation may provoke an air leak. Adjunctive studies are important if esophageal injury is suspected; missed esophageal injury is associated with a 20% mortality rate. Esophagoscopy is combined with esophagography; if water-soluble contrast does not demonstrate a leak, barium is used. Such studies may be falsely negative in 50% of cases. Patients with zone II or III injuries who are candidates for nonoperative management may not require additional studies.

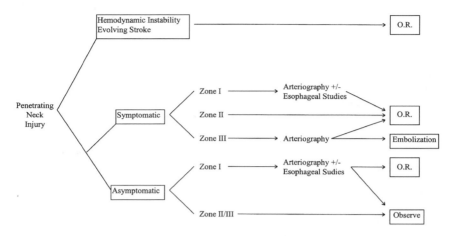

Management of penetrating neck trauma.

15. Should an asymptomatic patient with a penetrating neck wound be sent home from the emergency department?

No. Life-threatening penetrating neck wounds may be initially clinically occult; therefore, the safest policy is to observe all patients in the hospital for at least 24 hours.

BIBLIOGRAPHY

1. Asensio JA, Berne J, Demetriades D, et al: Penetrating esophageal injuries: Time interval of safety for pre-operative evaluation—How long is safe? J Trauma 43:319–324, 1997.
2. Back MR, Baumgartner FJ, Klein SR: Detection and evaluation of aerodigestive tract injuries caused by cervical and transmediastinal gunshot wounds. J Trauma 42:680–686, 1997.
3. Biffl WL, Moore EE, Rehse DH, et al: Selective management of penetrating neck trauma based on cervical level of injury. Am J Surg 174:678–682, 1997.
4. Demetriades D, Asensio JA, Velhamos G, et al: Complex problems in penetrating neck trauma. Surg Clin North Am 76:661–683, 1996.
5. Demetriades D, Theodorou D, Cornwell E, et al: Evaluation of penetrating injuries of the neck: Prospective study of 223 patients. World J Surg 21:41–48, 1997.
6. Sofianos C, Degiannis E, Van den aardweg MS, et al: Selective surgical management of zone II gunshot injuries of the neck: A prospective study. Surgery 120:785–788, 1996.

21. BLUNT THORACIC TRAUMA

Jeffrey L. Johnson, M.D., and Ernest E. Moore, M.D.

1. How often do patients with isolated blunt chest trauma need an emergent operation?

Rarely. Injuries to pulmonary, vascular, and mediastinal structures are surprisingly rare; only 5% of patients with isolated injuries to the chest require thoracotomy.

2. In a patient with a hemothorax after blunt chest injury, what is the most important guide for the decision to operate?

The clinical condition of the patient. Although chest tube output is a useful guide in patients with penetrating chest injuries, hemothorax after blunt injury most often is due to nonoperative lesions of the lung and chest wall. In a stable patient, therefore, evacuation of the hemothorax, re-expansion of the lung, and correction of coagulopathy should be the initial focus.

3. What is a tension pneumothorax?
Air in the pleural space under pressure due to a one-way valve mechanism. This is a life-threatening condition because air under pressure produces circulatory collapse from impaired right ventricular filling.

4. What are the clinical signs of tension pneumothorax?
Hypotension, absent breath sounds on the involved side, and distended neck veins. Tension pneumothorax should be treated upon clinical suspicion and without delay for radiographic confirmation.

5. How is tension pneumothorax treated?
For prehospital care, needle decompression via the 5th intercostal space in the midaxillary line. In the hospital setting, however, an experienced physician can completely decompress the pleural space just as rapidly with a tube thoracostomy.

6. What is a flail chest?
A flail chest occurs when a portion of the thoracic cage loses bony continuity with the rest of the chest. When multiple ribs are fractured in two or more places, the chest wall moves paradoxically ("flails") with respiration.

7. How does flail chest impact ventilation?
In spontaneously breathing patients, the portion of the thoracic cage that has lost bony continuity retracts *inward* during inspiration. This paradoxical motion results in impaired ventilation.

8. Does flail chest affect oxygenation?
Flail chest per se has little direct impact on oxygenation. However, virtually all patients with flail chest have an underlying pulmonary contusion. The severity of the pulmonary contusion is a more important determinant of outcome than the impaired mechanics of the chest wall. The pathophysiology of blunt injury to the chest with severe bony injury should be thought of as a single process (i.e., flail chest/pulmonary contusion).

9. What is the natural history of pulmonary contusion?
Like other tissues, the lung undergoes shearing of parenchyma and rupture of small blood vessels after a blunt injury or rapid deceleration. This tissue injury is followed by edema. Thus, patients with pulmonary contusion usually develop clinical deterioration in the first 48 hours. The initial chest radiograph may appear deceptively benign.

10. What is the most common initial presentation of blunt injury to the thoracic aorta?
Death in the field. Eighty-five percent of patients with a torn thoracic aorta die of exsanguination before they reach the hospital. Disruption of the heart and great vessels is second only to head injury as a cause of death due to blunt injury.

11. Of patients surviving to reach the hospital, where is the most common injury to the thoracic aorta?
A tear across the intima and media just distal to the takeoff of the left subclavian artery. Because the adventitia is intact, the patient does not immediately exsanguinate, and, if the lesion is detected promptly and treated, the survival rate is 85%.

12. What are the clinical signs of torn thoracic aorta?
There are no definitive signs and symptoms. Suspicion must be based on mechanism of injury (rapid deceleration). The signs associated with aortic disruption include upper extremity

hypertension, unequal upper extremity pressures, loss of lower extremity pulses, and expanding hematoma in the root of the neck.

13. What findings on chest radiograph are associated with rupture of the descending thoracic aorta?

Like physical signs, no initial radiographic signs are definitive. The signs that have been associated with torn thoracic aorta include indistinct aortic knob, widened mediastinum (> 8 cm at the level of the aortic knob), apical cap, left pleural effusion, depression of the left mainstem bronchus, lateral displacement of the esophagus (with nasogastric tube in place), first rib fractures, displacement of the trachea and loss of the aortopulmonary window. Approximately 15% of patients with torn aorta have a normal mediastinum, and 7% have a completely normal chest radiograph.

14. In the stable patient with a major mechanism of injury or chest radiographs consistent with aortic injury, how is the diagnosis made?

Dynamic helical computed tomography of the chest approaches 100% sensitivity for detecting aortic injury; it is widely available and applicable to all stable patients. The definitive test remains aortography because it more precisely identifies the site and extent of injury.

15. How is the diagnosis of cardiac contusion made?

It is not. Although a contusion of the myocardium may be evident on pathologic examination, this anatomic lesion has no reliable clinical, radiographic, chemical, or electrocardiographic markers.

16. If there is no reliable marker of cardiac contusion, how does one identify the patient with a blunt injury to the heart?

The most common manifestation of blunt cardiac injury is arrhythmia. Studies confirm that patients with an initial electrocardiogram (EKG) that is normal have an exceedingly small chance of developing clinically significant arrhythmias during their hospital course. Any EKG abnormality is an indication for admission and 24 hours of cardiac monitoring. Hemodynamic compromise from blunt cardiac injury is unusual.

17. Where do blunt injuries to the bronchus usually occur?

Within a few centimeters of the carina. The mainstem bronchi are splayed apart with severe anteroposterior compression of the chest. As the lungs are displaced laterally, the mainstem bronchi may tear near the site where they are fixed at the carina.

18. Can blunt trauma produce a rupture of the esophagus?

Almost never.

19. What are the indications for emergency department thoracotomy after blunt chest injury?

Cardiovascular collapse after arrival in the emergency department. The outcome, however, is typically dismal; less than 1% of patients survive neurologically intact.

20. What is traumatic asphyxia?

Traumatic asphyxia is the result of a protracted crush injury to the upper torso. In such an injury, venous hypertension is transmitted to the valveless veins of the upper body. Patients present with altered sensorium, petechial hemorrhages, cyanosis, and edema of the upper body. Although its initial presentation can be dramatic, with supportive care the outcome is usually good.

BIBLIOGRAPHY

1. Allen GS, Coates NE: Pulmonary contusion: A collective review. Am Surgeon 62:895–900, 1996.
2. Branney SW, Moore EE, Feldhaus KM, et al: Critical analysis of two decades of experience with postinjury emergency department thoracotomy in a regional trauma center. J Trauma 45:87–95, 1998.
3. Dyer DS, Moore EE, Mestak M, et al: Thoracic aortic injury—How predictive is mechanism and is chest CT a reliable screening tool? A prospective study of 1500 patients. J Trauma 1999 [in press].

4. Fabian TC, Richardson JD, Croce MA, et al: Prospective study of blunt aortic injury: Multicenter trial of the American Association for the Surgery of Trauma. J Trauma 42:374–383, 1997.
5. Hoff SJ, Shotts SD, Eddy VA, et al: Outcome of isolated pulmonary contusion in blunt trauma patients. Am Surgeon 60:138–142, 1994.
6. Richardson JD, Miller FB, Carrillo EH, et al: Complex thoracic injuries. Surg Clin North Am 76:725–747, 1996.
7. Shah R, Sabanathan S, Mearns AJ, et al: Traumatic rupture of the diaphragm. Ann Thorac Surg 60: 1444–1449, 1995.
8. Yeong EK, Chen MT, Chu SH: Traumatic asphyxia. Plast Reconstr Surg 93:739–744, 1994.

22. PENETRATING THORACIC TRAUMA

Jeffrey L. Johnson, M.D., and Ernest E. Moore, M.D.

1. How often do patients with penetrating chest wounds need a thoracotomy?

Most penetrating injuries seen in civilian practice are from knives and low-energy handguns. Consequently, although injuries to the chest wall and lung are common, the vast majority can be treated with tube thoracostomy alone. Formal thoracotomy or median sternotomy is required in less than 15% of isolated penetrating chest injuries.

2. What are the indications for emergency department thoracotomy (EDT) after penetrating chest wounds?

Patients who arrive with cardiac activity and have suffered circulatory collapse either en route or in the resuscitation area can benefit from EDT. Unlike blunt injury, a treatable cause is more commonly found (e.g., pericardial tamponade). EDT results in a survival of about 20%.

3. What is the "6-hour rule" for penetrating chest injuries?

In a patient with a penetrating chest injury, an upright chest radiography with no evidence of pneumothorax after 6 hours makes the likelihood of delayed pneumothorax or occult injury to an intrathoracic organ vanishingly small. The "6-hour rule" identifies patients who can be safely discharged.

4. How much blood in the pleural space can be detected by chest radiograph?

250 ml.

5. What are the indications for operation in a patient with hemothorax after penetrating chest injury?

Immediate return of over 1500 ml of blood from the pleural space or ongoing bleeding in excess of 250 ml/hr for 3 consecutive hours.

6. What is a "clam shell" thoracotomy?

Bilateral anterolateral thoracotomies with extension across the sternum. This procedure allows rapid access to pleural spaces, pulmonary hilae, and the mediastinum.

7. What is an open pneumothorax?

A defect in the chest wall that is open to the pleural space. In penetrating chest injuries, it most often is due to a close-range shotgun blast.

8. How is an open pneumothorax treated?

The defect in the chest wall should be covered with an occlusive dressing that is fixed on only three sides. This temporary fix prevents entry of air into the pleural space while allowing egress of air under pressure. A chest tube is then inserted. Formal repair of the chest wall can wait until other significant injuries are excluded.

9. Where is "the box"?

On the anterior chest between the midclavicular lines from clavicle to costal margin. Penetrating wounds are likely to cause cardiac injury in this region. Although the typical patient with a penetrating cardiac injury has a wound in the box, the heart also can be reached from the root of the neck, axilla, and epigastrium.

10. What is Beck's triad? How often is it present in patients with tamponade due to penetrating chest injuries?

Beck's triad consists of hypotension, distended neck veins, and muffled heart tones. These signs are difficult to appreciate in the trauma patient (particularly muffled heart sounds in a busy resuscitation room) and present in a minority of patients with tamponade from penetrating injuries (less than 40%). The absence of distended neck veins is to be expected, because most patients have concomitant hypovolemia.

11. In a stable patient with suspected penetrating cardiac injury, what is the most important initial study?

After completion of the primary survey (airways, breathing, circulation), bedside ultrasonography should be performed. This rapid, sensitive method for detecting pericardial fluid indicates cardiac injury. Although the initial study may be negative with a small effusion, serial exams detect virtually all cases.

12. What is the initial therapeutic maneuver in the patient with a penetrating cardiac wound who is not yet hypotensive?

Percutaneous pericardial drainage. Early pericardial tamponade does not appear immediately life-threatening; however, one of the early effects of tamponade is subendocardial ischemia, which puts the patient at risk for cardiac ischemia and refractory arrhythmias. Immediate decompression of the pericardium ensures safer transport to the operating room for definitive repair.

13. In a penetrating chest wound, how is injury to the diaphragm evaluated?

At end expiration the dome of the diaphragm reaches the level of the nipples. In principle, any patient with penetrating injury below the level of the nipples may have an injury to the diaphragm. Diagnostic peritoneal lavage is the preferred initial procedure. Red blood cell counts less than 1000/mm^3 are negative. Counts > 10,000 are positive; for counts of 1000–10,000, thoracoscopy is indicated to visualize completely the hemidiaphragm at risk.

14. Why is it important to detect a small diaphragmatic laceration?

Abdominal viscera herniate from the positive-pressure abdominal cavity into the negative-pressure pleural space. The morbidity of a strangulated diaphragmatic hernia is not trivial, often because of delay in diagnosis.

15. Does a patient with a gunshot wound traversing the mediastinum need an operation?

No. Surprisingly, not all wounds that pass completely through the mediastinum injure a critical structure. In fact, only about 35% of patients have an injury requiring exploration. The stable patient should be evaluated with history (odynophagia? hoarseness?), physical examination (deep cervical emphysema? expanding hematoma? pulseless extremity?), angiography, bronchoscopy, and esophagoscopy.

16. Are prophylactic antibiotics warranted to prevent empyema after tube thoracostomy?

Meta-analysis of currently published randomized studies on prophylactic antibiotics for tube thoracostomy suggests a benefit.

17. What is the most important risk factor for posttraumatic empyema?

Persistent hemothorax. Blood is an excellent incubation medium for bacteria; therefore, expedient evacuation of blood from the pleural space via tube thoracostomy for video-assisted thoracoscopic surgery is central in the management of traumatic hemothorax (starve the bugs).

18. What is a bronchovenous air embolism?

The classic presentation of bronchovenous air embolism is a patient with a penetrating chest injury who arrests after intubation and application of positive-pressure ventilation. The underlying pathophysiology is passage of air under pressure from a lacerated bronchus to an adjacent lacerated pulmonary vein. Air then travels to the left side of the heart and into the coronary arteries.

19. How is bronchovenous air embolism diagnosed and treated?

Diagnosis is based only on the typical history (see question 18). Therapy is directed toward removal of air from the left ventricle and coronary arteries: Trendelenberg (head down) position with right side down, immediate thoracotomy and aspiration of the apex of the left ventricle, the aortic root, and occasionally the coronary arteries.

20. What is Hamman's sign?

A crunching sound on auscultation of the chest, which indicates air in the mediastinum.

21. In a penetrating esophageal injury, where may air be evident on physical examination?

The deep subcutaneous tissues of the neck. In the upright position, air in the mediastinum dissects into a plane continuous with the deep cervical fascia.

22. How do penetrating tracheobronchial injuries present?

Laceration of the trachea and major bronchi presents with subcutaneous emphysema, hemoptysis and dyspnea. Chest radiographs reveal a pneumothorax and/or pneumomediastinum. After tube thoracostomy, continuous air leak and failure of the lung to reexpand ("dropped lung") should prompt suspicion of a major bronchial injury.

23. What does a blurry bullet on a chest radiograph indicate?

A bullet lodged in the myocardium. Movement of the heart causes the image to be blurry on the radiograph. Beware the blurry bullet.

BIBLIOGRAPHY

1. Aguilar MM, Battistella FD, Owings JT, et al: Posttraumatic empyema. Arch Surg 132:647–651, 1997.
2. Branney SW, Moore EE, Feldhaus KM, et al: Critical analysis of two decades of experience with postinjury emergency department thoracotomy in a regional trauma center. J Trauma 45:87–95, 1998.
3. Cornwell EEI, Kennedy F, Ayad IA, et al: Transmediastinal gunshot wounds. Arch Surg 131:949–953, 1996.
4. Mattox KL, Wall MJ, Pickard LR: Thoracic trauma: General considerations and indications for thoracotomy. In Feliciano DV, Moore EE, Mattox KL (eds): Trauma. Stamford, CT, Appleton & Lange, 1996, pp 345–354.
5. Nagy KK, Lohmann C, Kim DO, et al: Role of echocardiography in the diagnosis of occult penetrating cardiac injury. J Trauma 38:859–862, 1995.
6. Rhee PM, Foy H, Kaufmann C, et al: Penetrating cardiac injuries: A population-based study. J Trauma 45:366–370, 1998.
7. Wall MJ, Granchi T, Liscum K, et al: Penetrating thoracic vascular injuries. Surg Clin North Am 76:749–761, 1996.
8. Velmahos GC, Degiannis E, Souter I, et al: Outcome of a strict policy on emergency department thoracotomies. Arch Surg 130:774–777, 1995.

23. BLUNT ABDOMINAL TRAUMA

David J. Ciesla, M.D., and Ernest E. Moore, M.D.

1. What elements of the history are important in evaluating a patient with suspected blunt abdominal trauma (BAT)?

The mechanism of injury (fall, motor vehicle collision, automobile-pedestrian accident) provides the basic information in the history. In motor vehicle accidents it is important to note the position of the victim in the car, velocity of impact (high, moderate, low), type of accident (front, side, or rear impact, side swipe, rollover), and type of restraint used (lap belt, shoulder restraint, air-bag). Information about damage to the vehicle, such as a broken windshield or bent steering wheel, may raise suspicion of head and chest injuries. In a fall it is important to note the distance fallen and site of anatomic impact. Vertical landing on the feet or in a sitting position causes a different pattern of injury than lateral landing on the side. Field vital signs and mental status are important.

2. Is physical examination accurate in the diagnosis of intraabdominal injury?

Physical examination is neither sensitive or specific for diagnosis of intraabdominal injuries and may be normal in up to 50% of patients with acute intraabdominal bleeding. Signs of intraabdominal injury include abrasions and contusions over the lower chest and abdomen; subcutaneous emphysema or palpable rib fracture; clinically evident pelvic fracture; abdominal pain, tenderness, guarding, or rigidity; blood in the urine or urethral meatus; high-riding prostate or blood discovered on rectal exam; and microscopic hematuria.

3. Which organs are most frequently injured in BAT?

The frequency of organ injury among patients requiring laparotomy for BAT is as follows: spleen, 50%; liver, 50%; mesentery, 10%; urologic, 10%; pancreas, 10%; small bowel, 10%; colon, 5%; duodenum, 5%; vascular, 4%; stomach, 2%; and gallbladder, 2%.

4. What are the most common injuries associated with two-point fixation seatbelts?

The "seatbelt syndrome" is a complex of injuries caused by sudden deceleration and flexion of the upper body around the fixed lap belt. Injuries may include abdominal viscera (small bowel, mesentery, duodenum, pancreas) with concomitant fracture, distraction, or subluxation of the lumbar spine. Transverse abdominal ecchymosis is a common physical examination finding.

5. What diagnostic studies are helpful in BAT?

1. **Abdominal ultrasound:** reliably identifies peritoneal fluid (blood) and pericardial fluid but may fail to identify up to 25% of isolated solid organ injuries.

2. **Computed tomography (CT) scan:** identifies presence and severity of solid organ injury (liver and spleen), detects intraabdominal air and fluid (blood, mucus, urine), and aids in evaluation of pelvic fractures. CT scanning can also identify bowel, pancreatic, renal, and bladder injuries.

3. **Diagnostic peritoneal lavage (DPL):** grossly positive DPL (> 10 ml blood returned by aspiration of the catheter) indicates significant hemoperitoneum. Positive by cell count after infusion of 1 L of crystalloid fluid (> 100,000 red blood cells/mm^3, > 500 white blood cells/mm^3, presence of bile or fibers) indicates intraabdominal bleeding, injury to hollow viscus, or hepatobiliary system injury. Lavage fluid exiting through a chest tube or urinary catheter indicates diaphragmatic or bladder injury.

6. What are the limitations of DPL?

DPL is an invasive procedure that carries a small but real risk of complications, including stomach, bowel, and bladder perforation as well as injury to the major abdominal blood vessels.

DPL cannot assess retroperitoneal injuries. If performed early in the hospital course, DPL may miss a hollow organ injury, presumably because the degree of inflammation is insufficient to generate the peritoneal leukosequestration required to produce a positive DPL. Patients with prior abdominal operations are at increased risk of bowel perforation from catheter insertion.

7. What are the limitations of CT scan?

CT is time-consuming and contraindicated in hemodynamically unstable patients. Use of contrast media is associated with allergic reactions and renal damage.

8. How is hollow organ injury diagnosed?

CT findings include peritoneal fluid unassociated with solid organ injury, extravasation of oral contrast into the peritoneal cavity, and free intraabdominal air. Peritoneal lavage results suggestive of hollow organ injury include elevated amylase and alkaline phosphatase.

9. What are the indications for urgent operation in a patient with BAT?

Any hemodynamically unstable patient or any patient who exhibits significant hemoperitoneum requires emergent laparotomy. Other indications for urgent laparotomy include free intraabdominal air and evidence of hollow viscus injury.

10. What is the role of angiographic embolization?

Angiographic embolization may be effective for hemorrhage control in hemodynamically stable patients. Favorable embolization sites include liver, spleen, and kidney injuries, lumbar arteries with retroperitoneal hemorrhage, and pelvic blood vessels associated with pelvic fracture.

11. What is the "bloody viscous cycle"?

The bloody viscous cycle is a syndrome of hypothermia, acidosis, and coagulopathy that occurs with profound hemorrhage shock and massive transfusion. It represents a circular cascade of events in which severe hemorrhagic shock accompanied by acidosis provokes a coagulopathy that exacerbates further bleeding.

12. What is a staged or abbreviated laparotomy?

Staged laparotomy is terminated before all definitive procedures are completed with the intent to return to the operating room and complete the operation at a later (and safer) time. The purpose of this approach is to delay additional surgical stress until the patient is in a more favorable physiologic state. The objectives of the initial operation become (1) to arrest bleeding and correct coagulopathy, (2) to limit peritoneal contamination and the secondary inflammatory response (e.g., to control spillage), and (3) to enclose the abdominal contents to protect viscera and limit heat, fluid, and protein loss from an open abdomen.

13. When is staged laparotomy used in trauma patients?

1. Inability to achieve hemostasis due to recalcitrant coagulopathy (pack the bleeding)
2. Inaccessible major venous injury (retrohepatic caval injury)
3. Demand for nonoperative control of a life-threatening extraabdominal (head/thoracic) injury
4. Inability to close the abdominal incision due to extensive visceral reperfusion edema
5. Need to reassess abdominal contents because of questionable validity at the time of the initial operation

BIBLIOGRAPHY

1. Arrillaga A, Graham R, York JW, Miller RS: Increased efficiency and cost-effectiveness in the evaluation of the blunt abdominal trauma patient with the use of ultrasound. Am Surg 65:31–35, 1999.
2. Burch JM, Denton JR, Noble RD: Physiologic rationale for abbreviated laparotomy. Surg Clin North Am 77:779–782, 1997.
3. Davis KA, Fabian TC, Croce MA, et al: Improved success in management of blunt splenic injuries: Embolization of splenic artery pseudoaneurysms. J Trauma 44:1008–1013, 1998.

4. Feliciano DV, Moore EE, Mattox KL (eds): Trauma, 3rd ed. Norwalk, CT, Appleton & Lange, 1996.
5. Hirshberg A, Mattox KL: Planned reoperation for severe trauma. Ann Surg 222:3–7, 1995.
6. McAnena OJ, Moore EE, Marx JA: Initial evaluation of the patient with blunt abdominal trauma. Surg
   Clin North Am 70:495–515, 1990.
7. Moore EE: Staged laparotomy for the hypothermia, acidosis, and coagulopathy syndrome. Am J Surg
   172:405–410, 1996.
8. Rozycki GS: Abdominal ultrasound in trauma. Surg Clin North Am 75:175–191, 1995.
9. Velmahos GC, Tatavossian R, Demetriades D: The "seat belt mark" sign: A call for increased vigilance
   among physicians treating victims of motor vehicle accidents. Am Surg 65:181–185, 1999.

24. PENETRATING ABDOMINAL TRAUMA

Walter L. Biffl, M.D., and Ernest E. Moore, M.D.

1. Why is there a different approach to stab and gunshot wounds?

One-third of stab wounds to the anterior abdomen do not penetrate the peritoneum, whereas more than 80% of gunshot wounds violate the peritoneum. Furthermore, penetration of the peritoneum by a bullet is associated with visceral or vascular injuries in > 95% of cases, whereas only one-half of stab wounds violating the peritoneal cavity produce significant injury. The figure below outlines the decision algorithm for stab and gunshot wounds.

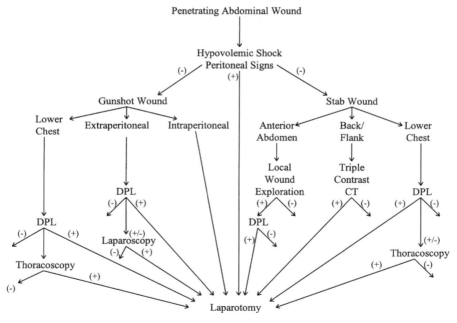

Decision algorithm for management of patients with penetrating abdominal trauma.

2. When is emergency department (ED) thoracotomy indicated for a penetrating abdominal wound?

Thoracotomy should be performed in the ED when patients present with cardiac arrest or profound hypotension (< 60 mmHg) refractory to initial resuscitation. Thoracotomy allows open cardiac massage and access to cross-clamp the descending aorta to improve coronary and cerebral perfusion as well as decrease subdiaphragmatic hemorrhage.

3. What are the appropriate initial studies?

The ABCs (airway, breathing, and circulation) are the first priority in every trauma patient. In stable patients, a chest radiograph excludes hemo- or pneumothorax and determines the position of intravenous catheters (endotracheal, nasogastric, and pleural tubes). Biplanar abdominal radiographs are helpful in locating retained foreign bodies and may reveal pneumoperitoneum. Injuries in proximity to the rectum obligate sigmoidoscopy (see chapter 28), whereas injuries in proximity to the urinary tract should be evaluated with intravenous pyelography (see chapter 31).

4. What is the secondary survey for a penetrating abdominal wound?

Tubes and fingers in every orifice. Important historical information includes the time of injury, type of weapon, length or caliber of the weapon, depth of penetration if the weapon was removed, and estimated blood loss at the scene. Each of these descriptors is included in the mechanism of injury. Physical examination must be comprehensive; in the heat of the battle it is easy to overlook synchronous injuries. Entrance and exit wounds should be identified with a radiopaque marker.

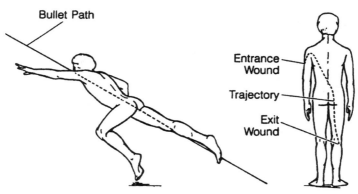

Illustrated is an example of how the path of a bullet through a contorted body can produce confusion when the patient is examined in the emergency department. An entrance wound will be found at the left upper arm and an exit wound at the medial aspect of the right knee. The bullet could have damaged any structure that was in between these two wounds when the patient's body was contorted.

5. What are the indications for prompt laparotomy in patients with stab wounds?

Abdominal distention and hypotension, overt peritonitis, and obvious signs of abdominal visceral injury (hematuria, hematemesis, proctorrhagia, evisceration; palpation of diaphragmatic defect on chest tube insertion; radiologic evidence of injury to gastrointestinal or genitourinary tracts) mandate immediate exploration.

6. What are the indications for immediate laparotomy in patients with gunshot wounds?

Because of the high incidence of visceral injury, immediate exploration is indicated for all gunshot wounds that violate the peritoneum.

7. What is the general plan for abdominal exploration in patients with penetrating trauma?

A midline abdominal incision provides rapid entry and wide exposure; it may be extended as a median sternotomy to access the chest or continued inferiorly into the pelvis. The aorta should be palpated to assess blood pressure. All findings, including a soft aorta and low blood pressure, should be communicated to the anesthetist. Evacuation of blood and placement of tamponade packs are followed by exploration of the wound tract. Actively bleeding areas are digitally controlled until the culprit vessel can be occluded. Hollow visceral injuries are temporarily isolated with noncrushing clamps. The entire abdomen is systematically explored before undertaking extensive repairs so that injuries can be addressed in the proper sequence.

8. What is the role for presumptive antibiotics?

Short courses (< 24 hr) of high-dose antibiotics are initiated only when the decision has been made to perform a laparotomy. Coverage of both anaerobic and aerobic flora is desirable. Tetanus prophylaxis should be given to all patients with penetrating injuries.

9. How is an anterior abdominal stab wound evaluated in asymptomatic patients?

The first step is local exploration of the wound to determine peritoneal penetration. If the tract clearly terminates superficially, no further evaluation or treatment is required. Confirmation of peritoneal penetration is followed by diagnostic peritoneal lavage (DPL) (see question 10). Double-contrast (oral and intravenous) computed tomography (CT) scanning is not useful because of its relative insensitivity for detecting hollow visceral injuries. Ultrasonography is useful primarily for detecting blood quickly and thus is helpful only if positive.

10. What constitutes a positive DPL after penetrating trauma?

A grossly positive tap (aspiration of > 10 ml of blood or gastrointestinal or biliary contents) mandates immediate exploration. A negative initial aspirate is followed by the instillation of 1000 ml of saline (15 ml/kg in children) into the abdomen through a dialysis catheter, followed by gravity drainage of the fluid back into the saline bag. The finding of > 100,000/mm^3 red blood cells or the combined elevation of amylase > 20 IU/L and alkaline phosphatase > 3 IU/L is an indication for exploration.

11. How are flank and back stab wounds evaluated?

The incidence of significant injuries is 10% for stab wounds to the back and 25% for stab wounds to the flank. However, evaluation of such wounds is problematic, because the retroperitoneum is not sampled by DPL and physical examination is even less sensitive. The major concern is missed colonic perforation. At present, triple-contrast (oral, intravenous, and rectal) CT and serial physical examination are the two primary modes of assessment.

12. How is a lower chest stab wound evaluated?

The lower chest is defined as the area between the nipple line (fourth intercostal space) anteriorly, the tip of the scapula (seventh intercostal space) posteriorly, and the costal margins inferiorly. Because the diaphragm reaches the fourth intercostal space during expiration, the abdominal organs are at risk after penetrating wounds to this region. Stab wounds to the lower chest are associated with abdominal visceral injury in 15% of cases, whereas gunshot wounds to the lower chest are associated with abdominal visceral injury in nearly 50%. Thus, wounds to the lower chest should be managed as abdominal wounds for the purposes of evaluating the abdomen. In the case of lower chest stab wounds, a red blood cell count of > 10,000/mm^3 warrants laparotomy; thoracoscopic exploration (not thoracotomy) is performed for counts of 1000–10,000/mm^3.

13. Which patients with abdominal gunshot wounds are managed nonoperatively?

Stable patients with tangential missile tracts or equivocal peritoneal penetration are candidates for DPL. The cut-off for red blood cell counts is reduced to 10,000/mm^3, above which laparotomy is indicated. Patients with a negative DPL are observed for 24 hours. For red blood cell counts of 100–10,000/mm^3, laparoscopy may be used to exclude peritoneal penetration. Selective management of gunshot wounds to the back and flank are generally based on triple contrast CT.

14. Should prehospital fluid resuscitation be withheld in patients with penetrating abdominal trauma?

Delaying resuscitation until major vascular injuries are under operative control has been proposed to improve outcome in patients after penetrating trauma. It is argued that the increase in perfusion pressure associated with resuscitation dislodges clots and overcomes hemostatic mechanisms, allowing uncontrolled hemorrhage. A large randomized clinical trial has corroborated animal studies to support this concept, but the study was flawed by excessive times in the ED and lack of patient stratification by degree of shock. Confirmation from other centers is required before widespread acceptance of this practice.

CONTROVERSY

15. What is the role of laparoscopy and thoracoscopy after penetrating abdominal trauma?

Although an intriguing diagnostic modality with additional therapeutic capabilities, laparoscopy thus far appears to have limited application after trauma. With the exception of the evaluation of suspected diaphragmatic injury, laparoscopy has yet to demonstrate advantages over the algorithm delineated above. The potential for missed injuries, poor evaluation of the retroperitoneum, and expense are major drawbacks. In patients with wounds to the lower chest with pneumothorax (and, thus, an indication for chest tube placement) thoracoscopy is a reasonable modality with which to exclude diaphragmatic injury.

BIBLIOGRAPHY

1. American College of Surgeons Committee on Trauma: Advanced Trauma Life Support for Doctors. Chicago, American College of Surgeons, 1997.
2. Bickell WH, Wall MJ Jr, Pepe PE, et al: Immediate versus delayed fluid resuscitation for hypotensive patients with penetrating torso injuries. N Engl J Med 331:1105–1109, 1994.
3. Biffl WL, Moore EE, Harken AH: Emergency department thoracotomy. In Mattox KL, Feliciano DV, Moore EE (eds): Trauma, 4th ed. Stamford Ct, Appleton & Lange, 1999.
4. Ginzburg E, Carrillo EH, Kopelman T, et al: The role of computed tomography in selective management of gunshot wounds to the abdomen and flank. J Trauma 45:1005–1009, 1998.
5. Nagy KK, Krosner SM, Joseph KT, et al: A method of determining peritoneal penetration in gunshot wounds to the abdomen. J Trauma 43:242–246, 1997.
6. Reber PU, Schmied B, Seiler CA, et al: Missed diaphragmatic injuries and their long-term sequelae. J Trauma 44:183–188, 1998.
7. Riddez L, Johnson L, Hahn RG: Central and regional hemodynamics during crystalloid fluid therapy after uncontrolled intra-abdominal bleeding. J Trauma 44:433–439, 1998.
8. Zantut LF, Ivatury RR, Smith RS, et al: Diagnostic and therapeutic laparoscopy for penetrating abdominal trauma: A multicenter experience. J Trauma 42:825–831, 1997.

25. HEPATIC AND BILIARY TRAUMA

Reginald J. Franciose, M.D., and Ernest E. Moore, M.D.

1. How often is the liver injured in trauma?

Because of its expansive mass and central location, the liver is the most common site of visceral injury after both blunt and penetrating abdominal trauma.

2. Do the liver and spleen respond similarly to injury?

No. The liver has a unique ability to establish spontaneous hemostasis even with extensive injuries. For this reason, the vast majority of liver injuries in hemodynamically stable patients can be managed nonoperatively. In contrast, major splenic fractures often continue to hemor-rhage; therefore, a greater percentage require operative intervention.

3. What are the determinants of mortality after acute liver injury?

Mechanism of injury and number of associated abdominal organ injuries are the major deter-minants of mortality. The mortality rate for stab wounds to liver is 2%; for gunshot wounds, 8%; and for blunt injuries, 15%. The mortality rate for isolated grade III hepatic injuries is 2%; for grave IV, 20%; and for grade V, 65%. Retrohepatic vena cava injuries carry mortality rates of 80% for penetrating trauma and 95% for blunt trauma.

4. What history and physical signs suggest acute liver injury?

Any patient sustaining blunt abdominal trauma with hypotension must be assumed to have a liver injury until proved otherwise. Specific signs that increase the likelihood of hepatic injury are contusion over the right lower chest, fracture of the right lower ribs (especially posterior frac-tures of ribs 9–12), and penetrating injuries to the right lower chest (below the fourth intercostal space, flank, and upper abdomen). Physical signs of hemoperitoneum may be absent in as many as one-third of patients with significant hepatic injury.

5. What diagnostic tests are helpful in confirming acute liver injury?

Diagnostic peritoneal lavage (DPL) is the most sensitive test for hemoperitoneum (99%). Currently there is enthusiasm among trauma surgeons for the use of emergency department ultra-sonography as an alternative to DPL. Ultrasound is highly sensitive in identifying more than 200 ml of intraperitoneal fluid. It is noninvasive and may be repeated at frequent intervals, but it is rela-tively poor for staging liver injuries. Abdominal CT scan is currently used only in hemodynamically stable patients who are candidates for nonoperative management. The major shortcoming of CT is the relatively poor correlation between hepatic CT staging and subsequent risk of hemorrhage.

6. What is the role of hepatic angiography and radionuclide biliary excretion scans in the diagnosis of liver injury?

Selective hepatic artery embolization is effective therapy for hepatic arterial bleeding both for avoidance of surgery and for recurrent postoperative bleeding.

SURGICAL ANATOMY OF THE LIVER

7. How many anatomic lobes are present in the liver? What is their topographic boundary?

The liver is divided into two anatomic lobes, the right and the left. Their boundary lies in an oblique plane extending from the gallbladder fossa anteriorly to the inferior vena cava posteri-orly. The three hepatic veins define the division between the lobar segments and the planes of surgical resection. Lobar segments are numbered I–VIII, according to Couinaud's nomenclature. (See figure at top of facing page.)

8. What is the blood supply to the liver and the relative contribution of each structure to hepatic oxygenation?

The hepatic artery supplies approximately 30% of the blood flow to the liver and 50% of its oxygen supply, whereas the portal vein provides 70% of the liver's blood flow and 50% of its oxygen. The relative significance of arterial flow in cirrhotic patients is greater; therefore, hepatic artery ligation is not recommended in patients with cirrhosis.

9. What are the most common variations in hepatic arterial supply to the right and left lobes of the liver?

In most people the common hepatic artery originates form the celiac axis and divides into right and left hepatic arterial branches within the porta hepatis. Approximately 15% of people have a replaced right hepatic artery (sole arterial supply to the right lobe) that originates from

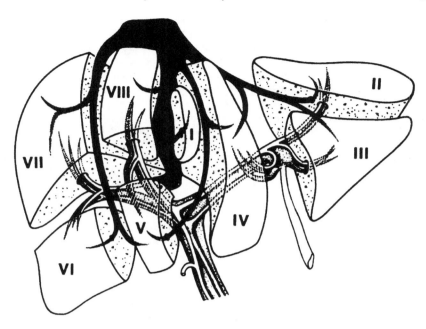

The functional division of the liver and the segments according to Couinaud's nomenclature. (From Bismuth H: Surgical anatomy and anatomical surgery of the liver. World J Surg 6:6, 1982, with permission.)

the superior mesenteric artery (SMA). A replaced right hepatic artery always supplies a cystic artery; thus, ligation should be followed by cholecystectomy. A replaced left hepatic artery (approximately 15% of people) arises from the left gastric artery; it may be the sole blood supply to the left lobe or may contribute to blood supply in conjunction with a normal left hepatic artery. In 5% of people, the hepatic arterial supply does not arise from the celiac axis. Either the right and left hepatic arteries are replaced, or a single main hepatic trunk derives from the SMA.

10. What is the venous drainage of the liver?

The right, middle, and left hepatic veins are the major venous tributaries and enter the inferior vena cava below the right hemidiaphragm.

OPERATIVE MANAGEMENT OF LIVER INJURY

11. How are acute liver injuries classified?

Liver wounds generally are graded on a scale of I to VI according the depth of parenchymal laceration and involvement of the hepatic veins or retrohepatic portion of the inferior vena cava. Optimal methods of obtaining hemostasis vary with the severity of the injury.

12. Do all patients with a traumatic liver injury require surgery?

No. Nonoperative treatment is the standard for victims of blunt trauma who remain hemodynamically stable (approximately 85% of patients). One-third of such patients require blood transfusions, but if volume exceeds 6 units in the first 24 hours angiography should be done. CT scan should be repeated in 5–7 days for grade IV and V injuries. Complications, including perihepatic infection, biloma, and hemobilia, have been reported in 10% of nonoperative patients.

13. What are the options for temporary control of significant hemorrhage in victims of hepatic trauma?

Hemorrhage may pose an immediate threat to life. Furthermore, ongoing hemorrhage leads to the vicious cycle of acidosis, hypothermia, and coagulopathy. Manual compression, perihepatic packing, and the Pringle maneuver are the most effective temporary techniques until the definitive techniques outlined below can be initiated.

14. What is the Pringle maneuver?

The Pringle maneuver is the manual or vascular clamp occlusion of the hepatoduodenal ligament to interrupt blood flow into the liver. Included in the hepatoduodenal ligament are the hepatic artery, portal vein, and common bile duct. Failure of the Pringle maneuver to control liver hemorrhage suggests either (1) injury to the retrohepatic vena cava or heptaic vein or (2) arterial supply from an aberrant right or left hepatic artery (see question 9).

15. What is the finger fracture technique?

Finger fracture hepatotomy or tractotomy is the method of exposing bleeding points deep within liver lacerations by blunt dissection. Pushing apart the liver parenchyma enables points to be identified and ligated. This method is required more commonly for penetrating injuries.

16. What is the role of selective hepatic artery ligation in securing hemostasis in patients with a major liver injury?

Deep lacerations of the right or left hepatic lobe may result in bleeding that cannot be completely controlled by suture ligation of specific bleeding points within the liver parenchyma. In this situation, either the right or left artery can be ligated for control of the bleeding with little risk of ischemic liver necrosis.

17. Why is retrohepatic vena caval laceration lethal?

The retrohepatic portion of the inferior vena cava is difficult to expose because it is enveloped by the liver. Exposure requires either extensive hepatotomy, extensive mobilization of the right lobe, right lobectomy, or transection of the vena cava. The large caliber and high flow of the inferior vena cava results in massive hemorrhage during surgical exposure, whereas clamping of the inferior vena cava often results in hypotension due to an abrupt fall in venous return to the heart.

18. What is the physiologic rationale for use of a shunt in attempted repair of retrohepatic vena caval injuries?

Hemorrhage control requires maintenance of venous return to the heart while both antegrade and retrograde bleeding through the laceration is stopped. These requirements are met by shunting blood through a tube spanning the laceration between the right atrium and lower inferior vena cava.

19. What is the intrahepatic balloon tamponading device?

For transhepatic penetrating injuries, a 1-inch Penrose drain is sutured around a red rubber catheter to form a long balloon that is threaded through the bleeding liver injury and inflated with contrast media through a stopcock in the red rubber catheter. The balloon tamponades liver hemorrhage. The catheter is brought out through the abdominal wall, deflated, and removed 24–48 hours later.

20. What are the indications for perihepatic packing?

Liver packing with planned reoperation for definitive treatment of injuries in patients who have hypothermia, acidosis, and coagulopathies is a life-saving maneuver. Laparotomy pads (up to 20) are packed around the liver to compress and control hemorrhage. The skin of the abdomen is then closed with towel clips (abbreviated laparotomy), and the patient's metabolic abnormalities are corrected with planned reoperation within 24 hours.

21. What is the abdominal compartment syndrome?
A potentially lethal complication of perihepatic packing is the abdominal compartment syndrome, which may occur when intraabdominal pressure exceeds 20 cmH_2O. Intraabdominal pressure increases because of bowel and liver edema secondary to ischemia and reperfusion injury or continued hemorrhage into the abdominal cavity. As pressure increases beyond 20 cmH_2O, venous return, cardiac output, and urine output decrease, whereas ventilatory pressures increase. Patients must return promptly to the operating room for decompression of the abdomen. A manometer attached to the Foley catheter is useful in following intraabdominal pressure.

BILIARY TRACT INJURY

22. Why are complications associated with bile duct leaks?
Bilomas (collections of bile) frequently become infected and may result in lethal peritonitis. Biliopleural fistula, a communication between the biliary system and pleural cavity, persists because of the relative negative pressure in the thorax and may result in a bile empyema.

23. What is the initial management of an established bile leak?
Endoscopic transampullary stenting frequently allows spontaneous resolution of bile duct injuries. Extensive injuries require hepaticojejunostomy for reconstruction.

BIBLIOGRAPHY

1. Burch JM, Ortiz VB, Richardson RJ, et al: Abbreviated laparotomy and planned reoperation for critically injured patients. Ann Surg 215:476, 1992.
2. Croce MA, Fabian TC, Menke PG, et al: Nonoperative management of blunt hepatic trauma is the treatment of choice for hemodynamically stable patients. Ann Surg 221:744, 1995.
3. Cue JI, Cryer HG, Miller FB, et al: Packing and planned reexploration for hepatic and retroperitoneal hemorrhage: Critical refinements of a useful technique. Trauma 30:1007, 1990.
4. Dawson DL, Jurkovich GJ: Hepatic duct disruption from blunt abdominal trauma—Case report and literature review. J Trauma 31:1698, 1991.
5. Hiatt JR, Gabbay J, Busutill RW: Surgical anatomy of the hepatic arteries in 1000 cases. Ann Surg 220:50, 1994.
6. Meldrum DR, Moore FA, Moore EE, et al: Cardiopulmonary hazards of perihepatic packing for major liver injury. Am J Surg 170:537, 1995.
7. Meredith JW, Young JR, Bowling J, Roboussin D: Nonoperative management of adult blunt hepatic trauma: The exception or the rule? J Trauma 36:529, 1994.
8. Moore EE: Staged laparotomy for the hypothermia, acidosis, and coagulopathy syndrome. Am J Surg 172:405, 1996.
9. Moore EE, Cogbill TH, Malangoni MA, et al: Organ injury scaling. Surg Clin North Am 75:2, 1995.
10. Pachter HL, Hofstetter SR: The current status of nonoperative management of adult blunt hepatic injuries. Am J Surg 169:442, 1995.
11. Poggetti RS, Moore EE, Moore FA, et al: Balloon tamponade for bilobar transfixing hepatic gunshot wounds. J Trauma 33:694, 1992.
12. Sheik-Gafoor M, Singh B, Moodley J: Traumatic thoracobiliary fistula: Report of a case with an overview of current diagnostic and therapeutic options. J Trauma 45:819, 1998.

26. SPLENIC TRAUMA

David J. Ciesla, M.D., and Ernest E. Moore, M.D.

1. What is the physiologic role of the spleen?

In fetal development the spleen serves as a major site for hematopoiesis. In early childhood the spleen produces immunoglobulin M. The spleen also functions as a filter, allowing resident macrophages to remove abnormal red blood cells, cellular debris, and encapsulated and poorly opsonized bacteria.

2. How is the spleen injured?

By direct blunt force, deceleration, and compression injuries to the left torso, which commonly occur with motor vehicle accidents and falls.

3. What are the signs and symptoms of splenic injury?

Splenic injury is associated with pain over the left upper torso that can be produced by stretching of the splenic capsule. Peritoneal irritation (rebound tenderness) from extravasated blood in the abdomen typically presents later in the course of injury. Fractures of the lower left ribs are commonly associated injuries in adults. Vital signs vary and are not specific for injuries to the spleen because a significant number of patients present with no signs or symptoms of splenic injury.

4. What is Kehr's sign?

Kehr's sign is left shoulder pain caused by diaphragmatic irritation from extravasated blood or splenic hematoma.

5. What studies help to diagnose splenic injury?

1. Ultrasound (US) performed in the emergency department allows the identification of intraabdominal fluid (blood) with volumes as small as 200 ml. When US is not available, diagnostic peritoneal lavage (DPL) provides an accurate and sensitive measure of intraabdominal bleeding.

2. Hemodynamic stability permits a more thorough evaluation. US is extremely sensitive for detecting significant intraabdominal bleeding, but computed tomography (CT) has the advantage of characterizing parenchymal injuries to intraabdominal organs (liver, spleen, pancreas, kidney) as well as detecting intraabdominal blood.

6. How are splenic injuries classified? Why is classification important?

Management is determined by the hemodynamic stability of the patient but is influenced by the CT grade of splenic injury. Nonoperative management is preferred for grades I–III, whereas operative intervention is required for grade IV and grade V injuries. Grade V injuries demand prompt operative intervention.

Grade I	Hematoma: nonexpanding, subcapsular, < 10% surface area
	Laceration: nonbleeding, capsular, < 1 cm parenchymal depth
Grade II	Hematoma: nonexpanding, subcapsular, < 50% surface area, or nonexpanding, intraparenchymal, < 5 cm diameter
	Laceration: bleeding, capsular, < 3 cm parenchymal depth
Grade III	Hematoma: subcapsular, > 50% surface area, expanding, ruptured with active bleeding, or intraparenchymal, > 5 cm diameter or expanding
	Laceration: capsular, > 3 cm parenchymal depth, involving trabecular vessel
Grade IV	Hematoma: ruptured, intraparenchymal, with active bleeding
	Laceration: involves segmental or hilar vessels with > 25% splenic devascularization

Grade V   Laceration: shattered spleen
                   Vascular: hilar avulsion or complete splenic devascularization

7. Do splenic injuries require laparotomy?

No. CT of the abdomen allows identification and grading of splenic injury, and patients that remain stable are selected for nonoperative management. Nonoperative management with observation is successful in approximately 95% of patients with grade I–III injuries. Stable patients with evidence of ongoing bleeding (requiring transfusion) may be candidates for selective arterial embolization if a bleeding site is identified on visceral angiography.

8. What are the contraindications to nonoperative management of splenic injuries?

1. Hemodynamic instability
2. Persistent coagulopathy
3. Additional intraabdominal injury requiring operative intervention
4. Confounding injury (additional injury that interferes with monitoring of the patient, such as pelvic fracture with ongoing bleeding)
5. Severe splenic injury (grade V and some grade IV)

9. When is nonoperative management considered a failure?

Any patient with signs of hemodynamic instability, persistent bleeding, worsening pain or tenderness, or progressive injury has failed nonoperative management.

10. What is delayed rupture of the spleen?

This rare complication occurs in < 1% of patients with splenic injury. Delayed splenic rupture must be distinguished from a delay in diagnosis of splenic injury and rupture of a known splenic injury. True delayed splenic rupture occurs after 48 hours in a patient with a history of abdominal trauma and no overt clinical evidence of intraabdominal injury on initial presentation.

11. What are the general principles of trauma splenectomy?

The first priority is to control bleeding, which usually can be done by packing and manual compression of the spleen. If this approach is successful, the abdomen is thoroughly explored for other injuries. Complete mobilization of the spleen by division of the splenocolic, splenorenal, phrenosplenic, and gastrosplenic ligaments is required for complete assessment. The short gastric vessels are ligated with division of the gastrosplenic ligament. The spleen may be repaired by application of hemostatic agents, direct repair of the splenic parenchyma, partial splenectomy, and construction of a splenic wrap using absorbable mesh. If splenectomy is required, the splenic artery and vein are ligated individually and the spleen is removed.

12. What is splenic autotransplantation?

Autotransplantation is accomplished by implanting splenic tissue homogenates or parenchymal slices into pouches created in the gastrocolic omentum.

13. Should the spleen be salvaged, removed, or autotransplanted?

Total splenectomy is warranted for patients who remain in shock, are coagulopathic, or have other potentially life-threatening injuries.

14. Does splenic autotransplantation preserve splenic function?

Autotransplantation after splenectomy is controversial. It is thought that at least 30% of the original splenic mass is needed to provide normal function after autotransplantation. However, it remains unclear whether autotransplanted splenic tissue is protective upon microbial challenge.

15. What early complications arise after splenectomy?

Bleeding, subphrenic abscess, acute gastric dilatation, gastric perforation pancreatitis (the splenic artery runs along the top of the pancreas), and thrombocytosis.

16. What is OPSS? How is it prevented?

Overwhelming postsplenectomy sepsis (OPSS) is a devastating bacteremia (typically due to encapsulated bacteria) that occurs in 2% of patients after splenectomy. The risk of OPSS is greatest when splenectomy is performed during infancy. The most common organisms are pneumococci (50%), menigococci, *Escherichia coli*, *Haemophilus influenzae*, staphylococci, and streptococci. Although rare, OPSS carries a mortality rate of 50% and has spurred interest in splenic preservatoin. OPSS is prevented primarily by vaccination. Pneumococcal and meningococcal vaccines must be given after splenectomy and are recommended every 5 years. Because sepsis may occur despite vaccination, long-term prophylaxis with oral penicillin is recommended, especially for children younger than 2 years.

17. How should a patient be followed after successful nonoperative treatment of a splenic injury?

Most patients who fail nonoperative management do so within 5 days. If initial management is successful, a follow-up ultrasound is usually obtained at 5 days to document nonprogression of injury. A postdischarge CT scan is obtained 6 weeks after injury to confirm complete healing. The patient should refrain from contact sports for 3 months.

BIBLIOGRAPHY

1. Cathey KL, Grady W Jr, et al: Blunt splenic trauma: Characteristics of patients requiring urgent laparotomy. Am Surg 64:450, 1998.
2. Cocanour CS, Moore FA, Ware DN, et al: Delayed complications of nonoperative management of blunt adult splenic trauma. Arch Surg 133:619, 1998.
3. Davis KA, Fabian TC, Croce MA, et al: Improved success in nonoperative management of blunt splenic injuries: Embolization of splenic artery pseudoaneurysms. J Trauma 44:1008, 1998.
4. Feliciano DV, Moore EE, Mattox KL (eds): Trauma, 3rd ed. Norwalk, CT, Appleton & Lange, 1996.
5. Goletti O, Ghiselli G, Lippolis PV, et al: The role of ultrasonography in blunt abdominal trauma: Results in 250 consecutive cases. J Trauma 36:178, 1994.
6. Kluger Y, Paul DB, Raves JJ, et al: Delayed rupture of the spleen—myths, facts and their importance: Case reports and literature review. J Trauma 36:568, 1994.
7. Krupnick AS, Teitelbaum DH, Geiger JD, et al: Use of abdominal ultrasonography to assess pediatric splenic trauma. Potential pitfalls in the diagnosis. Ann Surg 225:408, 1997.
8. Moore EE, Cogbill TH, Jurkovich GJ, et al: Organ injury scaling: Spleen and liver (1994 revision). J Trauma 38:323, 1995.
9. Pachter HL, Guth AA, Hofstetter SR, Spencer FC: Changing patterns in the management of splenic trauma: The impact of nonoperative management. Ann Surg 227:708, 1998.
10. Weber T, Hanish E, Baum RP, Seufert RM: Late results of heterotopic autotransplantation of splenic tissue into the greater omentum. World J Surg 22:833, 1998.

27. PANCREATIC AND DUODENAL INJURY

Reginald J.Franciose, M.D., and Jon M. Burch, M.D.

1. How often are the pancreas and duodenum injured in trauma?

Because of the relatively protected deep central retroperitoneal location of the pancreas and duodenum (except for the first portion of the duodenum), traumatic injuries are uncommon. Approximately 7% of patients undergoing laparotomy for trauma have a pancreatic injury. In large trauma centers fewer than 10 severe combined pancreaticoduodenal injuries are seen each year.

2. What are the determinants of mortality after pancreatic and duodenal injury?

The major determinants of outcome after pancreatic and duodenal injury are mechanism of injury, associated injuries, and combination of pancreatic and duodenal injury. Most early deaths are due to exsanguinating hemorrhage from associated vascular, hepatic, or splenic injuries. Ninety percent of patients with pancreatic or duodenal injuries have at least one associated injury, with an average of 3–4 associated intraabdominal injuries per patient. The single most important determinant of outcome with pancreatic injury is the presence of a major pancreatic ductal injury.

3. What mechanisms and patterns of injury are associated with trauma to the duodenum and pancreas?

Blunt pancreatic and duodenal injuries are caused primarily by deceleration injuries; in fact, at least 60% of blunt pancreatic injuries are due to steering wheel injuries. The three lesions associated with blunt injuries to the pancreas and duodenum are perforation of the duodenum, transection of the neck of the pancreas, and duodenal hematoma. Penetrating injuries to the pancreas and duodenum, most commonly caused by hand guns, result in complex localized tissue disruption with a high incidence of associated vascular injuries.

4. How are pancreatic and duodenal injuries diagnosed?

Because of the retroperitoneal position of the pancreas and duodenum, such injuries are hard to detect. A high index of suspicion based on mechanism of injury is necessary to prevent a delay in diagnosis. Screening abdominal ultrasonography is usually negative in blunt injury in the absence of associated splenic or hepatic injuries. Double-contrast computed tomography (CT) and soluble-contrast upper gastrointestinal studies may be helpful but require expert interpretation. Pancreatic ductal injuries may require endoscopic retrograde cholangiopancreatography (ERCP) or an intraoperative pancreatogram for diagnosis. The most reliable diagnostic maneuver is thorough exploration of the pancreas and duodenum at laparotomy.

5. What are the four portions of the duodenum and their surgical relationships?

The **first portion** of the duodenum starts at the pylorus of the stomach (intraperitoneally) and passes backward (retroperitoneally) toward the gallbladder (the remainder of the duodenum is retroperitoneal). The **second portion** descends 7–8 cm and is anterior to the vena cava. The left border of the duodenum is attached to the head of the pancreas, at the site where the common bile and pancreatic ducts enter; it shares a common blood supply with the head of the pancreas through the pancreaticoduodenal arcades. The **third portion** of the duodenum turns horizontally to the left, with its cranial surface in contact with the uncinate process of the pancreas, and passes posterior to the superior mesenteric artery and vein. The **fourth portion** continues to the left, ascending slightly and crossing the spine anterior to the aorta, where it is fixed to the suspensory ligament of Treitz at the duodenojejunal flexure.

6. What is the Kocher maneuver?

The Kocher maneuver is an incision of the lateral parietal peritoneal attachment of the second and third portions of the duodenum; blunt retroperitoneal dissection is carried medially to the level of the vena cava. This approach provides access to the posterior duodenum, distal common bile duct, and head of the pancreas.

7. What are the five parts of the pancreas and their relevant surgical anatomy?

The pancreas is a fixed retroperitoneal organ lying transversely between the duodenal sweep and the spleen. The **head** of the pancreas is firmly fixed to the medial aspect of the second and third portions of the duodenum and lies to the right of the superior mesenteric vessels. The **uncinate process**, an extension of the lower portion of the head, passes behind the portal vein and superior mesenteric vessels and in front of the aorta and vena cava. The **neck** of the pancreas, which overlies the superior mesenteric vessels, is the most common area for blunt traumatic transection. The **body** of the pancreas continues to the left of the superior mesenteric vessels. The body is the portion most readily visible through the lesser sac. The **tail** is relatively mobile and resides in the hilum of the spleen. The splenic artery runs along the upper border of the pancreas, and the splenic vein runs behind the pancreas.

8. How are duodenal perforations treated?

Approximately 80% of duodenal perforations can be treated by primary repair. The remaining 20% are severe injuries that require complex procedures such as pyloric exclusion, Roux-en-y duodenojejunostomy, vascularized jejunal graft, or, in rare cases, pancreaticoduodenectomy (Whipple procedure).

9. What is pyloric exclusion?

Pyloric exclusion is performed to protect tenuous duodenal repairs and to treat combined pancreaticoduodenal injuries. The pylorus is oversewn with a heavy suture via a gastrostomy on the greater curvature of the stomach near the pylorus. A gastrojejunostomy is then fashioned to divert the gastric contents away from the repair. The pylorus spontaneously opens within a few weeks in most patients.

10. What is a duodenal hematoma? How is it treated?

Duodenal hematomas are subseromuscular hematomas that cause duodenal obstruction associated with persistent vomiting. Although they may occur in adults after blunt injury, they usually are considered an injury of childhood or child abuse. They are diagnosed with an upper GI contrast study; the "coiled spring" sign is considered pathognomonic. The majority of duodenal hematomas can be treated nonoperatively with nasogastric suction and total parenteral nutrition.

11. How are pancreatic injuries treated?

Minor pancreatic injuries that do not involve the main pancreatic duct can be treated by external drainage or left alone. Injuries involving the neck, body, or tail of the pancreas can be treated with distal pancreatectomy. Extensive injury to the head of the pancreas or proximal main pancreatic duct requires complex reconstruction or, in rare cases, pancreaticoduodenectomy (Whipple procedure).

12. How much pancreas can be resected without subsequent endocrine or exocrine dysfunction?

In most people 80% of the pancreas can be resected without endocrine or exocrine dysfunction. A distal pancreatectomy at the level of the portal vein removes an average of 55% of the pancreas and thus is well tolerated.

13. What complications are specific to pancreatic and duodenal injuries?

Pancreatic injuries are associated with pancreatic fistulas, pancreatitis, and pancreatic pseudocysts. Duodenal injuries are associated with duodenal fistulas. One-third of patients who survive the first 48 hours have a complication related to the pancreatic or duodenal injury. Such complications contribute significantly to the sepsis and multiple organ failure that are responsible for most late deaths.

BIBLIOGRAPHY

1. Asensio JA, Demetriades D, Hanpeter DE, et al: Management of pancreatic injuries. Curr Probl Surg 36:325–419, 1999.
2. Bigattini D, Boverie JH, Dondelinger RF: CT of blunt trauma of the pancreas in adults. Eur Radiol 9:244–249, 1999.
3. Fleming WR, Collier NA, Banting SW: Pancreatic trauma: Universities of Melbourne HPB group. Aust N Z J Surg 69:357–362, 1999.
4. Holland AJ, Davey RB, Sparnon AL, et al: Traumatic pancreatitis: Long-term review of initial non-operative management in children. J Paediatr Child Health 35:78–81, 1999.
5. Jobst MA, Canty TG Sr, Lynch FP: Management of pancreatic injury in pediatric blunt abdominal trauma.J Pediatr Surg 34:818–823, 1999.
6. Patel SV, Spencer JA, el-Hansani S, Sheridan MB: Imaging of pancreatic trauma. Br J Radiol 71:985–990, 1998.
7. Wind P, Tiret E, Cunningham C, et al: Contribution of endoscopic retrograde pancreatography in management of complications following distal pancreatic trauma. Am Surg 65:777–783, 1999.

28. TRAUMA OF THE COLON AND RECTUM

Karin Cesario, M.D., and Jon M. Burch, M.D.

TRAUMA OF THE COLON

1. How do most colon injuries occur?

Nearly all (> 95%) colon injuries are due to penetrating trauma from gunshot, stab, iatrogenic, or sexual injury. Blunt colonic trauma is rare and usually results from misapplied seatbelts during motor vehicle accidents.

2. How are colon injuries diagnosed?

Most colonic injuries are diagnosed during laparotomy for penetrating trauma. For patients in whom the need for laparotomy has not been established, chest and abdominal radiographs should be obtained to evaluate for free free air or to detect the location of penetrating objects. Triple-contrast computed tomography (CT) or soluble-contrast radiographs (followed by barium, if necessary) may assist with diagnosing retroperitoneal colon injuries. Increased white cells or fecal material in diagnostic peritoneal lavage (DPL) is highly suggestive of a bowel injury.

3. What are three surgical options for managing a colon injury?

1. **Primary repair:** suturing of simple sidewall perforations or resection and primary anastomosis for more complex injuries.

2. **Colostomy:** injured colon is exteriorized as in a loop colostomy, or the injured area is resected and an end ileostomy or colostomy is formed.

3. **Exteriorized repair:** a repaired perforation or anastomosis is suspended on the abdominal wall. If after 10 days the suture line does not leak, it can be returned to the abdominal cavity under local anesthesia. If the repair breaks down, it is treated like a loop colostomy.

4. What are the advantages and disadvantages of each of these options?

1. **Primary repair** is desirable because definitive treatment is carried out at the initial operation. The disadvantage is that suture lines are created in suboptimal conditions; thus, leakage may occur.

2. **Colostomy** avoids an unprotected suture line in the abdomen but requires a second operation to close the colostomy. Stomal complications also may occur, including necrosis, stenosis, obstruction, and prolapse.

3. **Exteriorized repair** is similar to colostomy formation in that it avoids formation of an intraperitoneal suture line. Unfortunately, many patients require a colostomy closure, and stomal complications similar to those of colostomies may occur.

5. How are most colon injuries surgically managed?

Primary repair is safe and effective in most patients with colon trauma. Colostomy is appropriate in higher-risk patients, but selection criteria are controversial. Exteriorized repair is rarely indicated because most patients who were once candidates for this treatment can be managed successfully by primary repair.

6. What factors determine whether a patient with a colon injury should be managed with primary repair or colostomy?

Two theories address this issue: one is based on anatomic location of the injury and the other on systemic factors.

1. **Anatomic location of the injury.** All perforations that do not require resections should be treated by primary repair. If resection is required and the injury is proximal to the middle colic

artery, the damaged bowel is resected and a primary anastomosis is performed. If resection is required and the injury is distal to the middle colic artery, an end colostomy is created. This theory is based on the blood supply of the terminal ileum, which is vast; an anastomosis of the proximal colon reliably heals. Because distal colonic anastomoses have a marginal blood supply, healing is occasionally problematic, especially in trauma patients, who may be hypovolemic or in shock.

2. **Systemic factors.** All injuries should be repaired primarily unless the patient has protracted shock and extensive contamination, in which case a colostomy should be performed. This approach is based on the theory that systemic factors are more important than anatomic factors in determining whether a suture line heals.

7. What complications are associated with colonic injury and its treatment?
- Wound infection (as high as 40% if the skin incision is closed primarily)
- Intraabdominal abscess (10%)
- Stomal complications (5%)
- Anastomotic leak (3%)
- Fecal fistulas (1%)

TRAUMA OF THE RECTUM

8. How do rectal injuries occur?
Like colon injuries, most rectal injuries result from penetrating trauma. Blunt pelvic fractures, however, should be viewed with a strong index of suspicion for rectal (and urethral) injury.

9. How are rectal injuries diagnosed?
A thorough exam is crucial, and the diagnosis is suggested by the course of the projectiles and the presence of blood on digital rectal exam. If rectal trauma is suspected, the patient should undergo proctoscopy to look for hematomas, contusions, lacerations, or gross blood. If the diagnosis is in question, radiographs with soluble-contrast medium enemas should be performed.

10. How are intraperitoneal rectal injuries treated differently from extraperitoneal injuries?
The portion of the rectum proximal to the peritoneal reflection is called the intraperitoneal segment. Injuries of this portion are treated like colonic injuries.

11. What are the four basic principles for managing simple extraperitoneal rectal injuries?
1. **Diversion:** either a loop or an end-sigmoid colostomy is usually appropriate.
2. **Drainage:** a retroanal incision should be used to place Penrose or closed-suction drains near the perforation site.
3. **Repair:** appropriate, when possible.
4. **Washout:** irrigation of the distal rectum with isotonic solution until the effluent is clear. The role of washout remains controversial, but it may benefit patients whose rectum is full of feces.

12. How are complex extraperitoneal rectal injuries managed?
In patients with massive pelvic trauma and an associated rectal injury, an abdominoperineal resection may be required for adequate debridement and hemostasis. An abdominoperineal resection also is required in the rare instance in which anal sphincters have been destroyed.

13. What complications are associated with rectal trauma and its treatment?
Complications are similar in nature and frequency to those of colonic injuries. In addition, pelvic osteomyelitis may occur. In this case, debridement may be necessary, and culture-specific intravenous antibiotics should be administered for 2–3 months.

14. What is the role of antibiotics in colorectal trauma?

Antibiotics provide an important adjunct to therapy. They should be initiated preoperatively and ended quickly (12–24 hours postoperatively); the chosen antibiotics should provide a broad spectrum of coverage.

BIBLIOGRAPHY

1. Berne J, Velmahos G, et al: The high morbidity of colostomy closure after trauma: Further support for the primary repair of colon injuries. Surgery 123:157, 1998.
2. Burch J, Franciose R, Moore E: Trauma. In Schwartz S (ed): Principles of Surgery, 8th ed. New York, McGraw-Hill, 1999, pp 155–221.
3. Burch J, Martin R, et al: Evolution of the treatment of injured colon in the 1980s. Arch Surg 126:979, 1991.
4. Carrillo E, Somberg L, et al: Blunt traumatic injuries to the colon and rectum. J Am Coll Surg 183:548, 1996.
5. Chappius C, Frey D, et al: Management of penetrating colon injuries: A prospective randomized trial. Ann Surg 213:492, 1991.
6. Eshragi N, Mullins R, et al: Surveyed opinion of American trauma surgeons in management of colon injuries. J Trauma 44:93, 1998.
7. Ivatury R, Gaudino J, et al: Definitive treatment of colon injuries: A prospective study. Am Surg 59:43, 1993.
8. McGrath V, Fabian T, et al: Rectal trauma: Management based on anatomic distinctions. Am Surg 12:1136, 1998.
9. Pachter H, Hoballah J, et al: The morbidity and financial impact of colostomy closure in trauma patients. J Trauma 30:1510, 1990.
10. Sasaki L, Allaben R, et al: Primary repair of colon injuries: A prospective randomized study. J Trauma 39:895, 1995.
11. Taheri P, Ferrara J, et al: A convincing case for primary repair of penetrating colon injuries. Am J Surg 163:39, 1993.

29. PELVIC FRACTURES

Wade Smith, M.D., and Laurel Saliman, M.D.

1. What are the most important initial evaluation steps to undertake in the patient with a displaced pelvic fracture?

The ABCs (airway, breathing, and circulatory assessment). Trauma patients with displaced pelvic fractures have a high incidence of associated injuries to the head, chest, and abdomen.

2. What are the sources and potential volume of bleeding in the displaced pelvic fracture?

Pelvic fractures bleed from exposed cancellous bone surfaces, pelvic veins, and pelvic arteries. Cadaveric injection studies have demonstrated that 90% of trauma fatalities with pelvic fractures bleed from exposed bone and injured veins. Only 10% have bleeding from arteries. The total volume of the pelvis can hold 4–6 L of fluid before a tamponade effect slows venous and bone bleeding.

3. Should a Foley catheter be placed in trauma patients with displaced pelvic fractures?

Yes. Contraindications include urethral injuries, which should be suspected when blood is observed at the penile meatus or vaginal introitus. A manual rectal exam in men and a bimanual exam in women is mandatory to exclude an open fracture into the vagina or rectum or a high-riding prostate. If a urethral injury is present, a suprapubic catheter is inserted and a urethrogram or cystogram is performed.

4. What is the incidence of urologic injury associated with pelvic fractures?
The overall incidence of urologic injury is 16%.

5. What are the commonly used radiographic classification schemes for pelvic fractures?
The mechanistic classification describes pelvic fractures as anteroposterior compression (APC), lateral compression (LC), vertical shear (VS), or combined mechanism (CM). The Tile classification categorizes fractures into three groups, A, B, or C, with numbered subgroups based on increasing severity of ligamentous and bony disruption.

6. What is an open pelvic fracture?
An open pelvic fracture is exposure of the fracture to external or contaminated tissues through a laceration in the skin, vagina, or rectum. When an open pelvic fracture is suspected, patients should receive a rectal examination with an anuscope and a bimanual and speculum vaginal exam. With open fractures the morbidity and mortality rates are increased both in the acute period (due to hemorrhage) and in the delayed period (due to infection).

7. When is acute mechanical stabilization of a pelvic fracture indicated?
Open-book and vertical shear fractures with displacement may benefit from acute mechanical stabilization. When hemodynamic instability persists in the face of ongoing aggressive resuscitation, pelvic stabilization with a beanbag, external wrap, external fixator, or pelvic clamp may help to decrease pelvic bleeding by decreasing pelvic volume and stabilizing bony fragments.

8. What is the role of angiography in the acute pelvic fracture?
Angiography is used to identify and embolize arterial bleeding caused by pelvic fractures. Because a low percentage of pelvic bleeding is from arterial injury, suspicion should be increased when hypotension fails to respond to aggressive stabilization and fluid management.

9. Why do patients die from pelvic fractures?
Only 2% of patients with a pelvic fracture experience isolated trauma to the pelvis. Mortality is usually due to associated injuries rather than pelvic fracture. Early stabilization and mobilization, however, improve outcome significantly and have been shown to decrease the mortality rate from 26% to 6%.

10. What is external fixation?
External fixation by the use of pins placed into the iliac wings and connected to a frame or by pins placed into the bone just superior to the acetabulum and connected to a C-clamp can be used as a temporary method of fracture reduction and stabilization. External fixation does not prevent vertical and posterior displacement of the pelvis in the case of complete posterior disruption. The C-clamp is much quicker in application and can be pivoted out of the way for patient care and diagnostic imaging. In addition, the incisions for pin placement do not interfere with the approach for definitive operative fixation of the pelvis.

11. Is there a role for pneumatic antishock garments (PASGs) in the treatment of pelvic fractures?
Some controversy is associated with the use of PASGs in the treatment of pelvic fractures. Their potential role is limited to prehospital transportation and initial stabilization of patients with a complex pelvic fracture. They can reduce displacement of anteroposterior compression fractures but may increase the displacement of a lateral compression fracture. The garment also restricts access to the patient, compromises pulmonary reserve, and is associated with increased risk of compartment syndrome.

12. When can patients with a pelvic fracture ambulate?
Patients with fractures involving only the anterior pelvic ring, such as unilateral or bilateral pubic rami fractures, may bear weight as tolerated immediately. If the fracture pattern involves

the posterior structures, such as the sacroiliac joint or iliac wing, patients must not bear weight through that side of the pelvis for approximately 10 weeks.

13. What is the most common source of arterial bleeding associated with a pelvic fracture?
The internal iliac artery.

BIBLIOGRAPHY

1. Buehle R, Browner B, Morandi M: Emergency reduction for pelvic ring disruptions and control of associated hemorrhage using the pelvic stabilizer. Techn Orthop 9:258–266, 1995.
2. Burgess AR, et al: Pelvic ring disruptions: Effective classification system and treatment protocols. J Trauma 30:848–856, 1990.
3. Gruen GS, et al: The acute management of hemodynamically unstable multiple trauma patients with pelvic ring fractures. J Trauma 36:706–713, 1994.
4. Kellam JF, Browner BD: Fractures of the pelvic ring. In Browner BD, et al (eds): Skeletal Trauma, 2nd ed. Philadelphia, W.B. Saunders, 1997.
5. Perez JV, et al: Angiographic embolisation in pelvic fracture. Injury 29:187–191, 1998.
6. Poole GV, Ward EF: Causes of mortality in patients with pelvic fractures. Orthopaedics 17:691–696, 1994.
7. Routt ML, et al: A rational approach to pelvic trauma: Resuscitation and early definitive stabilization. Clin Orthop 318:61–74, 1995.
8. Tile M: Pelvic ring fractures: Should they be fixed? J Bone Joint Surg 70B:1–12, 1988.

30. UPPER URINARY TRACT INJURY

Norman E. Peterson, M.D.

1. When does one suspect renal trauma?
Any hematuria—gross or microscopic—that follows trauma signals the possibility of severe injury. Paradoxically, pedicle injuries (grade 4) may bleed little because of arterial interruption; therefore, an acute awareness of this connection is vital to possible renal salvage.

2. How is renal trauma investigated?
The traditional practice of routinely evaluating both the upper (intravenous pyelogram [IVP], computed tomography [CT]) and lower (cystourethrogram) urinary tracts after trauma is called into question by studies that disclose the rarity (< 0.5%) of coexisting significant renal and bladder/urethral injuries. Therefore, investigation should focus on the site of major trauma. Although urography (IVP) provides satisfactory information for early management, contrast CT scanning offers better imaging and less dependence on adequate hydration/perfusion (see question 3). Moreover, renal imaging is routinely included in emergency CT screening efforts, rendering IVP unnecessary.

3. What is a single-shot IVP?
A bolus (2 cc/kg contrast agent) is injected intravenously when circumstances permit (perhaps in transit to the operating room). The first film should be obtained at approximately 10 minutes, with additional films at 10-minute intervals as necessary for diagnosis. Hypotension or shock contraindicates urography. Intraoperative IVP is recommended when renal damage is first suggested (e.g., retroperitoneal hematoma) during emergency surgery for other injuries. Intraoperative arteriography also may be accomplished by injecting 10 ml of contrast agent directly into the renal artery with immediate film exposure.

4. How is renal trauma classified?
Renal injuries are consistently classified as grade I (contusion; 60%); grade 2 (superficial laceration; 20%); grade 3 (deep laceration or collecting system damage; 10%); grade 4 (pedicle

interruption; 5%); and grade 5 (stellate parenchymal fragmentation; 50%). Grades 1, 2, and 3 injuries are safely amenable to conservative nonoperative management, whereas grades 4 and 5 require operative intervention for repair or removal. Grade 4 injury (pedicle interruption) is reflected by ipsilateral urographic nonfunction and nominal bleeding. Grade 5 injury (parenchymal shattering) is manifested by urographic nonfunction and unrelenting gross hematuria. Likelihood of spontaneous resolution is closely allied with improving hematuria during the first several hours after injury.

5. Does the magnitude of renal bleeding alone reflect the significance or prognosis of injury?

The pattern of renal hemorrhage is the most reliable prognostic factor. Excluding pedicle interruption, which often is characterized by nominal hematuria, the status of renal bleeding within the first few hours after trauma effectively discriminates injuries amenable to spontaneous resolution from injuries requiring operative correction. Gross hematuria that subsides early (often before conclusion of emergency surgery for coexisting injuries) reliably identifies injury that may be exempted from emergency exploration. Conversely, unremitting hemorrhage or hemorrhage that subsides and recurs requires operative exploration or arteriography with selective therapeutic embolization.

6. Are there different kinds of renal pedicle trauma?

Yes. The renal pedicle may be interrupted by thrombosis or complete avulsion; both events are characterized by urographic nonvisualization and nominal hematuria. The most common site of arterial interruption is the junction of the proximal and middle thirds of the main renal artery. Although textbooks often claim absence of hematuria, transitory gross hematuria or microhematuria is the rule, underscoring the requirement for urinalysis in all circumstances. Left-sided pedicle avulsion produces little retroperitoneal bleeding because of prompt arterial retraction, whereas right-sided injuries often hemorrhage extensively because of avulsion of the vein from the vena cava. Reliable nonoperative distinction of pedicle thrombosis from avulsion is presently not available.

7. What is the time limit of renal tolerance of warm ischemia?

Four hours emerges as a valid standard. Revascularization usually cannot be accomplished within this period; we advocate vascular repair only for selected circumstances (solitary kidney and marginal renal function).

8. Both pedicle trauma and parenchymal shattering are characterized by nonvisualization on IVP. Do they need to be distinguished?

Distinction is characteristically not difficult. Pedicle injury results in minimal hematuria, whereas shattered kidneys produce extensive and unremitting bleeding in flank, retroperitoneum, and urine; nephrectomy is necessary to control bleeding, but pedicle interruptions are frequently managed conservatively.

9. What changes in renal function are anticipated after nephrectomy?

Trauma-related prerenal hypoperfusion (hypotension, hypovolemia) compromises renal function in accordance with degree and duration of perfusion deficit and also by preexisting compromise of nephron status (e.g., arteriosclerosis, diabetes, renal artery disease, chronic inflammatory disease). Variable azotemia (elevated serum creatinine) is common after trauma or nephrectomy despite adequate hydration, blood pressure, and urinary output; creatinine typically returns to normal after a few days, at which time renal function studies verify physiologic adjustments that increase function in the remaining kidney upward of 50%.

10. What is the significance of delayed gross hematuria?

Delayed gross hematuria signifies potentially unresolving arteriovenous injury. Fifty percent of cases resolve with temporary bedrest. The remainder are amenable to selective embolization. Exceptions require operative intervention, usually for partial nephrectomy.

11. What is the recommended response to unexpected intraoperative discovery of retroperitoneal bleeding?

Published reviews of retroperitoneal hematoma consistently refer to expansion and pulsation, both of which are rare. A pulsatile hematoma suggests a major vascular injury, and exploration should be preceded by vascular control and preparation for rapid blood replacement. Stable hematomas (above the pelvic brim), regardless of size, may be left undisturbed unless studies (preoperative or intraoperative) disclose severe ancillary damage. When doubt exists, exploration is justified, with awareness of high published nephrectomy rates associated with exploration in this setting.

12. What is the recommended response to posttraumatic urine extravasation?

When urine extravasation coexists with extensive persistent bleeding into flank and urine, major laceration into the collecting system is likely, and operative correction is advised. Otherwise, urine extravasation commonly resolves promptly. Reimaging at 48–72 hours defines cases requiring drainage, stenting, or operative repair.

13. What conditions predispose to traumatic renal injury?

Abnormal renal anatomy increases vulnerability to renal trauma. Preexisting abnormalities are dominated by hydronephrosis (50%) and ectopic positioning (pelvic, horseshoe). Renal tumors, particularly in children, must always be considered.

14. What is included in conservative management of renal trauma?

When clinical and radiographic appraisal endorses nonoperative management, bed rest is imposed until gross hematuria has subsided. Strenuous activity is avoided until microhematuria has subsided—usually within 3 weeks. Follow-up thereafter is often unnecessary. Patients followed for separated parenchymal fragments should undergo ultrasonography or urography at 6 weeks, at which time anatomic restoration is usually complete. Hospitalization is not required during these periods. Conditions responsible for delayed hemorrhage are typically *not* corrected by prolonged bed rest; therefore, early ambulation and limited activity are intended to unmask conditions that may require therapeutic embolization or operative correction.

15. What is the likelihood of subsequent hypertension?

Renal hypertension is a consequence of ischemia rather than infarction, thereby discouraging routine surgical responses to partial or total renal infarction. Authenticated posttraumatic hypertension occurs in under 2% of cases overall. Onset generally occurs within the first several months of injury; blood pressure is often controllable with salt restriction or diuretic therapy.

16. Do blunt and penetrating renal injuries pose different clinical challenges and demand different responses?

No.

17. Under what circumstances should ureteral injury be suspected?

Excluding overt operative and endoscopic mishap, gunshot is the usual mode of ureteral injury (90%). Conversely, 5% of abdominal gunshot wounds involve the ureter. Of all published cases of penetrating urologic trauma, the ureter is allegedly injured in 17%.

18. How is ureteral injury identified or verified?

Clinical manifestations are characteristically subtle and often obscured by coexisting injury and complaints. Up to 90% of gunshot wounds and 60% of stabbings that injure the ureter also injure bowel, colon, liver, spleen, blood vessels, or pancreas. Hematuria is almost exclusively microscopic (but rarely absent, as many publications promise). IVP within the first 36 hours of injury reveals urinary extravasation in 90% of cases. After 36 hours, the IVP more commonly demonstrates obstruction at the site of injury (no extravasation) with proximal ureterectasis; extravasation is then identified by retrograde ureterography. Bladder and ureteral extravasations are differentiated by comparing cystogram with ureterogram.

19. How is a ureteral injury identified during surgery?

When ureteral injury is suspected during laparotomy without radiographic assistance, retroperitoneal exposure with induced diuresis (Lasix, 20-mg IV bolus) may disclose the site of injury. Indigo carmine (1 vial IV bolus) may assist in locating the leak by coloring the extravasate.

20. What are the potential consequences of missed ureteral injury?

Complications may include fever, leukocytosis, azotemia, flank pain, ileus, flank mass (urinoma), or urinary fistula. Presentation is often delayed by 2 weeks or more after injury. Fistulous drainage is confirmed as urine by creatinine content exceeding serum levels.

21. What are the principles of ureteral repair?

The damaged ureter is debrided back to freely bleeding margins. The anastomosis must be a tension-free, spatulated closure with fine absorbable suture and internal ureteral stenting. Distal injuries are better served by direct implantation of the ureter into the bladder. Fat, omentum, or peritoneum should be interposed between repair site and adjacent muscle to prevent adhesion and obstruction. Drains should not abut anastomotic suture lines, because they may perpetrate urine leakage. Ureteral blood supply is provided from the kidney and bladder, rendering the central one-third most vulnerable to ischemic compromise. Rarely, ureteral loss prevents standard methods of reconstruction. Removal and distal renal reanastomosis (autotransplantation) are available to address this dilemma when renal sacrifice is unacceptable.

BIBLIOGRAPHY

1. Armstrong PA, Litscher LJ, Key DW, McCarthy MC: Management strategies for genitourinary trauma. Hosp Phys 34:19–25, 1998.
2. Campbell EW Jr, Filderman PS, Jacobs SC: Ureteral injury due to blunt and penetrating trauma. Urology 40:216–220, 1992.
3. Carroll PR, McAninch JW, Klosterman PW, et al: Renovascular trauma: Risk assessment, surgical management, and outcome. J Trauma 30:547–552, 1990.
4. McAninch JW: Traumatic and Reconstructive Urology. Philadelphia, W.B. Saunders, 1996.
5. Moore EE, Shackford SR, Pachter HL, et al: Organ injury scaling: Spleen, liver, and kidney. J Trauma 29:1664–1666, 1998.
6. Peterson NE: Genitourinary trauma. In Feliciano DV, Moore EE, Mattox KL (eds): Trauma, 3rd ed. Norwalk, CT, Appleton & Lange, 1996, pp 661–694.
7. Skinner EC, Parisky YR, Skinner DG: Management of complex urologic injuries. Surg Clin North Am 76:861–878, 1996.

31. LOWER URINARY TRACT INJURY AND PELVIC TRAUMA

Norman E. Peterson, M.D.

1. What clinical circumstances promote suspicion of bladder injury?

Trauma to the lower abdomen or pelvis that results in hematuria incriminates bladder injury. Other signs may include inability to void or incomplete recovery of catheter irrigation. Associated injuries are sustained in 90% of patients. Trauma need not be excessive; a full bladder is vulnerable to rupture from modest trauma. Penetrating wounds also may be responsible. Bladder injury without hematuria (usually gross) is rare because of the rich detrusor blood supply. Hematuria with a normal cystogram defines bladder contusion.

2. What types of bladder injury may occur?

Laceration or perforation may be either intra- or extraperitoneal. Extraperitoneal injuries constitute up to 85% of all bladder trauma, tend to concentrate at the bladder base or parasymphyseal area, and are generally not readily accessible to operative repair. Intraperitoneal rupture is typically blow-out of the dome of a distended bladder.

3. What is the likelihood of a bladder injury in patients with a fractured pelvis?

Bladder injury occurs in 10% of all pelvic fractures. Conversely, up to 83% of bladder injury results from (or coexists with) pelvic fracture. Intraperitoneal bladder rupture occurs with penetrating trauma or blunt blow-out of distended bladder; therefore, pelvic fracture is not a requirement. Bladder injuries occur more often with parasymphyseal pubic arch fractures and with bilateral than unilateral fractures. Isolated ramus fractures produce bladder laceration in 10% of cases.

4. How is bladder injury verified?

Retrograde urethrocystogram provides 95% diagnostic accuracy for bladder rupture. The radiograph should be taken after introduction of 300 ml of a 50% dilution of standard radiocontrast agent by catheter or meatal syringe. Extravasation is identified only by postevacuation films in some cases. When renal or distal ureteral injury is suspected, IVP should precede the cystogram. Diagnostic peritoneal lavage is unreliable (33% false-negative results).

5. What are the radiographic patterns of bladder injury?

Lateral contraction of the filled bladder ("teardrop") or elevation of the bladder out of the pelvis ("pie in the sky") indicates perivesical hemorrhage, but not necessarily a breach of bladder integrity. Extraperitoneal injury allows contrast to escape adjacent to the symphysis, but it is confined to the bladder base by the intact peritoneum. Intraperitoneal extravasation produces a "sunburst" appearance from the bladder dome, which may collect in the paracolic gutters, outline loops of bowel, or pool under liver or spleen. Gross hematuria without extravasation constitutes bladder contusion.

6. How is bladder rupture managed?

Conventional management of extraperitoneal lacerations is limited to indwelling catheter drainage for 7–10 days, at which time cystogram usually confirms resolution of extravasation. Intraperitoneal lacerations also frequently respond to catheter drainage, although many consultants routinely advocate operative repair. Bladder contusion requires catheter drainage until gross bleeding has subsided. Laparotomy that is necessary for other reasons provides opportunity for repair and eliminates possible nonresponse to simple catheter drainage.

7. What clinical settings mandate appraisal of urethral injury?

Proximal urethral trauma classically accompanies pelvic fractures (crushing or deceleration/impact); shearing forces focused at the prostatomembranous junction account for avulsion at this site. Straddle injuries produce bulbous urethral damage. Proximal urethral injury is heralded by blood at the urethral meatus, digital rectal disclosure of upward prostatic displacement, perineal ecchymosis, penile and/or scrotal swelling and ecchymosis, and inability to void or to pass a urethral catheter.

8. When a patient presents with a pelvic fracture, is concomitant urethral injury a major concern?

Yes. Urethral trauma occurs in 10% of pelvic fractures; it is more common with anterior disruption of the pelvic ring, including 20% of unilateral and 50% of bilateral parasymphyseal fractures. Posterior (prostatomembranous) avulsion is associated with potentially disabling sequelae and requirements for complex and challenging operative corrections. In contrast, more distal urethral injuries avoid impotence-incontinence issues and are more surgically accessible.

9. How is urethral injury best assessed?

Retrograde urethrography must always be performed before inserting a Foley catheter (see question 4). Incomplete urethral transection is reflected by local extravasation accompanied by bladder opacification. Total avulsion produces extensive local extravasation and prevents contrast from entering the bladder. Incomplete transection is more common with anterior (50%) than posterior (10%) urethral injuries.

10. How is urethral injury managed?

For incomplete transection regardless of site, either catheter stenting across the defect or diversion by suprapubic cystostomy permits gratifying spontaneous resolution. Complete urethral transection may be decompressed initially via suprapubic cystostomy if clinical conditions impede immediate restoration of continuity by placement of a bridging urethral catheter. A bridging catheter reduces complex scarring, avoids subsequent surgery in many patients, and is easily incorporated into laparotomy for associated injuries.

11. What conditions may complicate urethral rupture or repair?

Complications include stricturing (often correctable endoscopically), incontinence (uncommon), and impotence (statistically limited to traumatic prostatic displacement). Iatrogenic complications are associated with retropubic dissection or hematoma disturbance. Artificial remedies are available for patients who suffer permanent impotence.

12. What conditions may complicate pelvic fracture?

Extensive comminution and pelvic instability increase the likelihood of coexisting injury, blood loss, and morbidity/mortality. Destabilizing pelvic hemorrhage may persist despite all conservative efforts. Pelvic angiography may then disclose large-vessel involvement requiring operative intervention or bleeding from small hypogastric branches amenable to therapeutic embolization. Hemorrhage may become extensive when tamponade is attenuated by bony instability that increases pelvic capacity. Blood loss, transfusion requirements, and prognosis correlate with conditions producing expanded pelvic volume. Internal and external pelvic fixation and/or military antishock trousers (MAST) improve pelvic stability and tamponade.

BIBLIOGRAPHY

1. Armstrong PA, Litscher LJ, Key DW, McCarthy MC: Management strategies for genitourinary trauma. Hosp Phys 34:19–25, 1998.
2. Jacob TD, Gruen GS, Udekwu AO, Peitzman AB: Pelvic fracture. Surg Rounds Aug:583, 1993.
3. McAninch JW: Traumatic and Reconstructive Urology. Philadelphia, W.B. Saunders, 1996.
4. Peterson NE: Current management of urethral injuries. In Rous S (ed): 1998 Urology Annual. New York, Appleton-Century-Crofts, 1988, pp 143–179.
5. Peterson NE: Traumatic posterior urethral avulsion. Mongr Urol 7:61, 1986.
6. Spirnak JP: Pelvic fracture and injury to the lower urinary tract. Surg Clin North Am 68:1057, 1988.
7. Thomas CL, McAninch JW: Bladder trauma. In American Urological Association Update Series. Baltimore, American Urological Association, 1989, pp 242–247.

32. EXTREMITY VASCULAR INJURIES

Sandra C. Carr, M.D., and William H. Pearce, M.D.

1. What is the kinetic energy of a bullet? Why is it important?
The kinetic energy (K) of a bullet is determined by the following equation:

$$K = \tfrac{1}{2}\,mv^2$$

where m = mass and v = velocity. The tissue energy is related to the square of the velocity. A high-velocity bullet causes more damage and requires more extensive debridement than a bullet of smaller mass and lower velocity.

2. What are the four ways in which an arterial injury may manifest?
Hemorrhage
Thrombosis (with or without ischemia)
Pseudoaneurysm
Arteriovenous fistula

3. In the patient with a long bone fracture, what are the possible mechanisms by which arterial injuries occur?
Acute angulation, laceration, or longitudinal stretching with subsequent acute thrombosis.

4. What is the most common extremity artery to be injured?

Femoral	35%	Axillary	10%
Brachial	30%	Subclavian	5%
Popliteal	20%		

5. Which are the most commonly injured major veins in extremity trauma?

Superficial femoral vein	40%
Popliteal vein	20%
Common femoral vein	15%

6. Which two extremity fractures are associated with a significant risk of arterial injury?
Supracondylar humeral fracture—brachial artery
Posterior dislocation of the knee—popliteal artery

7. Which arterial injury bleeds more—a complete transection or an incomplete transection? Why?
The incomplete transection bleeds more because it does not have the ability to undergo retraction, vasoconstriction, and thrombosis as the complete transection often does.

8. What is the most common cause of brachial artery injuries?
Iatrogenic complications of arterial catheterization. The needle or catheter may cause intimal injury or dissection. Thrombosis of the brachial artery may result from an adherent clot being stripped off a catheter or sheath during removal.

9. What are the important risk factors for amputation in patients with blunt popliteal artery trauma?
• Severe soft tissue injury
• Deep soft tissue infection
• Preoperative ischemia

10. What is a pseudoaneurysm? How is it different from a true aneurysm?

A pseudoaneurysm is a disruption of the vessel wall that results in a pulsating hematoma covered by fibrous tissue. A true aneurysm is a localized dilation of an artery covered by all three layers of the vessel (intima, media, and adventitia).

11. What is the most common location for pseudoaneurysm? What is the most common cause?

Most pseudoaneurysms occur in the femoral artery and result from iatrogenic injury during diagnostic or interventional endovascular procedures.

12. What are the clinical signs of arteriovenous fistula?
- Bruit ("machinery murmur" over the lesion)
- Palpable thrill
- Venous hypertension (varicose veins, swelling, ulceration)
- Arterial ischemia distal to the fistula
- Widened pulse pressure
- High-output cardiac failure (tachycardia)

13. Which type of penetrating injury is more likely to create an arteriovenous fistula— those caused by low-velocity or by high-velocity mechanisms?

Arteriovenous fistulas are more likely after low-velocity trauma, such as small-caliber missiles, knife wounds, or iatrogenic catheter injury. High-velocity wounds tend to disrupt major vessels and lead to hemorrhage.

14. Can a patient with an arterial injury present with palpable distal pulses in the affected extremity?

Yes. Depending on the location of the injury, palpable pulses may be present even in the setting of a significant arterial injury. Pulses may be normal in up to 20% of operatively proven arterial injuries.

15. Does the presence of Doppler signals over an artery rule out an arterial injury?

No, nor does it indicate adequate perfusion.

16. What are the symptoms of complete acute arterial occlusion?

The six Ps: pain, pallor, pulse deficit, paresthesia, paralysis, and poikilothermia (coldness).

17. What are the hard signs of arterial injury?
- Pulsatile or expanding hematoma
- Pulsatile bleeding
- Bruit or thrill
- Extremity ischemia

18. What is the appropriate management of a patient with hard signs of arterial injury?

The patient should undergo prompt operative exploration (first, obtain proximal control) and appropriate repair. Arteriogram is usually not necessary and only delays appropriate treatment.

19. What are the soft signs of arterial injury?
- Unexplained shock
- Proximity
- Stable hematoma
- Injury to an adjacent nerve
- History of possible arterial bleeding

Arteriography is indicated in some patients with soft signs of arterial injury.

20. What is the most useful first-line screening test to exclude an occult vascular injury?

Measurement of the ankle-brachial index (ABI) using Doppler pressures at the bedside. An ABI less than 1.0 is a significant predictor of arterial injury.

21. How is the ABI measured?

The ABI is measured at the bedside using the hand-held Doppler to determine systolic pressure in both arms and at both ankles, dorsalis pedis and posterior tibial. The ABI for each leg is the ratio of the highest ankle pressure to the highest brachial pressure. A value less than 1.0 is abnormal.

22. In patients with subclavian artery injuries, how often are pulses in the involved upper extremity decreased or absent?

Only 20% of patients have decreased or absent pulses. A high index of suspicion and angiography are needed to diagnose these injuries reliably.

23. What is the most effective way to control hemorrhage from an extremity vascular injury in the emergency department?

Direct digital pressure is the most effective maneuver. Attempts at blind clamping with hemostats should be avoided because they may further damage the injured vessel and adjacent nerves.

24. Should tourniquets be used to control hemorrhage from an extremity vascular injury?

No. Tourniquets should be used only as a last resort because they may occlude collateral flow and increase tissue damage.

25. In the emergency department, how should one manage an embedded knife with a surrounding hematoma?

Neither an embedded weapon nor a hematoma should be removed until proximal control is obtained in the operating room.

26. If an arterial injury is ligated but not repaired, what is the chance of amputation?

It depends on which artery is ligated:

Common iliac	55%	Subclavian	25%
External iliac	50%	Axillary	50%
Femoral	50%	Brachial	25%
Popliteal	75%		

27. What is the initial step in the surgical management of vascular injuries?

Obtain proximal and distal control of the injured vessel.

28. What are the important steps involved in repair of an injured vessel?

- Debridement of ragged, devitalized vessel
- Removal of adjacent intravascular thrombus (often with an embolectomy catheter)
- Arterial reconstruction
- Soft tissue coverage of the arterial repair

29. What is the first choice of conduit for repairing an extensive arterial injury that cannot be closed primarily?

Vein from an uninjured extremity, usually greater saphenous vein from the contralateral leg.

30. Most injuries to major extremity veins in the hemodynamically stable patient should be repaired. Why?

Although the long-term patency for venous repair is not excellent, short-term patency is beneficial. It allows development of collateral venous drainage, increased arterial inflow during the acute postoperative period, and reduction in peripheral edema.

31. When is it appropriate to ligate a major venous injury?

When the venous repair is extremely complex or the patient is hemodynamically unstable, ligation is appropriate. Extremity elevation and elastic wrapping may control postoperative edema.

32. How often does nerve injury occur in association with extremity vascular injury? Why is it important?

Nerve injuries occur in about 50% of upper extremity and 25% of lower extremity vascular injuries. The nerve injury determines the long-term prognosis and ultimate functional status of the injured extremity.

33. What is reperfusion injury? Why is it important in patients with an extremity vascular injury?

Restoration of blood flow delivers oxygen to the ischemic muscle. Reperfusion injury is thought to be due to the formation of oxygen free radicals, which increase vascular permeability and lead to edema and further injury to the surrounding tissues.

34. What are the four compartments in the lower leg? Why are they important in arterial injuries to the extremity?

| 1. Anterior compartment | 3. Superficial posterior compartment |
| 2. Lateral compartment | 4. Deep posterior compartment |

Ischemia to the limb or massive soft tissue trauma may result in edema, leading to a compartment syndrome.

35. What are the local and systemic consequences of ischemia/reperfusion in patients with ischemia due to extremity vascular trauma?

Local	Systemic
Compartment syndrome	Acidosis
Neurologic injury	Hyperkalemia
Tissue necrosis/gangrene	Myoglobinuria
	Sepsis

36. What is the treatment for a suspected compartment syndrome?

Prompt four-compartment fasciotomy.

37. What clinical signs suggest the development of a compartment syndrome in a patient who is recovering from arterial repair of an extremity vascular injury?

Pain on passive stretch of the involved muscle is the most sensitive sign. Sensory changes may include decreased sensation in the first metatarsal space, and motor changes may include inability to dorsiflex the great toe or footdrop (late sign). Compartment syndrome and severe tissue damage may occur in the presence of palpable pulses. Loss of pulses is a late finding.

38. What factors suggest the need for a fasciotomy to prevent or treat compartment syndrome?

- Prolonged period between injury and restoration of perfusion (6 hr or more)
- Prolonged period of shock
- Massive crush injury with swelling
- Combined arterial and venous injury
- Postoperative sensory or motor changes
- Elevated compartment pressures (> 30 mmHg is abnormal)

HONORS

39. What is Branham's sign?

Branham's sign is a decrease in tachycardia when an arteriovenous fistula is occluded.

40. Who was the first to use a vein graft to repair an arterial injury?

Goyanes in 1906.

41. Who performed the first end-to-end arterial repair?
John B. Murphy in 1897.

BIBLIOGRAPHY

1. Callow AD, Ernst CB (eds): Vascular Surgery: Theory and Practice. Stamford, CT, Appleton & Lange, 1995, pp 985–1037.
2. Ernst CB, Stanley JC (eds): Current Therapy in Vascular Surgery, 3rd ed. St. Louis, Mosby, 1995, pp 625–656.
3. Frykberg ER: Advances in the diagnosis and treatment of extremity vascular trauma. Surg Clin North Am 75:207–723, 1995.
4. Modrall JG, Weaver FA, Yellin AE: Diagnosis and management of penetrating vascular trauma and the injured extremity. Emerg Med Clin North Am 16:129–144, 1998.
5. Moore WS (ed): Vascular Surgery: A Comprehensive Review, 4th ed. Philadelphia, W.B. Saunders, 1993, pp 630–647.
6. Rutherford RB (ed): Vascular Surgery, 4th ed. Philadelphia, W.B. Saunders, 1995, pp 713–735.
7. Schwartz SI (ed): Principles of Surgery, 7th ed. New York, McGraw-Hill, 1999, pp 158–177.
8. Weaver FA, Papanicolaou G, Yellin AE: Difficult peripheral vascular injuries. Surg Clin North Am 76:843–860, 1996.

33. FACIAL LACERATIONS

Lawrence L. Ketch, M.D.

1. What distinguishes facial from other lacerations?
Cosmesis (appearance) is clearly of primary importance. Quality of the final result depends on strict adherence to basic principles of wound management and painstaking technique. Copious irrigation, judicious debridement, gentle tissue handling, meticulous hemostasis, and minimization of sutures combined with early stitch removal are critical to an optimal result. Fine suture and sharp instruments are to be used; eversion of the wound margin with layered closure, obliteration of dead space and lack of tension are mandatory.

2. What factors influence choice of treatment for the wound?
The mechanism of injury, the clinical assessment of contamination, and the time elapsed since wounding dictate treatment. Clean lacerations, heavily contaminated wounds, crush injuries, and bites are treated differently.

3. How are clean lacerations repaired?
Clean lacerations should be irrigated with normal saline or Ringer's lactate. Only the surrounding skin should be prepared, and no antiseptic should be introduced into the wound. Regional anesthesia is preferred because of the potential for spread of contamination with direct injection of the wound margin. Epinephrine should be avoided because it devitalizes tissue and potentates infection. Wounds should be repaired in layers with absorbable suture in deep tissue. The smallest number of sutures necessary to overcome the natural resting wound tension should be used. Sutures should be removed within 3–5 days and the wound margin supported with Steri-strips subsequently.

4. How are dirty lacerations repaired?
In general, heavily contaminated wounds remain open after irrigation and debridement to undergo delayed closure. Because of cosmetic considerations, however, this approach is unacceptable in the face. For this reason, meticulous debridement of devitalized tissue and removal of

all foreign bodies are necessary. The wound should be cultured prior to copious irrigation, and a broad-spectrum antibiotic should be instituted prophylactically. The patient must be informed of the potential of a postrepair infection.

5. What factors influence suture selection?

Any method of suturing perpetuates tissue damage, impairs host defense, increases scar proliferation, and invites infection. Presence of a single silk suture in a wound lowers the infective threshold by a factor of 10,000. Therefore, fine, monofilament suture, just strong enough to overcome the resting wound tension, should be used. The amount of suture material placed in the wound should be minimized. Wounds with little or no retraction should be closed with tape, because this is the least injurious approach and produces the best scar.

6. Which wounds are suitable for closure with tissue adhesives?

N-butyl-2-cyanoacrylate has been used for cutaneous closure of low-tension lacerations in children and adults. This adhesive effectively closes selected lacerations, particularly those of low tension. The method is relatively painless and fast and may replace the need for suturing. It has become a preferred method for closure of pediatric facial lacerations in many emergency departments. It has a low complication rate and produces excellent cosmetic outcomes. In some instances, if initial wound orientation is against Langer's lines, it may, in fact, offer an advantage over conventional manual suturing.

7. Should eyebrows be shaved when facial lacerations are repaired?

No. They provide a landmark for realignment of disrupted tissue edges and do not always grow back.

8. How should crush avulsion injuries with associated skin loss be repaired?

Crush avulsion injuries result in irregular wound edges and devitalized tissue. Nonviable elements must be surgically excised because they predispose to infection and lead to excessive scarring. If viability is in doubt, the wound should be irrigated thoroughly and left open with continuous moist dressings. A delayed closure can be accomplished when the questionable areas have declared themselves. It is often prudent to close facial tissue as it lies; this technique often produces a less obtrusive scar than straight-line debridement and closure.

9. How should bites be treated?

Both animal and human bite wounds are highly contaminated and prone to infection. Again, because of cosmetic considerations, the wound should be treated as outlined above and closed meticulously. Antibiotic prophylaxis is indicated. If the wound becomes infected. the sutures must be removed and the wound allowed to heal. In this circumstance the patient should be informed that a scar revision will be necessary.

10. Should skin grafts or flaps be used for primary closure of a wound?

Complicated tissue transfer techniques have no place in the acute treatment of the facial wound. Closure should be achieved in the simplest way possible and complex reconstructive efforts should be deferred until the scar has matured. With tissue loss such that closure is impossible, it may be necessary to use a thin split-thickness skin graft.

11. When are antibiotics indicated in the treatment of facial lacerations?

Adherence to previously outlined principles of copious irrigation, debridement, and gentle tissue handling is more pertinent to the prevention of infection than the use of antibiotics in clean and clean-contaminated wounds. Antibiotic coverage is indicated, however, in crush avulsion injuries, bites ,and heavily contaminated injuries.

12. What determines the quality of the scar?

Location of the wound, age of the patient, and type and quality of skin are of great significance in the final outcome. Lesser determinants are the type and quantity of suture material and wound care. Final appearance depends little on the method of suture. Contusion, infection, retained foreign body, improper orientation of laceration, tension, and beveling of edges predict a poor outcome. Differences among suture materials are negligible; however, the technical factors of suture placement to produce wound eversion and time to removal affect the final result.

13. When should scars be revised?

A scar usually has its worst appearance at 2 weeks to 2 months after suturing. Scar revision should await complete maturation, which may take 4–24 months. A good rule of thumb is to undertake no revisions for at least 6–12 months after initial repair. The maturation of the wound may be assessed by its degree of discomfort, erythema, and induration.

CONTROVERSIES

There is little controversy about the care and repair of facial lacerations. Attention to basic principles of wound care usually produces a satisfactory scar. Because of the cosmetic considerations in facial trauma, primary repair in some instances is undertaken for the sake of appearance despite the risk of infection, which in other areas of the body would be deemed unacceptable.

BIBLIOGRAPHY

1. Amiel GE, Sukhotnik I, Kawar B, Siplovich l: Use of N-butyl-2-cyanoacrylate in elective surgical incisions—Longterm outcomes. J Am Coll Surg 189:21–25, 1999.
2. Keyes PD, Tallon JM, Rizos J: Topical anesthesia. Can Fam Physicians 44:2152–2156, 1998.
3. Adame N Jr, Bayless P: Carotid arteriovenous fistula in the neck as a result of a facial laceration. J Emerg Med 16:575–578, 1998.
4. Simon HK, Zempsky WT, Burns TB, Sullivan KM: Lacerations against Langer's lines: To glue or suture? J Emerg Med 16:185–189, 1998.
5. Hollander JE, Richman PB, WerBlud M, et al: Irrigation in facial and scalp lacerations: Does it alter outcome? Ann Emerg Med 31:73–77, 1998.
6. Quinn J, Wells G, Sutcliffe T, et al: A randomized trial comparing octylcyanoacrylate tissue adhesive and sutures in the management of lacerations. JAMA 277:1527–1530, 1997.
7. Manson PN: Facial injuries. In McCarthy JG (ed): Plastic Surgery, vol. 2. Philadelphia, W.B. Saunders, 1990, pp 889–916.
8. Davis PKB, Shaheen O: Soft tissue injuries of the face and scalp: Fractures of the larynx. In Rowe NL, Williams JI (eds.):Maxillofacial Injuries. New York, Churchill Livingstone, 1985, pp 184–200.
9. Junkiewicz MJ, Krizek TJ, Mathes SJ, Ariyn S: Principles and Practice in Plastic Surgery. St. Louis, Mosby, 1990.

34. BASIC CARE OF HAND INJURIES

Michael J.V. Gordon, M.D., and Lawrence L. Ketch, M.D.

1. What are the goals of hand repair?

Functional considerations override cosmesis in the treatment of hand trauma. There are no minor hand injuries. Initial diagnosis and management determine the final result; expert secondary repair cannot overcome primary neglect or errors in diagnosis or decision making.

2. What determines the final outcome of a hand injury?

Minimal sacrifice of tissue and primary healing accomplished by early wound closure are essential. Minimization of scar tissue by control of edema, prevention of infection, early wound closure, and vigorous physical therapy produce the optimal functional outcome.

3. What factors influence treatment of hand trauma?

Mechanism, location, and timing of injury and hand dominance, occupation, age, and general health of the patient help to determine treatment plans.

4. How common are occupational hand injuries?

Hand injuries result in more days lost from work than any other type of occupational injury.

5. What are the essentials of examination of the hand?

Inspection of position, color, and temperature often reveals the injury. Location suggests possible injury to underlying structures. Motor, sensory, and Doppler ultrasonic examination are confirmatory. All injuries must be x-rayed, and surgical exploration provides the definitive diagnosis.

6. How and where should hand injuries be explored?

Hand wounds should be explored under tourniquet control with adequate analgesia, using delicate instruments in a well-lighted surgery suite. Visual magnification is usually mandatory.

7. How is emergency hemostasis of the injured hand achieved?

In the acute setting, outside the operating suite, no tourniquet should be applied, and there should be no blind clamping of any structures within the injured part. Hemostasis may be achieved by elevation of the extremity with direct compression of the wound. This approach prevents injury to delicate underlying structures that cannot be identified under such circumstances.

8. How are fingertip injuries treated?

If less than 1 cm of pulp is disrupted, the wound will heal spontaneously with daily cleansing and dressing with nonadherent, moist gauze. Larger defects may require a skin graft, which often can be provided by defatting the amputated piece. Bone exposure necessitates flap coverage if digital length is to be maintained. Digital nerves cannot be repaired distal to the distal interphalangeal joint.

9. What is the classification system for fingertip amputations?

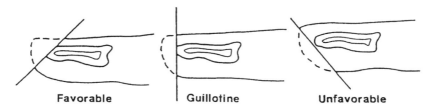

Favorable   Guillotine   Unfavorable

Classification for fingertip amputations based on the amount of remaining sensate volar skin. Although the favorably angulated amputation commonly removes some nail and bone, the volar skin is available for easy coverage. This amputation type is "favorable" for treatment by dressings only, allowing wound repair by contraction and epithelialization. The volarly angulated amputation angle is "unfavorable" for conservative management and usually requires a reconstructive procedure. (From Ditmars DM Jr: Fingertip and nail bed injuries. In Kasdan ML (ed): Occupational Hand and Upper Extremity Injuries and Disease. Philadelphia, Hanley & Belfus, 1991, with permission.)

10. How are nailbed injuries repaired?

Subungual hematomas should be evacuated by a hot-tipped paper clip or battery-powered electric cautery. Repair of the disruption of the sterile or germinal matrix must be meticulously approximated under magnification and the nailbed splinted, preferably with the avulsed part. The eponychial fold must be maintained for 3 weeks with Xeroform gauze or with the original nail. Often, nailbed disruption cannot be diagnosed without removal of the nail.

11. What is the initial management of flexor tendon laceration?

Flexor tendon laceration is not an emergency, and repair should not be undertaken in the emergency department by an unskilled person. If a hand surgeon is unavailable, the wound should be copiously irrigated and sutured and prophylactic antibiotics instituted. The patient should be referred for definitive repair.

12. What is the proper management of an open fracture?

Open fractures should be cultured and then undergo copious lavage with normal saline or Ringer's lactate. Broad-spectrum antibiotic coverage should be instituted, and the part should be splinted in the position of the function with a bulky dressing.

13. What is the proper treatment for hand infection?

The extremity should be immobilized and elevated, and parenteral antibiotics should be given. The patient should be referred immediately for possible surgical drainage.

14. What is the proper management of human bites?

Initial evaluation includes radiographs and cleansing of the wound. The wound should be left open—never closed. Antibiotics are started, and the wound is rechecked at 24 and 48 hours. If evidence of infection is present, parenteral antibiotics should be instituted and referral for possible surgical drainage should be made. The so-called "fight bite" occurs over the metacarpophalangeal (MCP) joint or proximal interphalangeal joint when a clenched fist is impaled on the front teeth of the adversary. This often inoculates the MCP joint with anaerobic streptococci. When infection is diagnosed, immediate arthrotomy and lavage should be performed.

15. How are injection injuries treated?

Despite their innocuous appearance, injection injuries may cause profound destruction of hand structures. Any such injury requires immediate hospitalization with prompt and extensive decompression and debridement.

16. What is carpal tunnel syndrome (CTS)?

CTS is the most common peripheral compression neuropathy; it is signaled by numbness and tingling of the hand.

17. Is CTS more common in older or younger people? Men or women?

CTS is more common in people over 40 years of age, but an increasing number of young people with CTS have been reported in recent years, usually those whose jobs involve repetitive manual labor. Women are affected approximately twice as often as men.

18. What are the most preventable causes of deformity in hand injuries?

Edema and infection lead to increased scarring and restricted function. Prolonged immobilization in poor position also impairs function, as does delayed skin closure. Failure to obtain a radiograph or a missed diagnosis with delay in recognition of an injury has severe consequences.

19. What is the proper emergency department treatment of all hand injuries?

The patients should be sedated and the wound cultured and irrigated. A thorough examination must be performed and a sterile compression dressing placed. The upper extremity should be splinted, tetanus prophylaxis should be administered, and broad-spectrum antibiotic coverage instituted for crush avulsion or heavily contaminated wounds. A radiograph should be obtained and blood drawn for preoperative laboratory tests.

20. What are the guidelines for replantation of an amputated part?

There are no absolute guidelines. A microsurgeon who is a member of a replantation team should be consulted. If replantation is planned, parts should not be immersed directly in water or put directly on ice or dry ice. The part should be copiously irrigated, wrapped in a moist sponge, and placed in a sterile plastic container; the plastic container should be placed in an ice-water slurry for transport.

BIBLIOGRAPHY

1. Hansen TB, Carstensen O: Hand injuries in agricultural accidents. J Hand Surg 24B:190–192, 1999.
2. McAuliffe JA: Hand care in the new millennium: Surgeons' perspective. J Hand Ther 12:178–181, 1999.
3. Riaz M, Hill C, Khan K, Small JO: Long term outcome of early active mobilization following flexor tendon repair in zone 2. J Hand Surg 24B:157–160, 1999.
4. Taras JS, Lamb MJ: Treatment of flexor tendon injuries: Surgeons' perspective. J Hand Ther 12:141–148, 1999.
5. Van der Molen AB, Matloub HS, Dzwierzynski W, Sanger JR: The hand injury severity scoring system and workers' compensation cases in Wisconsin, USA. J Hand Surg 24B:184–186, 1999.

35. BURNS

Paul Bauling, M.D.

1. Why do burn injuries often evoke an accentuated psychoemotional response in both the general population and medical care providers?
The physical injury severity score of a fractured femur exceeds that of a burn to the face and neck region, yet the psychoemotional response of the family and sometimes even physicians and nurses may be much more pronounced in the case of the facial burn. Every medical professional must be aware of the potential risk of an inappropriate emotional reaction and should attempt through mental preconditioning and behavior modification not to increase the level of anxiety or fear of the patient and family by words, actions, or body language.

2. How then can the medical professional avoid and overcome this reaction?
The key is knowledge. One needs to have a clear, well-digested understanding of the pathophysiology of burn wounds and their local and systemic effects on the patient. (Read on.)

3. Why does such a seemingly simple mechanism of injury pose so tremendous a threat to the well-being and the life of the patient?
Before reviewing the pathology of a burn injury, everyone needs to recall the immensely important and complex functions of the skin. The integument represents a uniquely flexible, selectively permeable envelope with immunologic, thermoregulatory, and neurosensory functions. It hosts its own microcosm of commensal bacterial but is able to prevent invasion by a wide variety of bacteriologic and other physicochemical intruders. But these few words do not do justice to the complex and vast number of other important functions of the skin, which is the largest single organ of the body. The skin envelopes a living entity that consists of about 70% water and receives 20% of cardiac output. A human can survive without one kidney or one-half of the liver and live quite well without one-half of the gut but will not survive for long without one-half of the skin.

4. What really happens in a burn injury?
Events occur locally at the injury site as well as systemically.

5. What happens locally?
The burn injury site and the ensuing local events may be divided into three zones: zone of necrosis, zone of stasis, zone of hyperemia. In the **zone of necrosis**, all proteins are denatured; cellular form, function, and integrity are destroyed; and most importantly, all microvascular and macrovascular structure and function are destroyed. Therefore, this segment of the skin is

structurally and functionally destroyed forever. Adjacent to and surrounding this zone of death, destruction, and desolation is a **zone of stasis**. Cellular morphology is intact when examined microscopically, but cells are swollen with microstructural changes. Histopathologists also report extravasation of leukocytes and red cells into the interstitial space, increased interstitial fluid, and capillary occlusion, both partial and complete, indicating low flow. Finally, on microscopy, these findings are surrounded by a third zone where cells appear intact, healthy, and show no intracellular microstructural changes. Minimal edema is seen in the extravascular space, with widely dilated capillary blood vessels and no signs of sludging or microvascular thrombosis. This **zone of hyperemia** then gently transitions into the adjacent normal tissues where no abnormalities are seen.

6. What changes occur systemically?

On a systemic level, two important abnormalities occur in burn patients: (1) a trend to fluid retention/ with generalized edema, partly caused by an increased systemic microvascular permeability, and (2) a definite and reproducible decrease in cardiac output. Immunochemical alterations involving cytokines, inflammatory mediators, and other humoral reactions are seen as the possible cause of the fluid leak and myocardial lesion. In summary, the pump is failing, and the hoses are leaking.

7. How can burn victims be managed in a rational way?

All of the key principles that underlie advanced trauma life support are of paramount importance to burn victims, in particular the management of the first (golden) hour after injury.

- Airway—look for soot in the mouth.
- Breathing—listen for breath sounds on both sides.
- Circulation—begin IV fluids; the Parkland formula is 4 ml/kg body weight/% body burn.

Uncontrolled extreme pain can act as a signal to perpetuate damaging cytokine pathway activity. Thus, pain management and psychoemotional support are vitally important. Finally, the constant appreciation of the catastrophic loss of skin integrity at the burn site must lead us to avoid all possible iatrogenic acts of microbial contamination; we must protect the patient against the medical team.

8. How is the severity of a burn injury determined?

The most important factor is the size of the burn. The size is usually expressed as a percentage of total body surface area (% TBSA). The palm of the hand represents one-half of a percent of the TBSA (palm size = 0.5% TBSA). This percentage is most useful on scattered small burns. When large burns are to be sized, use the rule of nines or a Lund & Browder chart. Note that adults and children differ most significantly by the difference in the relative size of the head (9% in adult, 15% in infant). The thighs, by contrast, are much smaller in infants than in adults.

Contrary to popular belief, the depth of a burn injury has much less impact on the severity of the injury. The depth of injury also remains an area in which accurate clinical diagnosis, even by experts, is lacking. Burn depth, however, does determine whether a wound will heal on its own or whether skin grafting has to be done.

9. What is the rule of nines?

The rule of nines is the most practical method of determining the size of a burn injury, although not the most accurate. The body surface is divided into sections, each of which represents 9% of the total surface area or multiples of 9. The entire head and neck equal 9%; each upper extremity equals 9%; the anterior trunk equals 2×9 (18%), as does the posterior trunk; both lower extremities equal 18% each; and the perineum makes up 1%, bringing the total to 100%.

10. How is the depth of burn injury graded?

The grading system for depth of burn injury revolves around whether the burn wound will heal on its own or require skin grafting. What makes this determination so difficult and inconsistent for the inexperienced clinician is the confounding factor of skin appendages that carry the basal layer deep into the dermis, from which reepithelialization may occur. The following table helps to elucidate the question.

DEPTH OF INJURY	CLINICAL SIGNS AND SYMPTOMS	OUTCOME
First degree (superficial injury limited to epidermis)	Erythema of the skin with mild-to-moderate discomfort.	Wounds heal spontaneously in 5–10 days; damaged epithelium peels off, leaving no residual effects.
Second degree Superficial (involves entirety of epidermis and superficial portion of dermis)	Wounds are blistered or weeping erythematous, and painful.	Wounds heal spontaneously within 3 weeks without residual scarring and with good quality skin; pigmentation may be altered.
Deep (involves deeper dermis but viable portions of epidermal appendages remain)	Skin is desiccated, blistered, with eschar often seen. Wounds are occasionally moist and difficult to distinguish from third-degree burn.	Wounds heal spontaneously beyond 3–4 weeks; hypotrophic scarring often occurs and, occasionally, unstable epithelium. For best results remove eschar by tangential excision and cover with split-thickness skin graft.
Third degree (all epidermal appendages destroyed)	Avascular, waxy, white, leathery brown or black, insensate eschar.	Unless small in size, wounds require removal of eschar and coverage with skin graft for healing.

11. What other significant prognosticators have been identified in burn injury survival?

A recently published multivariate analysis on burn injury survival revealed three risk factors with essentially equal weight in predicting mortality; 40% TBSA, age above 60 years, and presence of inhalation injury to the lungs.

0   Risk factor: mortality = 0.3%
1   Risk factor: mortality = 3%
2   Risk factors: mortality = 33%
3   Risk factors: mortality = 90%

12. What is meant by inhalation injury?

The external burn injury is a visible and somewhat quantifiable injury. On the other hand, the inhalation of heat, carbon monoxide, and toxic/noxious substances is less visible and less quantifiable yet very dangerous. The three separate mechanisms of injury to the airways are sometimes incorrectly grouped as inhalation injury. All three injuries may occur separately or in combination.

1. **Carbon monoxide (CO) intoxication.** CO is a product of incomplete combustion of organic or synthetic materials due to inadequate oxygen supply to the fire. CO has a 250 times greater affinity for hemoglobin than oxygen, causing a relative hypoxemia with possible hypoxic brain and kidney damage. Levels around 5% are found in cigarette smokers; burn victims become symptomatic around 15–20%; life is threatened around 30%. Management is by administration of 100% O_2, which reduces the half-life of carboxyhemoglobin from 250 to 40 minutes.

2. **Heat damage to upper airways.** A house fire can reach temperatures up to 1000° C. The countercurrent effect of blood flow in upper airway passage is able to cool down the air to temperatures below 100°C. Prolonged breathing of such air or superheated steam, however, may lead to heat damage to the naso-, oro-, and laryngopharynx and, most critically, the vocal cords. Furthermore, even a minimal amount of vocal cord edema presents as altered phonation or hoarseness and rapidly progresses to acute laryngeal edema, asphyxia, and death. Therefore, all patients with altered phonation need immediate endotracheal intubation.

3. **Inhalation of toxic smoke components** produced by the combustion of modern synthetic materials used in the interior decoration of houses, buildings, and cars. Examples include plastics,

paints, carpets, synthetic fabrics, and floor tiling. The overall mortality from this kind of injury (for which the term *inhalation injury* is reserved) remains at 35–50%, even in the best institutions.

13. After hemodynamic and other life-preserving issues have been addressed, how should the wound be managed acutely?

The wound needs simple coverage with a surgically clean or, if available, sterile sheet of linen or surgical drape. No ointment or specific antibacterial treatment is initially required, but this does not mean that the wound can be neglected or allowed to become contaminated, cool, or dry. Wound exposure leads to hypothermia, and wound surface cooling and desiccation deepen the wound and arrest wound healing.

If appropriate wound care is applied, healing should occur within 14–18 days in areas where germinal cells are present in sufficient numbers. Wherever and whenever an area of burn injury is identified as full-thickness, healing will never occur unless the wound area is very small (2-cm diameter). The only available cure is allogeneic skin grafting, if suitable and sufficient donor sites are available, or sheets of cultured epithelial cells and keratinocytes.

14. How is the site of a full-thickness skin burn managed before skin grafting?

Three options are to be considered: autolytic separation of necrotic tissues, exogenous enzymatic debridement, or surgical excision. The natural separation of devitalized tissue takes place through proteolytic enzymes generated by leukocytes, but this process is very slow.

15. What are the risks of circumferential burn injuries?

The human skin is an extremely elastic, pliable, and compliant envelope. When damaged by burns, the proteins and collagen fibers are denatured and the skin becomes a hard, leathery crust called eschar (pronounced *eskar*). The skin, therefore, becomes a rigid encasing shell with no elasticity. This change is compounded by interstitial fluid leak and edema, which lead to poor venous return. Needless to say, this process must be prevented or arrested at its inception. Escharotomy is a procedure of "cutting into" (otomy) the eschar so that the rigid shell is split in half to allow release of tissue pressure and to save limbs, digits, and extremities. It is sometimes required for circumferential torso burns that may impair breathing.

16. What are the properties of temporary synthetic skin substitutes?

When skin will or may heal spontaneously (i.e., clearly not third-degree burns), the application of synthetic skin substitutes is indicated. These products have repeatedly been shown to reduce healing time by 50%.

17. What is the impact of such a severe injury on the body? What demands are placed on the metabolism?

The metabolic response to injury in general is maximally stimulated in patients with large burns and peaks at 2½ times the basal metabolic rate. This maximal acceleration of the body's metabolism by burn injury leads to rapid and severe catabolism, further aggravated by periods of septicemia as well as heat loss through increased evaporation.

18. How can we best supply fuel to the metabolic furnace of the body?

The realization that nutritional support of the burn victim is paramount has been with us for several decades. However, the critical importance of maximal reliance on the gut as primary and sole route of nutritional support (as opposed to intravenous nutrition) has been slow to achieve acceptance. Enteral nutritional support (via a feeding tube as opposed to the intravenous parenteral route) supplies calories and sustains the gut mucosal barrier.

19. What major life-threatening complications may occur during the healing period?

The three most important potential complications that a burn victim may suffer during the hospital phase of recovery are septicemia, septicemia, and septicemia. However, this very knowledge has led to the abuse and misuse of antibiotics.

20. What is the role of antibiotics in burn care?

Antibiotics are *never* administered prophylactically for burn injuries. Less than 10% of all burn injuries require antibiotics during the entire course of treatment. However, few patients with major burns will survive hospitalization without one or several courses of antibiotics. Appropriate antibiotic therapy is a critically important and life-saving tool in the management of burns. The key to appropriate antibiotic therapy is the diagnosis of an infective/septic event and wise selection of the appropriate empirical drug(s) based on the unique infectious profile of burn victims.

The real dilemma of burn care, however, is that a raised core body temperature does not always indicate infection or sepsis. It is important to see abnormal temperature readings in conjunction with other contemporaneous aberrations in clinical, biochemical, and microbiologic data. Such warning signs include sudden changes in hemodynamic parameters, mental status, general appearance of the patient (he or she suddenly looks ill or is unwilling to cooperate), mental status changes, arterial blood gas changes, sudden intolerance of enteric feeding, thrombocytopenia, glucose intolerance, and many more that can be pathophysiologically traced to organ dysfunctions induced by sepsis.

21. How are chemical burn injuries approached?

Brush off all chemicals in powdered form. Thereafter, immediate (within seconds) copious and prolonged irrigation (20 minutes) of the contaminated skin with running tap water is indicated. Some chemicals may be absorbed; therefore, immediate contact with a poison control center is indicated.

22. How are electrical injuries approached?

Injuries due to electricity may be of several different types, such as electrical flash burns and electrical conduction injuries. In electrical conduction injury to the body, the mechanism of tissue damage is energy (amperage) transfer, leading to heat production with resultant protein denaturation and cell death or damage. Because different body structures have different compositions (bone, skin, muscle, nerve, tendon, lung) electrical conductivity is different, resulting in a totally erratic and unpredictable destruction of various structures, often with small skin lesions. Thus, the skin is often only minimally involved at entry point and exit site, with extensive muscle, nerve, tendon, and even bone necrosis in erratic patterns. Compartment syndrome and myoglobinuria are the significant complications that flow from this complex pattern, and rapid tissue decompression with early and repeated reexplorations to remove necrotic tissue is essential.

23. Once healed, what important issues remain to be addressed in the rehabilitation period?

The rehabilitation of a burn victim must begin on the day of admission. The rehabilitation of a burn victim is a total team effort involving occupational therapists, physical therapists, nutritionists, psychologists, social services, pulmonologists, microbiologists, pharmacists, speech therapists, and of course, nursing services. Rehabilitation of mind and body may require as long as 18–36 months, often with intervention by plastic, reconstructive, and hand surgeons in the final stages.

24. Are burnt children just small adults with burn injuries?

No. Many unique variations demand the involvement of a pediatric specialist to ensure appropriate care in children with serious burns.

25. Is this a complete and exhaustive, up-to-date overview of contemporary burn care?

No, this is just an hors d'oeuvre. Please review the bibliography below.

BIBLIOGRAPHY

1. Barnett S: Classic research: Moist wound healing. Wound Care 4:475–490, 1995.
2. Demling RH: Burns. In Wilmore DW, et al (eds): American College of Surgeons. Care of the Surgical Patient, vol 3. New York, Scientific American, 1999.
3. Herndon DN (ed): Total Barn Care. Philadelphia, W.B. Saunders, 1996.

36. PEDIATRIC TRAUMA

David A. Partrick, M.D., and Denis D. Bensard, M.D.

1. What is the leading cause of death in children?

Injuries cause more death and disability in children from ages 1 to 18 years than all other causes combined. Each year nearly one child in four receives medical treatment for an injury. The estimated annual cost is $15 billion.

2. What age groups are at particular risk for traumatic death?

Infants less than 2 years of age have a consistently higher mortality rate for the same level of injury. During adolescence, however, injury takes the greatest toll, accounting for nearly 80% of deaths.

3. What primary mechanisms account for pediatric traumatic injuries?

Blunt (86%), penetrating (12%), and crush injuries (2%). Motor vehicle accidents are the most common cause of injury and death in childhood.

4. What are the incidence and mortality rate of injuries by body region?

BODY REGION	INCIDENCE (%)	MORTALITY (%)
Extremities	19	0
Head and neck	17	6
External injuries	13	0
Abdomen	3	2
Face	2	0
Thorax	1	3
Multiple	44	5

5. Are boys and girls equally susceptible to injury?

No. Boys are injured twice as often as girls. Males are at a 4 times greater risk for suicide, 3 times greater risk for drowning, 2.5 times greater risk for homicide, and 2 times greater risk for motor vehicle-related trauma.

6. How is a child's airway different from an adult's?

Children are at increased risk of airway obstruction because of their large tongue, floppy epiglottis, increased lymphoid tissue, and short trachea with a small diameter. Uncuffed endotracheal tubes are appropriate in children weighing less than 60 pounds (younger than 6 years) to minimize vocal cord trauma, subglottic edema, and ulceration. The narrowest part of a child's airway is the cricoid ring, which functions as a seal for the uncuffed endotracheal tube.

7. What if oral endotracheal intubation cannot be accomplished?

A needle cricothyrotomy is preferable to surgical cricothyrotomy and can be performed with a 14-gauge catheter. This technique uses the same concept as jet insufflation in adults. Surgical cricothyrotomy is technically much more difficult in a small child than in an adult and has a high association with secondary subglottic stenosis.

8. Why are head injuries more common in children than adults?

Children lead with their heads. Until the age of 10 years, the head of a child is larger in relation to the body than the head of an adult.

9. What type of head injuries are more common in children?

Young children are more susceptible to epidural hemorrhage; subdural hemorrhage is relatively rare. Pediatric patients also tend to sustain injuries that produce diffuse edema rather than focal, spacy-occupying lesions.

10. Can children have significant chest trauma without rib fractures?

Absolutely. The chest wall is much more compliant in children than in adults; thus, kinetic energy is transmitted more readily to structures within the thorax. A child with significant blunt chest trauma is at increased risk of life-threatening contusion to the lungs or heart even with no or relatively few rib fractures. Furthermore, pneumothorax is poorly tolerated in children and can result in a rapidly fatal situation because children have a more mobile mediastinum than adults.

11. What is a child's total blood volume?

80 ml/kg (8% of body weight).

12. What is the first sign of significant blood loss in children?

Tachycardia. Young children have a remarkable tolerance to blood loss. Hemorrhage greater than 30% of blood volume may result in no blood pressure change, but such blood loss does cause a rapid increase in pulse rate. Children are predisposed to hypovolemic shock. Because cardiac output depends largely on heart rate, they have a limited capacity to increase stroke volume.

13. Why are children at increased for hypothermia during resuscitation?

The child's surface area is large relative to internal body mass. Using cold intravenous fluids and inhaled gases can exacerbate hypothermia, leading to pulmonary hypertension, hypoxia, and progressive metabolic acidosis. Particularly vulnerable are infants < 6 months of age who lack significant subcutaneous fat and an involuntary shivering mechanism.

14. What sites are preferred for venous access in children?

Two large-bore intravenous catheters should be inserted percutaneously in the upper extremities. The second choice is percutaneous access to the distal saphenous vein (or a cut-down).

15. What if you cannot establish an IV line?

The intraosseous route is safe and efficacious and actually requires less time than a venous cutdown. The anteromedial surface of the proximal tibia is used most commonly, with the needle placed 3 cm distal to the level of the tibial tuberosity. The proximal femur, distal femur, and distal tibia are also potential sites of intraosseous access. Saline, glucose, blood, bicarbonate, atropine, dopamine, epinephrine, diazepam, antibiotics, phenytoin, and succinylcholine have been administered successfully via the intraosseous route. Complications are rare and result primarily from infection or extravasation. Intraosseous volume resuscitation facilitates subsequent cannulation of the venous circulation.

16. What are the appropriate crystalloid and blood resuscitation volumes in children?

Administer 20 ml/lg of Ringer's lactate solution or normal saline by bolus. A response is manifest by a decrease in heart rate, increase in urinary output, and overall improvement in level of perfusion. The 20-ml/kg bolus should be repeated if assessment reveals inadequate tissue perfusion. If evidence of shock persists after two bolus infusions of crystalloid solution, 10 ml/kg of packed red blood cells (type-specific if available or O-negative) should be administered. An appropriate response to resuscitation does not exclude abdominal injury.

17. What is the frequency of abdominal organ injury in blunt trauma compared with penetrating trauma?

In decreasing order of frequency, spleen, kidney, liver, intestine, pancreas, and urinary bladder.

18. How accurate is physical examination in the evaluation of pediatric blunt abdominal trauma?

Poor. Physical examination may prove misleading in up to 50% of injured children.

19. What are the advantages and disadvantages of diagnostic peritoneal lavage (DPL) in children?

DPL is 96% accurate in detecting intraabdominal injury. However, it may lead to nontherapeutic laparotomy rates of 15%.

20. What are the advantages and disadvantages of computed tomography (CT) in children?

Abdominal CT scan is safe, noninvasive, and able to evaluate retroperitoneal structures as well as identify specific organ injuries. It can aid in the decision to manage children nonoperatively. Disadvantages include insensitivity for hollow visceral injury and the need for intravenous and enteral contrast agents. In addition, CT is time-consuming, requires patient transport and sedation, and may leave patients vulnerable during the scanning period. Thus, CT is risky in unstable patients.

21. Is ultrasonography effective in the evaluation of children with abdominal trauma?

Abdominal ultrasound examination is simple, fast, and readily available; it can be performed at the bedside. In addition, it is noninvasive and easily repeatable. The sensitivity and specificity of a focused abdominal ultrasonographic examination for traumatic injury exceed 95%. Abdominal ultrasound is best used as a triage tool for detecting significant intraperitoneal fluid, thus identifying patients who require laparotomy for hemodynamic instability.

22. Is there a reliable method to diagnose hollow visceral injury in children?

No. Serial physical examinations remain the gold standard for diagnosing pediatric gastrointestinal perforation.

23. What are the "soft signs" of pediatric intraabdominal injury?

- Lap-belt ecchymosis corresponds to a high incidence of solid organ injury, hollow viscus injury, and lumbar spine injury.
- Gross hematuria has a 30% risk for significant intraabdominal injury not involving the genitourinary system.
- Elevation of the liver enzymes aspartate aminotransferase (> 250) or alanine aminotransferase (> 450) corresponds to a 50% risk for significant liver injury.
- Children with documented pelvic fracture have at least a 20% risk for associated intraabdominal injury.
- Children with severe neurologic impairment (Glasgow Coma Scale score < 8) frequently suffer concurrent intraabdominal injury.

24. What should be suspected in children with seat-belt or handlebar injuries?

The **seat-belt complex** consists of ecchymosis of the abdominal wall, a flexion-distraction injury to the lumbar spine (Chance fracture), and intestinal injury. Approximately 30% of children with the seat-belt sign have an associated intestinal injury.

A **handlebar** injury classically causes disruption of the pancreas at the junction of the body and tail, where the pancreas crosses the vertebral column and is vulnerable to anterior blunt compression.

25. Do all children with solid organ injuries require operative repair?

No. Selective nonoperative management of solid organ injuries has revolutionized the management of pediatric trauma and has gained further acceptance as safe and efficacious in the management of solid organ injuries in adults.

26. When is nonoperative management of solid organ injury in children appropriate?

When the vital signs remain stable, less than one-half of the blood volume is replaced, and no other significant intraabdominal injuries are present. The decision for nonoperative management versus laparotomy should be based on the child's physiologic condition and not on the extent of injury as documented radiographically.

27. What are the indications for operative intervention for solid organ injuries?

Massive bleeding on presentation and transfusion of more than one-half of blood volume (40 ml/kg) within 24 hours of injury.

28. What is SCIWORA?

Spinal cord injury without radiologic abnormalities (SCIWORA) is a problem unique to children. A child's spine has increased elasticity, shallow and horizontally oriented facet joints, anterior wedging of the vertebral bodies, and poorly developed uncinate processes. The spinal cord can be completely disrupted in young children without apparent disruption of the vertebral elements. However, most patients have evidence of spinal cord injury on magnetic resonance imaging. Two-thirds of SCIWORA cases are seen in children ≤ 8 years of age.

29. What is the hallmark of SCIWORA?

A documented neurologic deficit that may have changed or resolved by the time the child arrives in the emergency department. The danger is that immediate reinjury of the same area may produce permanent disability. Many children with SCIWORA tend to develop neurologic deficits hours to days after the reported injury. Therefore, spinal immobilization should continue, and thorough neurosurgical evaluation is essential in any child with reliable evidence of even a transient neurologic deficit.

30. What percentage of pediatric deaths due to injury are caused intentionally?

Approximately 75% of all injury-related deaths in children are due to unintentional injuries, and the rest are due to violence. More than 80% of deaths from head trauma in children younger than 2 years of age result from intentional abuse.

31. What signs are suspicious for nonaccidental trauma (NAT)?

- History of failure to thrive
- Delay in obtaining medical care
- Multiple previous injuries
- Absent or uninterested caregiver
- Fluctuating or conflicting histories
- History inconsistent with the injury or developmental level of the victim

Suspicious physical findings include bite, pinch, slap, or cord marks or bruises in various stages of healing; multiple or bilateral skull fractures; a skull fracture in a fall < 4 feet; and retinal hemorrhages (from shaking).

32. List the characteristics of "shaken-baby" syndrome.

- Retinal hemorrhage
- Subdural or subarachnoid hemorrhage
- Little evidence of external trauma
- Age < 2 years

33. What fracture patterns are suspicious for NAT?

- Multiple rib fractures of different ages
- Extremity fractures such as metaphyseal "chip" or "bucket-handle" fractures
- Diaphyseal spiral fracture in children < 9 months of age
- Transverse midshaft long-bone fracture

- Femur fracture in an infant < 2 years of age
- Fracture of the acromion process of the scapula
- Proximal humerus fracture

34. What percentage of NAT cases involve burn injuries? What are their characteristics?
Approximately 20% of abuse cases involve burns. Scalding by hot water is the most common. Specific patterns of injury may raise suspicion of abuse, including burns involving the buttock and perineum (bathing trunk distribution), back, dorsum of the hand, and stocking-glove distribution. Cigarette burns also may be observed as circular, punched-out ulcers of similar size.

35. What are the necessary steps in evaluation of children with suspected NAT?
Any child with suspected NAT should have a detailed physical examination, head CT scan, skeletal survey (babygram), and retinal fundoscopic examination. The appropriate child protective services should be contacted immediately.

BIBLIOGRAPHY

1. American College of Surgeons Committee on Trauma: Recognition of Physical Child Abuse. Chicago, American College of Surgeons, 1997.
2. Bensard DD, Beaver BL, Besner GE, Cooney DR: Small-bowel injury in children after blunt abdominal trauma: Is diagnostic delay important? J Trauma 41:476–483, 1996.
3. Fallat ME, Casale AJ: Practice patterns of pediatric surgeons caring for stable patients with traumatic solid organ injuries. J Trauma 43:820–824, 1997.
4. Grabb PA, Pang D: Magnetic resonance imaging in the evaluation of spinal cord injury without radiographic abnormalities in children. Neurosurgery 35:406–414, 1994.
5. National Pediatric Trauma Registry: Children and Adolescents with Disability Due to Traumatic Injury: A Data Book. Boston, Department of Physical Medicine and Rehabilitation, New England Medicine Center, 1996.
6. Orlowski JP: Emergency alternatives to intravenous access: Intraosseous, intratracheal, sublingual, and other-site drug administration. Pediatr Clin North Am 41:1183–1199, 1994.
7. Partrick DA, Bensard DD, Moore EE, et al: Ultrasound is an effective triage tool to evaluate blunt abdominal trauma in the pediatric population. J Trauma 45:57–63, 1998.
8. Pigula FA, Wald SL, Shackford SR, Vane DW: The effect of hypotension and hypoxia on children with severe head injuries. J Pediatr Surg 28:310–316, 1993.
9. Ruess L, Sivit CJ, Eichelberger MR, et al: Blunt abdominal trauma in children: Impact of CT on operative and nonoperative management. Am J Roentgenol 169:1011–1014, 1997.
10. Shafi S, Gilbert JC, Carden S, et al: Risk of hemorrhage and appropriate use of blood transfusions in pediatric blunt splenic injuries. J Trauma 42:1029–1032, 1997.

III. Abdominal Surgery

37. APPENDICITIS

Alden H. Harken, M.D.

1. What is the classic presentation of acute appendicitis?
Periumbilical pain that migrates to the right lower quadrant (RLQ).

2. Where is McBurney's point?
One-third the distance between the anteroposterior iliac spine and the umbilicus.

3. What is McBurney's point?
The point of maximal tenderness in acute appendicitis.

4. Was McBurney a cop from Boston?
Probably. Another McBurney was a surgeon from New York who, in collaboration with a surgeon named Fitz, coined the term "appendicitis" in classic papers published in 1886 and 1889.

5. What are the typical laboratory findings of a patient with appendicitis?
• White blood cell count: 12,000–14,000
• Negative urinalysis (no white cells)
• Negative pregnancy test

6. What layers does the surgeon encounter on exposing the appendix through a Rockey-Davis incision?
Skin, subcutaneous fat, aponeurosis of the external oblique muscle, internal oblique muscle, transversalis fascia and muscle, and peritoneum.

7. Was Rockey-Davis a prize fighter from Philadelphia?
Probably. Another Rockey-Davis was a pair of surgeons—A.E. Rockey and G.G. Davis— who developed RLQ transverse, muscle-splitting incisions that extend into the rectus sheath.

8. What is the blood supply to the appendix and right colon?
The ileocolic and right colic arteries.

9. Does surgery for appendicitis involve a risk of mortality?
No surgical procedure is devoid of risk.

	Mortality rate
Nonperforated appendix	< 0.1%
Perforated appendix	As high as 5%

10. What patient groups are at higher risk of perforated appendicitis?
1. Very young patients (less than 2 years old).
2. Elderly patients (over 70 years old), who exhibit dampened abdominal innervation and present late.
3. Diabetic patients, who present late because of diabetic visceral neuropathy.
4. Patients taking steroids. Steroids mask everything.

11. What is the role of ultrasound in the diagnosis of acute appendicitis?

Ultrasound can be both negatively and positively helpful. It is nice to see a perfectly normal right fallopian tube and ovary (to rule out an ectopic pregnancy and tuboovarian abscess). It is also reassuring to see an inflamed, edematous appendix.

12. Is laparoscopic appendectomy replacing the traditional approach?

Surgeons are now facile with laparoscopic cholecystectomy, colectomy, and hiatus herniorrhaphy. The normal appendix can be removed easily and safely via the laparoscope, but the inflamed/perforated appendix is tougher. Laparoscopic appendectomy probably should be reserved for the normal appendix.

13. What is a "white worm"?

A normal appendix.

14. What is the differential diagnosis of right lower quadrant pain?

- Meckel's diverticulitis
- Diverticulitis
- Ectopic pregnancy
- Crohn's disease
- Tuboovarian abscess
- Pelvic inflammatory disease
- Carcinoid tumor
- Cholecystitis

15. What is a Meckel's diverticulum?

Meckel's diverticulum is a congenital omphalomesenteric mucosa remnant that may contain ectopic gastric mucosa. It is found in 2% of the population, 2 feet upward from the ileocecal valve. It becomes inflamed in 2% of patients.

16. Can chronic diverticulitis masquerade as appendicitis?

Yes. Fifty percent of patients aged 50 years have colonic diverticula. The appendix is just a big cecal diverticulum. Thus, it makes sense that appendicitis and diverticulitis should look, act, and smell alike.

17. Can a woman with a negative pregnancy test present with an ectopic pregnancy?

Yes. The fallopian tube must be inspected for a walnut-sized lump. Appropriate surgical therapy is a longitudinal incision to "shell out" the fetus with subsequent repair of the tube. This approach (as opposed to salpingectomy) is designed to preserve fertility.

18. Can Crohn's disease initially present as appendicitis?

Indeed, this presentation is typical. Crohn's disease is boggy, edematous, granulomatous inflammation of the distal ileum. Traditional surgical dictum suggests that it is appropriate to remove the appendix in patients with Crohn's disease unless the cecum at the appendiceal base is involved.

19. Is it possible to confuse appendicitis with a tuboovarian abscess (TOA)?

Of course. An ovarian abscess buried deep in an inflamed, edematous, matted right adnexa can be treated successfully with intravenous antibiotics alone. Do not drain pus into the free peritoneal cavity—this will only make the patient sicker.

20. How about pelvic inflammatory disease (PID)?

PID can look exactly like appendicitis except for a positive "chandelier" sign. On pelvic examination, manual tug on the cervix moves the inflamed, painful adnexae, and the patient hits the chandelier. PID should be treated with antibiotics (either orally or intravenously, depending on how sick the patient is).

21. How does one deal with an appendiceal carcinoid tumor?

Carcinoid tumors may present anywhere along the GI tract; 60%, however, are in the appendix. An obstructing carcinoid tumor, like a fecalith, can lead to appendicitis—and in 0.3% of appendectomies, carcinoid tumors are the culprit. Most carcinoid tumors are small (< 1.5 cm) and benign; 70% are located in the distal appendix. They are effectively treated with appendectomy alone. A large carcinoid tumor (> 2.0 cm) at the appendiceal base, especially with invasion of the mesoappendix, must be considered malignant and mandates a right hemicolectomy.

22. Can appendicitis be mistaken for acute cholecystitis?

Occasionally, yes. Both entities reflect acute, localized, intraperitoneal inflammation. Laboratory studies may be identical: white blood cell count of 12,000–14,000, negative urinalysis, and negative pregnancy test. Thus, if one is thinking "appendicitis," the major difference may be only right upper vs. right lower quadrant pain. Laparoscopic cholecystectomy is possible for acute cholecystitis, but conversion to an open procedure should be more frequent.

BIBLIOGRAPHY

1. Fitz RH: Perforating inflammation of the vermiform appendix with special reference to its early diagnosis and treatment. Trans Assoc Am Physicians 1:107, 1886.
2. Lane JS, Sarkar R, Schmit PJ, et al: Surgical approach to cecal diverticulitis. J Am Coll Surg 188:629–634, 1999.
3. Meakins JL: Appendectomy and appendicitis. Can J Surg 42:90, 1999.
4. Rice HE, Arbesman M, Martin DJ, et al: Does early ultrasonography affect management of pediatric appendicitis? A prospective analysis. J Pediatr Surg 34:754–785, 1999.
5. Rockey AE: Transverse incisions in abdominal operations. Med Rec 68:779, 1905.
6. Shah DR, Dev VR, Brown CA: The utilization of a neural network system in the diagnosis of appendicitis. MD Comput 16:65–67, 1999.
7. Tehrani HY, Petros JG, Kumar RR, Chu Q: Markers of severe appendicitis. Am Surg 65:453–455, 1999.
8. Urbach DR, Cohen MM: Is perforation of the appendix a risk factor for tubal infertility and ectopic pregnancy? An appraisal of the evidence. Can J Surg 42:101–108, 1999.

38. GALLBLADDER DISEASE

Jeff Cross, M.D.

1. What is the prevalence of gallstones in Western society for women and men 60 years of age?

Women, 50%; men, 15%,

2. What percentage of asymptomatic stones convert to symptomatic stones?

10% at 5 years, 15% at 10 years, and 18% by 15 years.

3. What is the incidence of gallbladder perforation in patients with acute cholecystitis?

5%.

4. What organisms should be covered by antibiotic therapy?

Escherichia coli, Klebsiella species, *Streptococcus faecalis, Clostridium welchii, Proteus* species, *Enterobacter* species, and anaerobic *Streptococcus* species.

5. What percentage of patients with common duct stones have positive bile bacterial cultures?

90%.

6. Has the incidence of cholecystectomy increased in the laparoscopic era?

Yes. Previously the incidence was stable at 500,000 operations per year. Recently there has been an increase to over 700,000 per year.

7. What percentage of patients undergoing cholecystectomy have missed common duct stones?

2%,

8. What is the difference between retained common duct stones and choledocholithiasis in patients after laparoscopic cholecystectomy?

Stones found within 2 years of cholecystectomy are considered retained stones. The patient who develops choledocholithiasis more than 2 years after cholecystectomy is arbitrarily defined as having recurrent rather than retained common duct stones.

9. What is the incidence of acalculus cholecystitis?

10% of all cases of cholecystitis.

10. How does laparoscopic intraoperative ultrasound (LUS) compare with laparoscopic intraoperative cholangiography (LIOC)?

The sensitivity of LUS is high (90%) and comparable to that of LIOC. Potential advantages of LUS include less time and less dissection than LIOC. Disadvantages include less sensitivity in detecting stones in the intrapancreatic portion of the common bile duct.

11. What is postcholecystectomy syndrome?

Unexplained pain, similar to that noted preoperatively, occurred in 20% of patients in previous decades. The incidence has decreased recently with the advent of newer modalities that diagnose specific conditions more accurately.

12. What are the potential causes of postcholecystectomy pain?

- Common duct stone
- Retained gallbladder
- Traumatic stricture
- Cystic duct remnant
- Stenosing papillitis
- Biliary dyskinesia

13. What is the conversion rate from laparoscopy to the open approach in acute cholecystitis and in symptomatic cholelithiasis?

10% for acute cholecystitis, > 5% for symptomatic cholelithiasis.

14. Is there a difference in mortality and morbidity rates in cholecystectomy performed early compared with cholecystectomy performed late after the initial onset of symptoms in patients with acute cholecystitis?

No.

15. What is the incidence of common bile duct injury in the laparoscopic era?

0.7% for laparoscopic cholecystectomy vs. 0.5% for open cholecystectomy.

16. When, if ever, should laparoscopic cholecystectomy be performed during pregnancy?

Because of the risk of spontaneous abortion and the fact that most attacks of acute biliary colic during pregnancy resolve spontaneously, cholecystectomy should be performed after delivery except for patients with complicated disease. If surgery is necessary, the second trimester is preferred.

17. What is the prevalence of gallbladder carcinoma found incidentally during cholecystectomy?
Open era, 1%; laparoscopic area, 0.1%.

18. Why is cholecystectomy increasing in the pediatric population?
Gallstone identification has increased because of the more liberal use of ultrasonography in patients with abdominal pain.

19. Should patients with asymptomatic stones undergo laparoscopic cholecystectomy?
No. The risk of observation of patients with asymptomatic gallstones is less than or equal to the risk of operation.

20. In what groups of patients with asymptomatic stones is prophylactic cholecystectomy beneficial?
1. Patients with congenital hemolytic anemia how have gallstones at the time of splenectomy.
2. Obese patients undergoing bariatric surgery who have already developed gallstones.

21. What is the optimal timing for laparoscopic cholecystectomy in acute cholecystitis?
Laparoscopic cholecystectomy optimally should be performed within 72 hours of the onset of symptoms. Procedures performed within the first 20 hours generally are easier, because the area of dissection remains within the edematous phase. Fibrosis and increased blood vessel proliferation have not yet occurred.

BIBLIOGRAPHY

1. Adamsen S, Hansen OH, Funch-Jensen P, et al: Bile duct injury during laparoscopic cholecystectomy: A prospective nationwide series. J Am Coll Surg 184:571–578, 1997.
2. Bender JS, Zenilman ME: Immediate laparoscopic cholecystectomy as definitive therapy for acute cholecystitis. Surg Endosc 9:1081–1084, 1995.
3. Grace P, et al: Management of gallstones in pregnancy. Br J Surg 84:1646, 1997.
4. Hooper KD, Landis JR, Meilstrup JW, et al: The prevalence of asymptomatic gallstones in the general population. Invest Radiol 26:939–945, 1991.
5. Kolecki R, Schirmer B: Intraoperative and laparoscopic ultrasound. Surg Clin North Am 78:251–271, 1998.
6. Koo KP, Thirlby RC: Laparoscopic cholecystectomy in acute cholecystitis: What is the optimal timing for operation? Arch Surg 131:540–545, 1996.
7. Machi J, Tateishi T, Oishi A, Furumoto N, et al: Laparoscopic ultrasonography versus operative cholangiography during laparoscopic cholecystectomy: Review of the literature and a comparison with open intraoperative ultrasonography. J Am Coll Surg 188:361–367, 1999.
8. Mirza DR, Narsimhan KL, Ferraz Neto BH, et al: Bile duct injury following laparoscopic cholecystectomy. Referral pattern and management. Br J Surg 84:786–790, 1997.
9. Moody F: Post cholecystectomy problems. In Cameron J (ed): Current Surgical Therapy. St. Louis, Mosby, 1998, pp 434–438.
10. Rattner DW, Ferguson E, Warshaw AL: Factors associated with successful laparoscopic cholecystectomy for acute cholecystitis. Ann Surg 217:233–236, 1993.
11. Sharp K, Peach S: Common bile duct stones. In Cameron J (ed): Current Surgical Therapy. St. Louis, Mosby, 1998, pp 410–415.
12. Waldhausen J, Benjamin D: Cholecystectomy is becoming an increasingly common operation in children. Am J Surg 177:364–367, 1999.

39. PANCREATIC CANCER

Nathan W. Pearlman, M.D.

1. What are the presenting signs of pancreatic cancer?
1. Painless jaundice (40% of patients)
2. Pain (epigastric, right upper quadrant, back) with jaundice (40%)
3. Metastatic disease (e.g., hepatomegaly, ascites, lung nodules) with or without jaundice

2. Why is there such a high rate of advanced disease at diagnosis?
The pancreas is retroperitoneal and relatively insensate. Symptoms of disease are uncommon unless the pancreatic or biliary duct is obstructed or the process (pancreatitis, cancer) extends outside the gland.

3. A previously healthy 73-year-old patient presents with pruritus, dark urine, and icteric sclerae after recent overseas travel. What is a reasonable differential diagnosis?
1. Biliary tract stones
2. Cancer of the extrahepatic bile ducts
3. Cancer of the pancreas
4. Hepatitis

4. What is the first step in evaluating the patient?
Liver function tests and ultrasound. Liver function tests determine the degree of jaundice and hepatic dysfunction. Ultrasound detects dilated extrahepatic bile ducts and stones in the gallbladder or common duct with about 95% accuracy; it detects a mass in the head of the pancreas with 80% accuracy. If the bile ducts are normal and alkaline phosphatase, aspartate aminotransferase, and alanine aminotransferase are elevated, the patient has intrahepatic cholestasis, probably from hepatitis.

5. What if ultrasound shows dilated extrahepatic bile ducts?
Proceed to endoscopic retrograde cholangiopancreatography (ERCP) or transhepatic cholangiogram to determine whether the obstruction is high or low in the common bile duct and its likely cause (stricture, stone, tumor). The biliary tract can be decompressed with an internal stent at this time, allowing liver function to improve before major surgery. If stones are present, endoscopic sphincterotomy should be performed, allowing the stones to pass and simplifying future surgery.

6. What about computed tomography (CT) scan instead of ERCP?
ERCP findings are more diagnostic. Intraluminal filling defects mean stones, gradual narrowing of the bile duct means stricture, and a sharp cut-off of the dye column means tumor. CT scan provides other information, such as size of the tumor (if one is present), its relationship to other structures, such as portal vein, and presence or absence of liver metastases.

7. In this case, ultrasound, ERCP and CT scan show dilated extrahepatic bile ducts from a mass in the head of the pancreas. The tumor seems separate from the portal vein, and there are no liver metastases. What now?
If the patient is a poor operative risk, one should consider percutaneous fine-needle aspiration (FNA) to document cancer and avoid surgery. However, if the patient is a good operative risk, FNA adds no useful information. If no malignant tissue is obtained, surgery is still indicated because the needle may have missed the lesion, sampling only the pancreatitis that surrounds all

such tumors. In addition, FNA often causes hemorrhage in the pancreas, adding to the difficulty of tumor removal. In this patient, proceed to the operating room.

8. We are in the operating room, the abdomen is open, and the discussion revolves around taking the tumor out. What is a "Whipple procedure"?

Removal of the gallbladder, distal common duct, duodenum, and the portion of pancreas to the right of the portal vein—in essence, a proximal pancreatectomy. In some centers, it is also routine to remove the gastric antrum, with or without a vagotomy.

9. What is distal pancreatectomy? A total pancreatectomy?

Distal pancreatectomy removes the portion of gland to the left of the portal vein, along with the spleen. Total pancreatectomy combines both procedures—again, with antrectomy in some centers.

10. Why remove gallbladder, duodenum, and stomach if the problem is in the pancreas?

Once the ampulla of Vater is removed, the gallbladder does not function well and forms stones. The second and third portions of the duodenum share a blood supply with the pancreas and are usually devascularized when the pancreas is removed. Historically, the gastric antrum was removed to improve resection margins. Vagotomy was added to reduce the incidence of marginal ulceration at the site where the gastric remnant was anastomosed to small bowel.

Removing the antrum adds little to the scope of the operation, however, and marginal ulceration can be prevented by placing the gastroenterostomy downstream from where bile and pancreatic secretions enter the gut. Thus, many surgeons now perform a pylorus-preserving/vagus-preserving Whipple procedure whenever possible; survival is the same as with more radical procedures and long-term function somewhat better.

11. How does one determine whether to perform a Whipple procedure, distal pancreatectomy, or total pancreatectomy?

Whipple procedures are used for mobile tumors confined to the head of the pancreas with no signs of lymph node metastases at the celiac axis or root of mesentery. Distal pancreatectomies are used for mobile lesions in the tail of the pancreas, unaccompanied by signs of spread. Total pancreatectomy is generally reserved for special situations in which cancer involves most of the gland, but nowhere else.

12. What if there are nodal metastases at the celiac axis or root of mesentery?

The patient cannot be cured with surgery. The goal now is palliation. If obstructive jaundice is present, a biliary-enteric bypass should be performed. Some surgeons feel gastroenterostomy also should be done at this time because of a 30% chance of future duodenal obstruction.

13. Are there any other signs of inoperability that we should know about?

Most pancreatic tumors lie near the portal vein and adhere to or invade the vein as they expand. Most surgeons consider attachment to the portal vein a sign of incurability. Some, however, remove the affected portion of vein, if this is the only sign of inoperability, and bridge the gap with a graft.

14. What is the cure rate with this operation?

About 20% 5-year survival.

15. With cure rates so low, why are surgeons so eager to do a Whipple?

Unfortunately, the Whipple procedure represents the only chance for cure. If the patient has unresectable disease, median survival is 8–12 months, with or without chemotherapy and/or radiation, and there are essentially no 5-year survivors. Thus, although survival figures with surgery certainly are not impressive, they are considerably better than results with any other treatment.

BIBLIOGRAPHY

1. Bluemke DA, Fishman EK: CT and MR evaluation of pancreatic cancer. Surg Oncol Clin North Am 7:103–124, 1998.
2. Cameron JL, Pitt HA, Yeo CJ, et al: One hundred and forty-five consecutive pancreaticoduodenectomies without mortality. Ann Surg 217:430–438, 1993.
3. Fuhrman GM, Leach SD, Staley CA, et al: Rationale for en bloc resection in the treatment of pancreatic adenocarcinoma adherent to the superior mesenteric-portal vein confluence. Ann Surg 223:154–162, 1996.
4. Harrison LE, Klinstra D, Brennan MF: Portal vein resection for adenocarcinoma of the pancreas: A contraindication for resection? Ann Surg 224:342–349, 1996.
5. Neuberger TJ, Wade UP, Swope TJ, et al: Palliative operations for pancreatic cancer in the hospitals of the U.S. Department of Veterans Affairs from 1987–1991. Am J Surg 166:632–637, 1993.
6. Peters JH, Carey LC: Historical review of pancreaticoduodenectomy. Ann J Surg 161:219–225, 1991.
7. Yeo CJ: Pylorus-preserving pancreaticoduodenectomy. Surg Oncol Clin North Am 7:143–156, 1998.

40. ACUTE PANCREATITIS

Clay Cothren, M.D., and Jon M. Burch, M.D.

1. What are the common causes of acute pancreatitis?
Gallstones (45%) and alcohol (35%).

2. What are the uncommon causes?
Hyperlipidemia, hypercalcemia (hyperparathyroidism, multiple myeloma), iatrogenic factors (endoscopic retrograde cholangiopancreatography), drugs (didanosine, thiazide diuretics), H_2 blockers, tetracycline, azathioprine), infections (mumps, coxsackievirus), and scorpion bites (favorite pimp question on rounds). Approximately 10% of cases are considered idiopathic.

3. What are the characteristic symptoms?
Moderate-to-severe epigastric pain that is described as boring in nature and often radiates to the back. Pain frequently is accompanied by nausea and vomiting.

4. What may be found on physical examination?
Diffuse abdominal tenderness, abdominal distention, and hypoactive bowel sounds may be appreciated on exam. Patients may be febrile, tachycardic, and dehydrated. Evidence of jaundice is associated with gallstone pancreatitis.

5. What is the appropriate therapy for mild-to-moderate pancreatitis?
Fluid resuscitation to maintain urine output (place a Foley catheter), nasogastric tube in presence of vomiting, meperidine or other pain medications, alcohol withdrawal prophylaxis, and avoidance of oral ingestion until amylase levels decrease and abdominal pain resolves.

6. Which is the better lab test: amylase or lipase?
Serum lipase has somewhat greater sensitivity and specificity; however, an isolated elevation of lipase with a normal amylase is unlikely to be due to pancreatitis. Serum amylase levels tend to peak sooner than lipase levels, which may remain elevated for 4–5 days. About 10–30% of patients with pancreatitis have normal amylase levels, most notably alcoholics with chronic "burned-out" pancreatitis.

7. What other disease states cause hyperamylasemia?

Perforated peptic ulcers, small bowel obstruction, parotid inflammation or tumor, and ovarian tumors are associated with elevations in amylase.

8. What are Ranson's indices?

Ranson's indices are 11 measurements that are useful in predicting the occurrence of severe pancreatitis.

On admission	**After the initial 48 hours**
Age > 55	Blood urea nitrogen > 5 mg/dl
White blood cell count > 16,000	Hematocrit > 10%
Glucose > 350	Calcium < 8
Lactate dehydrogenase > 350	PaO$_2$ < 60 mmHg
Aspartate aminotransferase > 250	Base deficit > 4
	Fluid sequestration > 6 L

9. How do Ranson's indices relate to mortality?

Number of criteria	Mortality rate (%)
0–2	5
3–4	15
5–6	50
7–8	100

10. What is necrotizing pancreatitis?

The inflammation and edema of acute pancreatitis may progress with subsequent devitalization of pancreatic and peripancreatic tissue. Pancreatic necrosis occurs in approximately 20% of acute episodes.

11. Why is it important to differentiate acute pancreatitis from necrotizing pancreatitis?

The presence and extent of necrosis are key determinants of the clinical course. Approximately 70% of patients with pancreatic necrosis develop infected pancreatic necrosis; infection accounts for 80% of all deaths from pancreatitis and is an absolute indication for surgery.

12. What is the optimal method for diagnosing pancreatic necrosis with or without associated infection?

Dynamic computed tomography (CT) scans with contrast allow visualization and differentiation of healthy perfused parenchyma from patchy, poorly perfused necrotic tissue. CT-guided aspirate of the necrotic tissue is sent for Gram stain and culture to determine the presence of infection.

13. When should one add antibiotic therapy?

Mild cases of pancreatitis should be treated with supportive measures, because antibiotics do not alter the course or septic complications of the disease. In cases of necrotizing pancreatitis, randomized trials have shown a decreased incidence of sepsis in patients treated with the broad-spectrum antibiotic imipinem. Patients who have > 3 Ranson's criteria or are at high risk should be considered for early antibiotic treatment.

14. What is the most common complication of acute pancreatitis?

About 2–10% of patients develop pancreatic pseudocysts. Such patients typically present with persistent abdominal pain, nausea and vomiting, and an abdominal mass. One should wait 6–12 weeks for the pseudocyst to "mature" before undertaking operative or endoscopic drainage.

15. What is the significance of hypoxemia early in the course of pancreatitis?

Patients with necrotizing pancreatitis may develop respiratory failure requiring mechanical ventilation. In addition, they may become hemodynamically unstable and progress to multiple organ failure. Hypoxemia is an ominous sign.

16. What is the natural history of gallstone pancreatitis?

Attacks recur. Cholecystectomy is curative.

17. What is the natural history of alcoholic pancreatitis?

Attacks recur. Abstinence from alcohol should be encouraged because many patients develop chronic pancreatitis.

BIBLIOGRAPHY

1. Bosscha K, Hulstaert PF, et al: Fulminant acute pancreatitis and infected necrosis: Results of open management of the abdomen and "planned" reoperations. J Am Coll Surg 187:255–262, 1998.
2. Bradley EL: A clinically based classification system for acute pancreatitis. Arch Surg 128:586–590, 1993.
3. Bradley EL: A fifteen year experience with open drainage for infected pancreatic necrosis. Surg Gynecol Obstet 177:215–222, 1993.
4. Branum G, Galloway J, et al: Pancreatic necrosis: Results of necrosectomy, packing, and ultimate closure over drains. Ann Surg 227:870–877, 1998.
5. Bradley EL, Murphy F, Ferguson C: Prediction of pancreatic necrosis by dynamic pancreatography. Arch Surg 210:495–504, 1989.
6. Chase CW, Barker DE, et al: Serum amylase and lipase in the evaluation of acute abdominal pain. Am Surg 62:1028–1033, 1996.
7. Folsch UR, Nitsche R, et al: Early ERCP and papillotomy compared with conservative treatment for acute biliary pancreatitis. N Engl J Med 336:237–242, 1997.
8. Luiten EJT, Hop WCJ, et al: Controlled clinical trial of selective decontamination for the treatment of severe acute pancreatitis. Ann Surg 222:57–65, 1995.
9. Pederzoli P, Bassi C, et al: A randomized multicenter clinical trial of antibiotic prophylaxis of septic complications in acute necrotizing pancreatitis with imipinem. Surg Gynecol Obstet 176:480–483, 1993.
10. Powell JJ, Miles R, Siriwardena AK: Antibiotic prophylaxis in the initial management of severe acute pancreatitis. Br J Surg 85:582–597, 1998.
11. Rau B, Pralle U, et al: Management of sterile necrosis in instances of severe acute pancreatitis. J Am Coll Surg 181:279–288, 1995.
12. Schoenberg MH, Rau B, Beger HG: New approaches in surgical management of severe acute pancreatitis. Digestion 60(Suppl S1):22–26, 1999.
13. Steinberg W, Tenner S: Acute pancreatitis. N Engl J Med 330:1198–1210, 1995.
14. Takeda K, Matsuno S, et al: Continuous regional arterial infusion of protease inhibitor and antibiotics in acute necrotizing pancreatitis. Am J Surg 171:394–398, 1996.

41. CHRONIC PANCREATITIS

Clay Cothren, M.D., and Jon M. Burch, M.D.

1. What is chronic pancreatitis?

The classic syndrome consists of abdominal pain and evidence of pancreatic insufficiency. Histologically, chronic inflammation of the pancreas results in destruction of the parenchyma and associated fibrosis.

2. What is the most common cause?

Alcohol abuse accounts for 75% of cases.

3. Is chronic pancreatitis the result of acute pancreatitis?

Many patients have not had acute pancreatitis, although alcoholism is common to both. The average age for chronic pancreatitis is 13 years less than for acute disease.

4. What are the signs of pancreatic insufficiency?

Insulin-dependent diabetes mellitus (found in up to 30% of patients) and steatorrhea (in 25%).

5. How much of the pancreas must be destroyed before diabetes develops?

Approximately 90%.

6. What is steatorrhea? How does one confirm the diagnosis?

Steatorrhea is soft, greasy, foul-smelling stools. A 72-hour fecal fat analysis may be done to confirm the diagnosis. The D-xylose test is normal and the Schilling test insensitive for pancreatic insufficiency. Steatorrhea is treated with a variable combination of low-fat diets, pancreatic enzymes, antacids, and cimetidine.

7. Is serum amylase elevated in chronic pancreatitis?

No. Serum amylase is usually normal in cases of "burned-out" pancreatitis.

8. What are the complications of chronic pancreatitis?

Pancreatic pseudocyst, abscess, or fistula may occur. Obstruction of the biliary tree with resultant jaundice may be caused by areas of fibrosis. Malnutrition and narcotic addiction are more likely to coexist than actual complications.

9. What is a possible source of upper gastrointestinal bleeding (UGIB) in a patient with chronic pancreatitis?

Although gastritis and peptic ulcer disease are perhaps more commonly associated with UGIB, splenic vein thrombosis with associated gastric varices and hypersplenism also should be considered. (Your attending will love this answer!)

10. What is the "chain of lakes"?

In performing endoscopic retrograde cholangiopancreatography, dye is introduced into the pancreatic duct; sequential areas of narrowing of the duct cause the appearance of a "string of beads" or "chain of lakes."

11. What are the indications for surgery?

There are no steadfast rules. Relative indications include unabating pain refractory to medical management, biliary obstruction, and suspicion of malignancy.

12. Which operative procedures are commonly performed?

The Peustow procedure may be used for the "chain of lakes" duct to provide longitudinal head-to-tail drainage via a Roux-en-Y pancreaticojejunostomy. Distal pancreatectomy may be used for isolated distal disease or retrograde drainage into a pancreaticojejunostomy. A modified Whipple approach also may be considered.

13. What is the result of such operations?

Pain relief occurs in 70% of patients at the end of 1 year and in 50% of patients at the end of 5 years.

BIBLIOGRAPHY

1. American Gastroenterological Association: AGA technical review: Treatment of pain in chronic pancreatitis. Gastroenterology 115:765–776, 1998.
2. Beger HG, Schlosser W, et al: The surgical management of chronic pancreatitis: Duodenum-preserving pancreatectomy. Adv Surg 32:87–104, 1999.
3. Fernandez-del Castillo C, Rattner DW, Warshaw AL: Standards for pancreatic resection in the 1990s. Arch Surg 130:295–300, 1995.
4. Mergener K, Baillie J: Chronic pancreatitis. N Engl J Med 332:1379–1385, 1995.
5. Steer ML, Waxman I, Freedman S: Chronic pancreatitis. N Engl J Med 332:1482–1490, 1995.
6. Wiersema M: Diagnosing chronic pancreatitis: Shades of gray. Gastrointest Endosc 48:102–106, 1998.

42. PORTAL HYPERTENSION AND ESOPHAGEAL VARICES

Greg Van Stiegmann, M.D.

1. What is the blood supply to the liver?

Total hepatic blood flow is roughly 1500 ml/mm or about one-fourth of cardiac output. The hepatic artery normally supplies about 30% of blood flow and delivers 50% of oxygen. The hepatic portal vein supplies 70% of blood flow and delivers 50% of oxygen. In patients with cirrhosis and portal hypertension, the contribution of the hepatic artery increases.

2. What is hepatopedal flow?

When cirrhosis is really bad and hepatic vascular resistance increases, portal venous flow may actually reverse (hepatopedal). The hepatic artery supplies virtually all of the blood flow to the liver.

3. What is portal hypertension?

Normal portal venous pressure is less than 10 mmHg. Portal venous pressure over 20 mmHg constitutes portal hypertension.

4. What are the four anatomic connections between the portal and venous systems?

1. Left gastric (coronary) vein to esophageal vein (leads to esophageal varices)
2. Inferior mesenteric vein to superior hemorrhoidal vein to hypogastric vein (leads to rectal varices)
3. Umbilical vein to superficial veins of the abdominal wall (leads to caput medusae).
4. Mesenteric veins to perilumbar veins of Retzius to inferior vena cava.

5. What causes portal hypertension?

1. **Prehepatic:** portal vein thrombosis, portal vein compression by tumor or schistosomiasis
2. **Hepatic:** cirrhosis
3. **Posthepatic:** hepatic vein thrombosis (Budd-Chiari syndrome) or right heart failure

6. What are the most common causes of portal hypertension?

1. In the United States, Laennec's (alcoholic) disease
2. In the word, schistosomiasis
3. In children, extrahepatic portal venous occlusion usually due to thrombosis of the portal vein (results in "cavernous transformation")

7. What are the common complications of portal venous hypertension?

1. Hemorrhage from esophageal varices (most catastrophic)
2. Hypersplenism
3. Rectal varices
4. Portal hypertensive gastropathy
5. Portosystemic encephalopathy

8. How common are esophageal varices?

Hemorrhage from varices occurs in 30% of patients within 1 year of diagnosis. A 20% mortality rate is associated with a variceal bleed; mortality is related directly to liver function (Child's class; see question 17).

9. Is upper GI bleeding in cirrhotic patients (even with documented varices) always from varices?

No. Twenty-five percent of cirrhotic patients bleed from another source (e.g., superficial gastric erosions).

10. What is the initial treatment of patients with suspected esophageal variceal hemorrhage?

Aggressive fluid resuscitation followed by early endosocpy to confirm (and possibly treat) the variceal bleeding.

11. What is a Sengstaken-Blakemore tube?

The Sengstaken-Blakemore tube is used for mechanical tamponade of variceal hemorrhage. It consists of a nasogastric tube with two large balloons at the distal end. The tube is positioned in the stomach, and tube position must be confirmed by radiograph before inflating the balloons. The distal gastric balloon is inflated with 250 ml of air and then pulled up tight against the gastroesophageal junction (traction is accomplished by attaching the proximal end of the tube to the face mask of a football helmet). If the gastric balloon alone does not control hemorrhage, the proximal esophageal balloon is inflated to a pressure that equals portal venous pressure (25 mmHg). Balloon tamponade is a method of buying time. Fifty percent or more of patients rebleed after balloon deflation.

12. What drugs are used in the treatment of variceal bleeding?

Vasopressin (0.4–0.8 U/min IV) is a potent vasoconstrictor that decreases splanchnic blood flow. Watch out for concurrent coronary vasoconstriction leading to myocardial ischemia. Nitroglycerin may be used to counteract coronary artery trouble.

Glypressin (2 mg IV every 4 hours) is a synthetic analog of vasopressin with a longer half-life, simpler administration, and fewer systemic side effects. Nitroglycerin also may be used in conjunction with this vasoconstrictor.

Somatostatin (250 µg IV bolus, then 250 µg/hr IV) decreases portal blood flow by selective splanchnic vasoconstriction and is free from systemic side effects.

Octreotide (250 µg IV bolus, then 50 µg/hr IV) is the synthetic analog of somatostatin and appears equally effective.

13. What endoscopic treatments are available?

Sclerotherapy: intravariceal injection of a sclerosant (sodium morrhuate).

Endoscopic band ligation (EBL): strangling varices with rubber bands is an extension of ligating anal hemorrhoids.

14. What are the results of endoscopic therapy?

Acute variceal hemorrhage is controlled with a single endoscopic treatment in 75% of cases.

15. Is one form of endoscopic therapy superior?

Yes. EBL is safer, faster, and cheaper.

16. What is TIPS?

Transjugular intrahepatic portosystemic shunt (TIPS) is a radiologic technique for shunting portal blood across the liver into the vena cava. An 8-mm stent is placed fluoroscopically from the hepatic venous system through the hepatic parenchyma into the portal vein. The goal of TIPS is relief of ascites and variceal bleeding. Rebleeding is usually due to shunt thrombosis and occurs in 10% of cases.

17. What is the Child's classification?

The Child's classification assesses the severity of liver failure and is associated with both operative risk and survival:

Child's A: both albumin and bilirubin are on the correct side of 3 (serum albumin > 3 and serum bilirubin < 3); the patient is a good risk.

Child's C: serum albumin < 3 and serum bilirubin > 3; such patients are poor risks.

Child's B: between the two above extremes.

18. What are the surgical shunt operations?

Central (nonselective) shunt: portacaval and mesocaval central shunts nonselectively decompress the portal venous system. They may result in reversal of portal venous flow, thus worsening hepatic failure. They also dump large volumes of portal blood into the systemic circulation, thus risking encephalopathy.

Selective splenorenal (Warren) shunt: anastomosis of the distal (splenic side) splenic vein into the left renal vein with ligation of the coronary (left gastric) vein.

As a rule, the more central the shunt, the better the portal decompression and the worse the encephalopathy. Thus, if a shunt works well, it is likely to produce encephalopathy.

19. What is the operative mortality rate for elective protosystemic shunts?

The operative mortality rate depends on the Child's classification: 5% for Child's A, 10% for Child's B, and 40% for Child's C.

20. Are there any indications for an emergency portacaval shunt for the treatment of variceal bleeding?

Probably not. Radiologic shunt insertion (TIPS) has replaced surgical shunts at most hospitals for patients whose bleeding cannot be controlled with endoscopic methods.

21. What is the role of liver transplantation in the treatment of portal hypertension?

Liver transplantation is the only therapy that cures portal hypertension and underlying liver disease. All Child's B and C patients should be assessed as potential transplant recipients. Because organ supply is limited, however, the selection process is stringent.

22. Do prior TIPS or portosystemic shunt procedures preclude liver transplantation?

No.

CONTROVERSY

23. Should patients with esophageal varices that have not bled be treated?

Prophylactic shunt surgery aimed at preventing a first variceal bleed results in a greater chance of dying than doing nothing. Prophylactic endoscopic sclerotherapy results in either no benefit or a deleterious effect compared with no treatment. EBL prophylaxis has reduced bleeding and lessened mortality in several studies, but further confirmation is needed. Prophylactic treatment with nonselective beta-blocking agents reduces the risk of a first variceal bleed and appears to improve survival. Patients most likely to experience a first variceal bleed are those with large varices. Such patients should be considered for preventative therapy.

BIBLIOGRAPHY

1. Cameron J (ed): Current Surgical Therapy. St. Louis, Mosby, 1998, pp 373–389.
2. Henderson JM, Barnes DS, Geisinger MA: Portal hypertension. Curr Probl Surg 35:379–452,m 1998.
3. Rikkers LF: The changing spectrum of treatment for variceal bleeding. Ann Surg 228:536–546, 1998.
4. Shahi HM, Sarin S: Prevention of a first variceal bleed: An appraisal of current therapies. Am J Gastroenterol 12:2348–2358, 1998.
5. Tait KS, Krige J, Terblanche J: Endoscopic band ligation of esophageal varices. Br J Surg 86:437–446, 1999.

43. GASTROESOPHAGEAL REFLUX DISEASE

Lawrence W. Norton, M.D., and Michael E. Fenoglio, M.D.

1. What symptoms suggest gastroesophageal reflux disease (GERD)?

Substernal burning discomfort after meals or at night, associated occasionally with regurgitation of gastric juices, is a frequent symptom of GERD. Discomfort is relieved by standing or sitting. Dysphagia, a late complication of GERD, is caused by mucosal edema or stricture of the distal esophagus.

2. What is the difference between heartburn and GERD?

Heartburn is a lay term for mild, intermittent reflux of gastric content into the esophagus without tissue injury. It is relatively common among adults. GERD implies esophagitis with varying degrees of erythema, edema, and friability of the distal esophageal mucosa. It occurs in 5% of the population.

3. What causes GERD?

The underlying abnormality of GERD is functional incompetence of the lower esophageal sphincter (LES), which allows gastric acid, bile, and digestive enzymes to damage the unprotected esophageal mucosa.

4. Is hiatal hernia an essential defect in GERD?

Not all patients with GERD have a hiatal hernia, and not all patients with a hiatal hernia have GERD. However, they are frequently associated (50% of patients with GERD have an associated hiatal hernia).

5. What studies are useful to diagnose GERD?

Endoscopy with biopsy is the essential element in diagnosing GERD. Barium swallow with or without fluoroscopy can diagnose reflux but frequently cannot identify esophagitis. Twenty-four hour esophageal pH testing associates reflux with symptoms and is useful in some but not all patients. Manometry of the esophagus and LES is required whenever an esophageal motility disorder is suspected and prior to any surgical intervention.

6. What is the initial management of a patient suspected of having GERD?

- Change diet to avoid foods known to induce reflux (e.g., chocolate, coffee).
- Avoid large meals before bedtime.
- Stop smoking.
- Do not wear tight, binding clothes.
- Elevate the head of the bed 4–5 inches.
- Take antacids when symptomatic.
- Weight loss can be highly effective in reducing GERD symptoms.

7. If initial treatment fails, what should be recommended?

About 50% of patients show significant healing with H_2 blockers. Only a small number of such patients (10%) remain healed over the course of 1 year. Metoclopramide or cisapride may be prescribed to stimulate gastric emptying. Neither agent relieves symptoms consistently in the absence of acid reduction.

8. What is the role of proton pump inhibitors (PPI) in GERD?

PPIs (omeprazole, lanasoprazole) irreversibly inhibit the parietal cell hydrogen ion pump and are over 80% successful in healing severe erosive esophagitis. Two-thirds of patients who continue the medication remain healed. A concern in prolonged PPI therapy is hypergastrinemia secondary to alkalinization of the antrum. The fact that gastrin is trophic to gastrointestinal mucosa initially raised the fear of later neoplasia, but this fear has not been borne out by follow-up studies.

9. When should operation for GERD be recommended?

Current recommendations for surgical intervention include (1) failed medical therapy (intractable disease, intolerance and allergy to medications, noncompliance, and recurrence of symptoms while on medical therapy); (2) complications (stricture, respiratory symptoms, dental erosions, medico-social changes, and premalignant mucosal changes); and (3) patient preference (cost or lifestyle issues).

10. What is the goal of surgical treatment?

Operations for GERD attempt to prevent reflux by mechanically increasing LES pressure and, in most procedures, to restore a sufficient length of distal esophagus to the high-pressure zone of the abdomen. Hiatal hernia, when present, is reduced simultaneously. The crura of the diaphragm sometimes can be approximated to act as a pinchcock on the LES.

11. What procedures can accomplish this goal? How are they done?

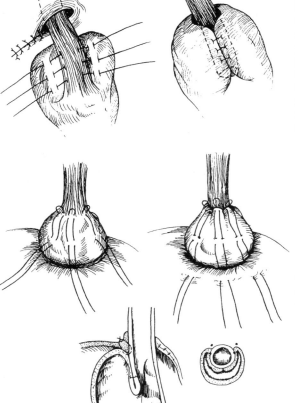

1. In the **Nissen fundoplication**, which is used in over 95% of patients, the fundus of the stomach is mobilized, wrapped around the distal esophagus posteriorly, and secured to itself anteriorly. The procedure alters the angle of the gastroesophageal junction and maintains the distal esophagus within the abdomen to prevent reflux. The operation is done transabdominally by either laparotomy or laparoscopy.

2. The **Belsey Mark IV operation** accomplishes the same anatomic changes but is done via a thoracotomy.

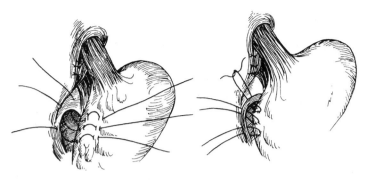

3. The **Hill gastropexy** restores the esophagus to the abdominal cavity by securing the gastric cardia to the preaortic fascia.

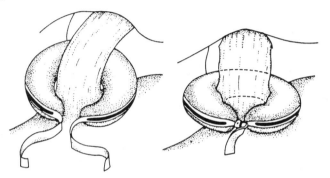

4. The **Angelchik prosthesis** is a silicone-filled collar placed around the distal esophagus within the abdominal cavity.

5. The **Toupet (partial) fundoplication** is used in patients with associated motility disorders. Because the wrap is not circumferential, the incidence of postoperative dysphagia is significantly reduced with a partial wrap compared with a full 360° wrap (Nissen fundoplication). However, long-term results may not be as good as with a Nissen fundoplication. This operation can be done transabdominally by either laparotomy or laparoscopy.

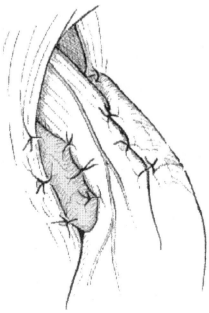

12. What are the success rates for such procedures?

All of the procedures described in question 11 eliminate GERD in about 90% of patients who are followed for 10 years. The Nissen fundoplication is considered to be the most effective in comparison studies.

13. What are the long-term complications of such procedures?

The repair may fail, with recurrence of reflux, after each operation. Incorrect placement or slippage of the stomach wrap can complicate Nissen fundoplication and the Belsey Mark IV procedure. Dysphagia and the inability to belch (gas-bloat syndrome) result from too tight a wrap. The Angelchik prosthesis may erode into a viscus or become displaced.

14. How can stricture from GERD be managed?

Pliable (unfixed) strictures can be dilated. Fixed strictures require surgical repair. One such operation is to patch the narrowed esophagus with stomach wall (Thal).

CONTROVERSIES

15. Is GERD better treated in the long-term by PPI therapy or Nissen fundoplication?

The effectiveness of PPI therapy in resolving esophagitis and eliminating symptoms of GERD is excellent, but the side effects of the medication over years are not fully known. Fundoplication frees the patient from the need for daily medicine but causes morbidity in about 5% of the patients.

16. Is Nissen fundoplication better done by laparoscopy or laparotomy?

Exactly the same procedure can be accomplished by either approach. The incidence of postoperative morbidity and mortality is comparable. The distinct advantages of laparoscopy are less postoperative pain, shorter hospitalization, and earlier return to work.

BIBLIOGRAPHY

1. Bremmer RM, DeMeester TR, Crookes F, et al: The effect of symptoms and nonspecific motility abnormalities on outcomes of surgical therapy for gastroesophageal reflux. J Thorac Cardiovasc Surg 107:1244, 1994.
2. Collard JM, Verstraete L, Otte JB, et al: Clinical, radiological and functional results of remedial antireflux operations. Int Surg 78:298, 1993.
3. DeMeester TR, Peters JH, Bremner CG, Chandrasoma P: Biology of gastroesophageal reflux disease: Pathophysiology relating to medical and surgical treatment. Annu Rev Med 50:469–506, 1999.
4. Hetzel DJ, Dent J, Reed WED, et al: Healing and relapse of severe peptic esophagitis after treatment with omeprazole. Gastroenterology 95:903, 1988.
5. Hinder RA, Filipi CJ, Wetscher G, et al: Laparoscopic Nissen fundoplication is an effective treatment for gastroesophageal reflux disease. Ann Surg 220:472, 1994.
6. Lagergren J, Bergstrom R, Lindgren A, Nyren O: Symptomatic gastroesophageal reflux as a risk factor for esophageal adenocarcinoma. New Engl J Med 340:825–831, 1999.
7. Liegermann DA: Medical therapy for chronic reflux esophagitis: Long-term follow-up. Arch Intern Med 147:1717, 1987.
8. Peters JH, DeMeester TR (eds): Minimally Invasive Surgery of the Foregut. St. Louis, Quality Medical Publishing, 1994.
9. Spechler SJ: Comparison of medical and surgical therapy for complicated gastroesophageal reflux disease in veterans. N Engl J Med 326:786, 1992.
10. Spivak H, Lulcuk S, Hunter JG: Laparoscopic surgery of the gastroesophageal junction. World J Surg 23:356–367, 1999.
11. Trus TL, Laycock WS, Waring JP, et al: Improvement in quality of life measures after laparoscopic antireflux surgery. Ann Surg 229:331–336, 1999.
12. Urschel JD: Complications of antireflux surgery. Am J Surg 166:68, 1993.
13. Watson DI, Jamieson JG, Pike GK, Davies N, et al: Prospective randomized double-blind trial between laparoscopic Nissen fundoplication and anterior partial fundoplication. Br J Surg 86:120–130, 1999.

44. ESOPHAGEAL CANCER

James R. Mault, M.D.

1. What are the risk factors for developing esophageal cancer?

Both alcohol and tobacco abuse increase the risk of developing carcinoma of the esophagus by a factor of ten. Additional risk factors include Barrett's esophagus with dysplasia as well as vitamin and trace element deficiencies and chemical toxins.

2. What is the epidemiology of carcinoma of the esophagus?

Esophageal cancer accounts for 1% of all cancers and 2% of cancer-related deaths. The incidence of carcinoma of the esophagus is 500 times greater in Asian countries than in Western countries.

3. What is Barrett's esophagus?

Barrett's esophagus, which results from chronic reflux of gastric fluid, is a histologic change in the esophageal mucosa in which the normal squamous mucosa is replaced with a glandular gastric type of mucosa. If the metaplasia progresses to high-grade dysplasia, patients with Barrett's esophagus have a 40-fold increased risk of developing adenocarcinoma. The relative incidence of adenocarcinoma of the esophagus compared with squamous cell carcinoma has increased dramatically over the past 20 years because of the comparable increase in the incidence of Barrett's esophagus.

4. What are the most common presenting symptoms of esophageal cancer?

Dysphagia	85%
Weight loss	60%
Pain	25%
Reflux	25%
Hoarseness	5%
Cough	3%

5. What is the anatomic distribution of esophageal cancer?

The esophagus is divided into three anatomic segments: upper, middle, and lower thirds. Fifteen percent of these cancers arise in the upper-third, 50% in the middle third, and 35% in the lower third.

6. What is the diagnostic work-up for patients presenting with the above symptoms?

1. Careful history and physical exam
2. Upper GI series
3. Upper endoscopy with biopsies of all concerning luminal structures
4. CT scan of chest and abdomen to define nodal and potential metastatic disease
5. Endoscopic ultrasound to define the T-stage (size) of the primary mass

7. What is neoadjuvant chemotherapy? What are its advantages and disadvantages?

Chemotherapy and/or radiation therapy to the primary lesion prior to surgical resection. The advantages of neoadjuvant strategies include:

1. Potential downstaging of the primary lesion
2. Early treatment of micrometastatic disease
3. Better tolerated and improved patient compliance (before surgery)
4. Preoperative stress test
5. Verification of primary tumor's sensitivity to the neoadjuvant regimen

The disadvantages of neoadjuvant strategies include:

1. The possibility of delay in treatment of the primary lesion, particularly when the primary tumor progresses despite neoadjuvant therapy

2. The theoretical disadvantage of selection for chemoresistant cell lines

8. What are the options for treatment of carcinoma of the esophagus?

Treatments include chemotherapy, radiation, resection, laser ablation, esophageal stenting, and dilation. Chemotherapy, radiation, and surgery are primary modes of therapy, which may be directed at complete resection and the occasional chance for cure. The surgical options include transabdominal resection of lesions located at the gastroesophageal junction; left thoracoabdominal (Sweet) procedure; combined abdominal (midline) and right thoracotomy (Ivor-Lewis procedure) with intrathoracic anastamosis; or transhiatal esophagectomy with cervical anastomosis. Laser therapy, esophageal stenting procedures, and dilation are reserved for palliation.

9. What major risk factors are associated with resection for carcinoma of the esophagus?

1. Death	5. Anastomotic stricture
2. Hemorrhage	6. Local recurrence of cancer
3. Anastomotic leak	7. Dysphagia
4. Empyema and sepsis	

10. What is the natural history of esophageal cancer?

In a collected series of almost 1,000 untreated patients, the 1- and 2-year survival rates were 6% and 0.3%, respectively. Untreated patients typically succumb to progressive malnutrition complicated by aspiration pneumonia, sepsis, and death. Formation of a fistula between the aorta or pulmonary artery and the esophagus or pulmonary tree is a somewhat more dramatic or perhaps merciful mode of exit.

11. After traditional esophagogastrectomy, what is the survival rate by stage?

Survival Rates after Surgery by Stage

	2 YEARS(%)	5 YEARS(%)
Stage I	29	12
Stage II	20	6
Stage III	6	0

12. Which sites are most commonly involved in distant metastatic spread of esophageal cancer?

Lung, liver, and bone.

BIBLIOGRAPHY

1. Orringer M: Multimodality therapy for esophageal carcinoma-update. Chest 103:406–409, 1993.
2. Reed C: Techniques of esophageal surgery. Chest Surg Clin North Am 5:379–574, 1995.
3. Walsh T: A comparison of multimodal therapy and surgery for esophageal adenocarcinoma. N Engl J Med 335:462–467, 1996.
4. Meluch AA: Preoperative (neoadjuvant) chemotherapy plus radiation therapy for esophageal carcinoma. Cancer J Sci Am 5:84–91, 1995.
5. Kelsen DP: Chemotherapy followed by surgery compared with surgery alone for localized esophageal cancer. N Engl J Med 339:1979–1984, 1998.
6. Smith A: Role of laparoscopic ultrasonography in the management of patients with oesophagogastric cancer. Br J Surg 86:1083–1087, 1999.
7. Jonker D: Neoadjuvant chemotherapy before surgery for resectable carcinoma of the lower esophagus. Dis Esoph 12:144–148, 1999.
8. Swaroop VS: Re: Practice guidelines for esophageal cancer. Am J Gastroenterol 94:2319–2320, 1999.

45. ACID-PEPTIC ULCER DISEASE

Frank H. Chae, M.D.

DUODENAL ULCER DISEASE

1. What is the incidence of duodenal ulcers?

Duodenal ulcers occur most frequently between ages 20–60 years, with peak incidence in the fourth decade. The lifetime risk for duodenal ulcer is about 1 in 14 for both genders.

2. What is the cause of duodenal ulcer?

Helicobacter pylori, a gram-negative bacillus, is strongly associated with peptic ulcer disease. Ulcers may occur in the setting of hyperacid secretion, normal acid secretion, or after acid reduction operations such as vagotomy. Recurrent or multiple ulceration may indicate an underlying endocrine disease. Breakdown of duodenal mucosal barrier is also thought to contribute to ulcerogenesis.

3. Is acid hypersecretion necessary for the onset of peptic ulcer disease?

No. Gastric hypersecretion of acid and pepsin plays an important role in ulcer formation; however, only 40% of ulcer sufferers manifest hypersecretion.

4. What are the clinically important complications of *H. pylori* infection?

Peptic ulcer disease. *H. pylori* is present in more than 90% of peptic ulcers. Up to one-half of the general population may harbor this organism, but only a small percentage develops ulcer disease. *H. pylori* may be part of the indigenous human gastric flora; antigens were detected in South American mummies as old as 1700 years.

Gastric carcinoma. *H. pylori* is strongly linked to gastric cancer and is now classified as a group I carcinogen. It also may cause mucosa-associated lymphoid tissue-lymphoma.

Barrett's esophagus is a possible *H. pylori*-associated as well as gastroesophageal reflux disease.

H. pylori probably exacerbates gastropathy and ulcer associated with nonsteroidal anti-inflammatory drug (NSAID) use.

5. What is the most commonly used test for *H. pylori*?

The **CLO test** is used most commonly to detect the presence of *H. pylori*. *H. pylori* releases urease, which breaks down urea to ammonia and bicarbonate, thus increasing the pH reading. The CLO test can be performed at the time of endoscopy by obtaining scrapings from the antral mucosa.

If endoscopy is not available, the **enzyme-linked immunosorbent assay** (ELISA) may be used to detect anti-*H. pylori* IgA and IgG antibody titers.

Direct culture of the organism should be reserved for cases in which antibiotic resistance becomes the issue.

6. What other risk factors are associated with duodenal ulcer disease?

1. Cigarette smoking is a major risk factor; its cessation is a key component of ulcer therapy.

2. Blood group O is associated with higher incidence of duodenal ulcer than other blood types, as are leukocyte antigens HLA-B5, B12, and BW35.

3. NSAIDs promote ulcer formation by suppressing systemic prostaglandin production.

4. Chronic pancreatitis, cirrhosis, emphysema, and alpha-1 antitrypsin deficiency.

7. Which endocrine disorder is associated with severe ulcer disease?

Patients with multiple endocrine neoplasia (MEN type I) have a 50–85% incidence of gastrinoma with severe ulcer diathesis.

8. What other endocrine disorders should be screened?

Pituitary tumor and hyperparathyroidism should be suspected when MEN type I is considered.

9. What are the clinical presentations of peptic ulcer disease?

1. Pain is usually epigastric in origin, although radiation to the back may indicate pancreatic involvement. It is often relieved by food or antacid ingestion. Nausea and vomiting may occur.
2. Upper GI bleeding
3. Gastric outlet obstruction (GOO) may result from pyloric spasm, inflammatory mass constriction, duodenal scarring, or fibrosis.
4. Perforation is a surgical emergency with a mortality rate of 5–10%. Perforation may occur without prior history of peptic ulcer disease, especially if the ulcer is situated on the anterior surface of the duodenum.

10. How does the location of the ulcer affect its clinical presentation?

Anterior wall ulcers (usually first portion of duodenum) may perforate and cause peritonitis with free air in the abdomen. Posterior ulcers may erode into the gastroduodenal artery or pancreas.

11. What are the differential diagnoses of epigastric pain?

In addition to peptic ulcer disease, gastroesophageal reflux disease, gastritis, gastric carcinoma, biliary tract disease, pancreatitis or pancreatic carcinoma, and myocardial ischemia should be considered.

12. What tests should be performed to evaluate epigastric pain? When?

Patients presenting with recurrent upper abdominal pain should be investigated. Flexible esophagogastroduodenoscopy (EGD) is preferred, although the upper GI contrast study with barium may be acceptable. The CLO test can be performed at the time of the EGD if indicated. Ultrasound should be performed if gallbladder disease is suspected, and a baseline electrocardiogram should be obtained if ischemic heart disease is in question.

13. How do you treat duodenal ulcer?

Diet: aspirin and NSAIDs must be discontinued. Alcohol, caffeine, and especially nicotine via smoking or chewing should be avoided.

Antacids: neutralizing gastric pH may alleviate symptoms, but its impact on ulcer healing is not well defined.

H_2 receptor antagonists: cimetidine or ranitidine prevents gastric acid secretions by blocking H_2 histamine receptor.

Sucralfate: a protective-barrier medicine that adheres to the ulcer base, providing a protective coating. Medications that decrease acid secretion should not be used because sucralfate requires an acidic environment to be activated.

Proton pump inhibitors: omeprazole blocks the hydrogen-potassium adenosine triphosphatase pump in the gastric parietal cells to inhibit hydrogen ion release. It usually is reserved for failures of first-line therapy (i.e., H_2 receptor antagonists).

***H. pylori* eradication:** if *H. pylori* infection is diagnosed, the combination of triple therapy (bismuth, tetracycline, and metronidazole) with an H_2 receptor antagonist regimen appears to provide a 90% cure rate. Erythromycin, amoxicillin-omeprazole, or erythromycin-omeprazole may be added for initial failures.

14. What are the recurrence rates after medical therapy?

Approximately 75–95% of duodenal ulcers heal in 4–6 weeks. The recurrence rate within 1 year of treatment is 70%; thus, repeated courses of treatment may be necessary.

15. What complications are associated with medical therapy?

H_2 receptor antagonists may induce mental status changes and gynecomastia. Cimetidine, in particular, may affect hepatic metabolism of warfarin, phenytoin, theophylline, propranolol, and digoxin, leading to abnormal serum levels. Omeprazole may cause hypergastrinemia by blocking gastric acid secretion. *H. pylori* resistance to antibiotics may develop, especially to metronidazole; hence, a triple combination of at least two antimicrobials with an acid inhibitory drug is recommended as initial therapy.

16. How should recurrent or multiple ulcers be evaluated?

In addition to the previously mentioned work-up, serum gastrin levels should be obtained to evaluate for possible endocrine disorder. Patients should be off omeprazole when tested for gastrin. In Zollinger-Ellison syndrome, gastrin hypersecretion from the pancreatic islet tumor results in multiple or intractable ulcers (normal serum gastrin, < 200 pg/ml; Zollinger-Ellison syndrome, usually > 500 pg/ml).

17. How do you evaluate a borderline gastrin value (200–500 pg/ml)?

The secretin stimulation test may be used to diagnose Zollinger-Ellison syndrome. An intravenous bolus of secretin (2 U/kg) should result in a rise of gastrin level of 150 pg/ml within 15 minutes.

18. What are the indications for operative treatment of duodenal ulcers?

Failure of medial management to control bleeding (> 6 units of packed red blood cell transfusions in 24 hours), obstruction, and intractability are the usual indications. Perforation of the ulcer is usually treated surgically unless the patient presents 24 hours after the event without peritonitis and the gastrograffin upper GI series confirms that the perforation has been well sealed.

19. What operations are used to treat duodenal ulcers?

1. Truncal vagotomy and pyloroplasty or gastrojejunostomy
2. Truncal vagotomy and antrectomy with Billroth I or II anastomosis
3. Subtotal gastrectomy with Billroth I or II anastomosis
4. Highly selective vagotomy
5. Total gastrectomy

20. What are Billroth I and Billroth II anastomoses?

The **Billroth I** operation refers to an anastomosis between the duodenum and the gastric remnant (gastroduodenostomy). The **Billroth II** is constructed by sewing a loop of jejunum to the gastric remnant (gastrojejunostomy). Either method is acceptable.

21. Which procedure is preferred, Billroth I or Billroth II?

Billroth I has the advantages of eliminating the duodenal stump and requiring only one suture line instead of two (as in Billroth II). Duodenal stump blowout is a critical surgical emergency requiring immediate laparotomy. Afferent loop syndrome is also a complication of Billroth II. Bile reflux gastritis may occur in both procedures. Billroth I is more physiologic; thus, it results in better protein and fat digestion. Billroth I has the disadvantage of being more liable to gastric outlet obstruction with ulcer or tumor recurrence; therefore, Billroth I is generally not recommended for gastric carcinoma.

22. What is the afferent loop syndrome?

Postprandial abdominal pain often is relieved by bilious vomiting. A narrowing at the junction of the stomach and duodenal side of a Billroth II anastomosis leads to biliary and pancreatic fluid build-up within the afferent limb of the intestine. Pain is relieved when the fluid content is emptied into the stomach, which may result in bilious vomiting and severe reflux gastritis.

23. How is the afferent loop syndrome prevented?

Prevention requires avoidance of a long or twisted afferent limb with too narrow an anastomosis during Billroth II reconstruction. The use of Billroth I eliminates this factor.

24. What are the rates of ulcer recurrence after surgical treatment?

Vagotomy and pyloroplasty: 10%
Vagotomy and antrectomy: 2–3%
Highly selective vagotomy: 10–15%
Subtotal gastrectomy: 1–2%
Total gastrectomy: < 1%

25. What is the mortality rate of these operations?

Vagotomy and pyloroplasty: 1%
Vagotomy and antrectomy: 1–3%
Highly selective vagotomy: 0.1%
Subtotal gastrectomy: 1–2%
Total gastrectomy: 2–5%

26. How do you treat a perforated duodenal ulcer?

The patient must be resuscitated first, following the ABCs of airway, breathing, and circulation. Stomach content is emptied via nasogastric tube. Surgical closure by omental patch (Graham closure) is widely practiced. For hemodynamically stable patients, oversewing of the ulcer followed by highly selective vagotomy may be added. Vagotomy and antrectomy to remove the ulcer are another alternative if the patient has a history of recurrent or intractable peptic ulcer disease.

27. What is the long-term result after Graham closure of a perforated ulcer?

One-third of patients remain asymptomatic, one-third have symptoms controlled by medical treatment, and one-third require an additional ulcer operation.

28. Who was Billroth?

Christian Albert Theodor Billroth (1829–1894) was an Austrian surgeon credited with performing the first gastric resection in 1881 and introducing innovations to intestinal bypass operations. The American surgeon William Halstead was an apprentice to Billroth when he was training in Vienna.

29. What are the complications of surgery for duodenal ulcers?

1. **Duodenal stump leakage** may occur within the first week after antral resection and Billroth anastomosis. Treatment consists of prompt reoperation to drain and control the leak. Total parenteral nutrition may be required as an adjunct to treatment.

2. **Gastric retention** may occur because of edema at the anastomosis or atony of the stomach after vagotomy. It usually resolves spontaneously in 3–4 weeks.

3. **Bleeding** may occur from a suture line, a missed ulcer, or other gastric mucosal lesions. Most postgastrectomy bleeding ceases spontaneously, but endoscopy may be necessary in some cases.

30. Where do ulcers recur after operation?

Ulcers usually recur adjacent to the gastric anastomosis on the intestinal side (jejunum, duodenum).

31. Why do they recur?

The responsible factors are inadequate gastric resection, incomplete vagotomy, inadequate drainage of the gastric remnant (stasis of gastric contents proximal to the anastomosis), or retained gastric antrum (Billroth II anastomosis).

32. How does alkaline or bile reflux gastritis recur?

Reflux of bile and pancreatic secretions into the stomach after a Billroth II anastomosis may cause marked gastric irritation, leading to chronic postprandial pain. Persistent pain should be evaluated with endoscopy, and surgical reconstruction should be considered, usually with a Roux-en-Y gastrojejunostomy from a 40-cm efferent jejunal limb.

33. What is the dumping syndrome?

Truncal vagotomy removes the vagal innervation to the stomach and pylorus, leading to uncontrolled, rapid emptying of hyperosmolar gastric contents into the proximal small bowel. The osmotic and glucose shifts produce symptoms of palpitation, sweating, flushing, weakness, nausea, abdominal cramps, and syncope. Ingesting a small, dry, low-carbohydrate meal may alleviate the symptoms. Anticholinergic drugs also may help. About 10–20% of patients experience the dumping syndrome in the early postoperative period, but 1–3% develop chronic problems.

34. How do you treat pyloric stenosis?

Fluid resuscitation and nasogastric tube decompression should be initiated. Metabolic alkalosis may be present as a result of prolonged vomiting (loss of hydrogen ions) and should be corrected with normal saline infusion. Either vagotomy with gastrojejunostomy or resection of the stenosis with a Billroth II bypass is acceptable. Partial gastrectomy is another option.

GASTRIC ULCER DISEASE

35. What is the most important factor to consider in managing gastric ulcers?

All gastric ulcers must be evaluated for malignancy. The incidence of malignancy is about 10%.

36. How do you investigate for gastric ulcer?

Esophagogastroduodenoscopy (EGD) with multiple biopsies of the ulcer crater is the best method. Upper GI series may be helpful but is not diagnostic. Biopsy is mandatory. The CLO test can be performed at the time of the EGD to detect *H. pylori*.

37. How are gastric ulcers classified?

Type I	At the incisura or most inferior portion of the lesser curvature
Type II	Gastric ulcer + duodenal ulcer
Type III	Prepylorus
Type IV	Gastroesophageal junction/proximal cardia
Type V	Any ulcer from NSAID or aspirin use

38. Which is the most common type of gastric ulcer?

Type I.

39. How do benign gastric ulcers differ from duodenal ulcers?

Benign gastric ulcers are difficult to treat and have a higher rate of recurrence and complications. Gastric ulcer disease and gastric carcinoma have a probable common etiologic factor, which is atrophic gastritis induced by *H. pylori*. By contrast, factors associated with duodenal ulcer may protect against gastric cancer.

40. How is *H. pylori* related to gastric ulcer disease?

H. pylori colonization induces chronic active gastritis, which is associated with ulcer formation, although a direct cause-and-effect link has not been clearly established. Other factors such as focal defect in acid neutralization that allows acid diffusion into the stomach mucosa or hypersecretion of acid (in cases of type II and III ulcers) may play important roles.

41. What is a "trial of healing"?

A combination of H_2 receptor antagonists or hydrogen pump inhibitors with anti-*H. pylori* medications, if indicated, may be tried for 6–12 weeks. A second EGD should be performed to evaluate the ulcer. An additional trial of 12 weeks is acceptable provided that no malignancy is detected.

42. What is the aim of *H. pylori* eradication in the setting of gastric ulcer?

Therapy aimed at *H. pylori* eradication is associated with increased ulcer healing and decreased ulcer relapse rates. Several series have shown decreases in recurrences from 50% to < 10% with *H. pylori* eradication. *H. pylori* is strongly linked to gastric cancer and is now classified as a group I carcinogen. It also may cause mucosa-associated lymphoid tissue-lymphoma.

43. How do you treat *H. pylori* infection?

A triple therapy of bismuth, metronidazole, and tetracycline, usually supplemented with an H_2 receptor antagonist.

44. Does gastric ulcer healing imply a benign state?

No. Gastric ulcers with foci of malignancy may heal completely on medical therapy.

45. What are the indications for operative therapy of benign gastric ulcers?

Indications are hemorrhage, perforation, obstruction, and intractability.

46. What is the definitive procedure for benign gastric ulcers?

Hemigastrectomy or antrectomy (including the ulcer) without vagotomy is the standard procedure.

47. What are the options under emergent (hemorrhage/perforation) conditions?

Hemodynamically stable: truncal vagotomy and distal gastrectomy

Unstable: truncal vagotomy and drainage procedure with biopsy and excision/oversewing of ulcer

48. What is the rebleeding rate if the ulcer is left in situ?

20–40%.

49. What is giant gastric ulcer?

An ulcer > 3 cm in diameter, usually located along the lesser curvature. The malignancy risk is about 30% and increases with the size of the diameter. Early surgical resection is indicated because of the malignancy risk. Vagotomy may be added.

50. What is a Cushing ulcer?

An ulcer found in a critically ill patient with central nervous system injury.

51. What is a Curling ulcer?

An ulcer found in a critically ill patient with burn injury.

52. What is a Dieulafoy ulcer?

Erosion of the gastric mucosa overlying a vascular malformation, which often leads to hemorrhage. Chronic inflammation is not associated with this lesion.

53. What is a marginal ulcer?

An ulcer found near the margin of the gastroenteric anastomosis, usually on the small bowel side.

BIBLIOGRAPHY

1. Correa P, Willis D, Allison MJ, et al: *Helicobacter pylori* in pre-Columbian mummies. Gastroenterology 114(Suppl 4):A956, 1998.
2. Donahue PE, Griffith C, Richter HM: A 50-year perspective upon selective gastric vagotomy. Am J Surg 172:9–12, 1996.
3. Emas S, Grupcev G, Eriksson B: Six-year results of a prospective, randomized trial of selective proximal vagotomy with and without pyloroplasty in the treatment of duodenal, pyloric, and prepyloric ulcers. Ann Surg 217:6–14, 1993.
4. Hansson LE, Nyren O, Hsing AW, et al: The risk of stomach cancer in patients with gastric or duodenal ulcer disease. N Engl J Med 335:242–249, 1996.
5. Jordan PH: Type I gastric ulcer treated by parietal cell vagotomy and mucosal ulcerectomy. J Am Coll Surg 182:388–393, 1996.
6. Lee WJ, Wu MS, Chen CN, et al: Seroprevalence of *Helicobacter pylori* in patients with surgical peptic ulcer. Arch Surg 132:430–433, 1997.
7. Malliwah JA, Tabaqchali M, Watson J, Venables CW: Audit of the outcome of peptic ulcer disease diagnosed 10 to 20 years previously. Gut 38:812–815, 1996.
8. Peura D: *Helicobacter pylori:* Rational management options. Am J Med 105:424–430, 1998.

46. SMALL BOWEL OBSTRUCTION

Joyce A. Majure, M.D.

1. Name three mechanisms of bowel obstruction. Give examples of each type.

1. **Extrinsic compression:** adhesions (60%), malignancy (20%), hernias (10%), volvulus, and others

2. **Internal blockage of the lumen** (usually at the ileocecal valve) by abnormal materials (obturation): bezoars, gallstones, worms, or foreign body

3. **Mural disease** encroaching on the lumen: inflammatory bowel disease (5%); fibrous structure secondary to trauma, ischemia, or radiation; or intussusception

2. What are the most common symptoms of small bowel obstruction (SBO)?

1. Abdominal pain: initially nonspecific; often colicky, coinciding with waves of peristalsis trying to pass the point of obstruction

2. Bloating: the more distal the obstruction, the more severe the abdominal distention due to proximal bowel dilation

3. Vomiting: bilious, frequent, and profuse with proximal obstruction; less frequent but larger volume and often feculent with distal obstruction

4. Obstipation: failure to pass gas or stool; occasionally patients have a few loose stools early in the course of disease because the bowel distal to the obstruction empties

3. What are the pertinent factors in the patient's history?

1. Previous abdominal or pelvic surgery

2. Previous SBO

3. History of cancer: type and treatment (radiation?)

4. Previous abdominal infections or inflammation (including pelvic inflammatory disease, appendicitis, diverticulitis, inflammatory bowel disease, perforation, and trauma)

5. History of gallstones

6. Current medications, particularly anticoagulants, anticholinergics, chemotherapy, or diuretics

4. What are the findings of the physical exam?

Patients often are dehydrated and may have a low-grade fever, postural hypotension, and abdominal distention. Bowel sounds may be hyperactive with tinkles and rushes or totally silent if the patient has delayed seeking treatment. Percussion usually reveals diffuse tympani, and thin elderly patients may even have visible loops of distended small bowel. Palpation may increase the abdominal pain, but localized tenderness or peritoneal signs indicate likely strangulation or another diagnosis.

5. Do I need to do a rectal exam?

Absolutely. The rectal exam may reveal signs of cancer, such as a rigid rectal shelf from carcinomatosis. Blood on hemoccult exam may herald ischemia or strangulation or indicate inflammatory bowel disease. An obturator hernia is best palpated transrectally or transvaginally.

6. Where should I look for obstructing hernias?

Examine the groin near the pubic tubercle and along the inguinal floor. Check the femoral triangles for bulging or tenderness. Do a rectal exam to check for obturator hernias (see above), and palpate all existing incisions. Check all trocar sites from previous laparoscopic surgeries.

7. What is the least expensive way to confirm the diagnosis?

The four-way abdominal series (flat and upright abdominal films plus posteroanterior and lateral chest radiographs) is diagnostic in about 75% of cases. Look for:

1. Air-fluid levels in dilated small intestine (also known as stair steps or string-of-pearls sign).

2. Absent or minimal air in the distal colon and rectum.

3. "Ground-glass" appearance and obscuring of the psoas shadows by extraperitoneal fluid.

4. Sometimes a single distended loop of small bowel with a "beak" at each end indicates a closed loop obstruction in an otherwise gasless abdomen, or a single fixed loop may remain in the same location on both supine and upright films.

5. Chest radiograph may demonstrate an infiltrate with accompanying ileus rather than SBO. The lateral chest radiograph is the most sensitive for identifying free air in the abdomen, which necessitates urgent laparotomy for perforated viscus.

8. What other imaging studies can be used?

1. Oral contrast studies with barium or water-soluble contrast help to distinguish partial from complete obstruction, intraluminal tumor or foreign body, and inflammatory bowel disease; they also may define the point of obstruction.

2. The accuracy of computed tomography (CT) scan is approximately 95%. CT may help to distinguish SBO from paralytic ileus; to identify tumor, abscess, hematoma, and occasionally a missed hernia; and to help identify strangulation and level of obstruction.

3. Ultrasound and magnetic resonance imaging (MRI) have been used with varying success when abdominal films are inconclusive but are *not* often used because of inaccuracy (ultrasound) or expense (MRI).

9. What laboratory studies are indicated?

1. Complete blood count to check for leukocytosis or unexpected anemia.

2. Urinalysis to look for urinary tract infection (which also may cause an ileus and present with a picture similar to SBO) and to assess hydration (urine specific gravity).

3. Chemistry panel to check for electrolyte abnormalities such as hypokalemic or hypochloremic metabolic alkalosis, hyponatremia, and prerenal azotemia (elevated blood urea nitrogen and creatinine).

4. Amylase levels to rule out pancreatitis (also may be elevated, although not as high, with ischemic bowel).

10. What are the initial steps in treatment?

Initiate nasogastric (NG) suction and IV fluids to restore electrolyte and fluid balance; use a Foley catheter to monitor urine output. As soon as resuscitation is complete, prompt surgical intervention is mandatory for complete obstructions.

11. How can I distinguish between complete and partial obstruction?

1. **Clinical features:** patients with partial obstruction may continue to pass small amounts of gas or stool. Pain and distention decrease rapidly with NG suction.

2. **Radiographic features:** radiographs show gas moving into the colon in patients with partial obstruction.

3. **Oral contrast studies:** barium or water-soluble contrast given via the NG tube shows passage of contrast into the colon in partial obstructions.

12. What conditions should be included in the differential diagnosis?

• Ileus from other causes (e.g., urinary tract infection, pneumonia, hypokalemia)
• Viral gastroenteritis
• Appendicitis (usually with perforation)
• Ureteral stone
• Diverticulitis
• Mesenteric thrombosis
• Obstructing colon cancer

13. What are the three types of SBO based on bowel viability?

Simple obstruction: nothing passes the point of obstruction, but the vascular supply is not compromised. The obstruction may be partial and resolve with nonoperative management.

Strangulated obstruction: the mesenteryis twisted, or the bowel is so dilated that arterial or venous flow is cut off and the bowel becomes ischemic. Urgent surgery is mandatory.

Closed-loop obstruction: the bowel is obstructed proximally and distally, usually for a short segment. The obstructed segment becomes massively dilated and susceptible to strangulation as well as perforation. Urgent surgery is mandatory.

14. What are the five classic signs of strangulation? How accurate are they?

1. Continuous pain (not colicky)
2. Fever
3. Tachycardia
4. Peritoneal signs (localized guarding or tenderness, rebound tenderness)
5. Leukocytosis

These signs usually indicate irreversible ischemia. Persistent pain, progressive fever, or leukocytosis, therefore, is an indication for surgery.

15. What is the mortality rate of SBO?

Simple obstruction: about 5% if surgery is performed within 24 hours.

Strangulated obstruction: about 25%, depending on the patient's resiliency (comorbid disease).

16. What operative interventions may be needed for treatment of SBO?

• Open or laparoscopic lysis of adhesions at the point of obstruction
• Reduction and repair of hernia
• Resection of obstructing lesions with primary anastomosis
• Resection of strangulated segment with primary anastomosis
• Bypass of obstructing lesions (used mostly for carcinomatosis)
• Placement of a long tube (Baker tube is the most commonly used)

17. Describe the criteria for distinguishing viable from dead bowel at the time of operation.

Color, peristalsis, and arterial pulsations are the most obvious ways to identify viable intestine. In questionable cases, Doppler ultrasound can detect arterial pulsations, but the most reliable method is intravenous injection of fluorescein dye with use of a Wood's lamp. Viable bowel fluoresces purple.

18. What is the risk of development of SBO after initial laparotomy? After previous laparotomy for SBO? Which operations are associated with high rates of SBO?

- Approximately 15% of all patients undergoing laparotomy eventually develop SBO.
- About 12% of patients with a prior SBO develop another obstruction. The more recurrences, the higher the recurrence rate.
- Total or subtotal colectomy has an SBO rate of 11% at 1 year and 30% at 10 years. Hysterectomy also carries a high rate of SBO: about 5% for routine procedures and up to 15% after radical hysterectomy.

19. What can the surgeon do to decrease the risk of SBO?

1. Use powderless gloves, or at least wash powder from gloves.
2. Avoid suturing through the peritoneum at closure.
3. Use barrier film between the incision and small intestine.

20. What is the role of laparoscopy in SBO?

Laparoscopic lysis of adhesions usually is reserved for patients who have not had multiple previous laparotomies. Approximately one-third can be treated successfully by laparoscopy alone, one-third require a minimal laparotomy ("lap-assisted"), and about one-third require a full open laparotomy.

21. What can be done for patients with multiply recurrent bowel obstructions due to adhesions?

Long tube placement, either NG or via gastrostomy or jejunostomy, with the tube advanced to the ileocecal valve. The long tube is left in position for approximately 7 days and reportedly allows the bowel to reform adhesions in more gentle curves. Many other techniques have been tried and abandoned, including Noble plication (suturing the bowel in orderly loops) and adding various irrigants (heparin, Dextran, saline) to the peritoneal cavity before closure.

22. Name five complications associated with surgery for SBO.

1. Enterotomy	4. Abscess
2. Prolonged ileus	5. Recurrent obstruction
3. Wound infection	

23. Name three new barrier products designed to decrease adhesion formation.

1. Oxidized cellulose (Interceed)
2. Polytetrafluoroethylene (PTFE better known as Gore-Tex)
3. Sodium hyaluronate and carboxymethylcellulose (Seprafilm)

BIBLIOGRAPHY

1. Bass KN, Jones B, Bulkley GB: Current management of small-bowel obstruction. Adv Surg 31:1, 1997.
2. Beck DE, Opelka FG, Bailey HR, et al: Incidence of small-bowel obstruction and adhesiolysis after open colorectal and general surgery. Dis Colon Rectum 42:241, 1999.
3. Chen SC, Lin FY, Lee PH, et al: Water-soluble contrast study predicts the need for early surgery in adhesive small bowel obstruction. Br J Surg 85:1692, 1998.
4. DeCherney AH, diZerega GS: Clinical problem of intraperitoneal postsurgical adhesion formation following general surgery and the use of adhesion prevention barriers. Surg Clin North Am 77671, 1997.
5. Donciker V, Closset J, Van Gansbeke D, et al: Contribution of computed tomography to decision making in the management of adhesive small bowel obstruction. 85:1071, 1998.

6. Frager DH, Baer JW: Role of CT in evaluating patients with small bowel obstruction. Semin Ultrasound CT MRI 16:127, 1995.
7. Helton WS: Intestinal obstruction. Scientific American Surgery, Vol. 2, Section VII. Scientific American, 1996, p 3.
8. Leon EL, Metzger A, Tsiotos GG, et al: Laparoscopic management of small bowel obstruction: Indications and outcome. J Gastrointest Surg 2:132, 1998.

47. INTESTINAL ISCHEMIA

Patrick L. McConnell, M.D.

1. What is the arterial supply to the gut?

The foregut (stomach and duodenum) receives its blood supply from the **celiac artery**, the midgut (jejunum to the proximal descending colon) from the **superior mesenteric artery** (SMA), and hindgut (the remainder of the intraperitoneal gut) from the **inferior mesenteric artery** (IMA).

2. What are the major collaterals that may develop in response to gradual occlusion of one or more these vessels?

The **superior** and **inferior pancreaticoduodenal arteries** form the major collaterals between the celiac artery and the SMA. The IMA and SMA have more than one collateral communication. The **arc of Riolan** (meandering mesenteric artery) is larger and more central and connects the middle colic branch of the SMA and the left colic branch of the IMA. The **marginal artery of Drummond** is also made up of branches from the SMA and IMA, but it is more peripheral and usually is found within the mesentery near the splenic flexure (Griffith's point).

3. Name the arterial causes of acute intestinal ischemia.

The compromise of blood flow to one of the major vessels of the gut may result from thrombotic occlusion associated with atherosclerosis; embolic occlusion, most commonly of cardiac origin; or extrinsic compression, as occurs in a strangulated hernia or celiac compression syndrome (see Controversies). Nonocclusive mesenteric ischemia (NOMI) accounts for 20–30% of acute ischemic cases; arterial spasm is the most common etiology. Arterial spasm usually results, paradoxically, in response to systemic hypoperfusion. In such cases of hypoperfusion, this mechanism reduces splanchnic visceral blood flow during shock, preserving cardiac and cerebral blood flow.

4. What are the possible nonarterial causes of acute intestinal ischemia?

In cases of bowel wall distention, secondary to various mechanical etiologies or idiopathic (Ogilvie's syndrome), a point may be reached at which intraluminal pressure exceeds capillary filling pressure, resulting in ischemic colitis. By preventing adequate venous outflow, mesenteric venous thrombosis (MVT) may limit arterial inflow, resulting in hemocongestion. Hypercoagulable states such as polycythemia vera represent the greatest risk factor for MVT.

5. Does acute occlusion of one major artery cause bowel infarction? Which vessel is most likely to be affected?

Yes. Sudden occlusion of the SMA from an embolus is the most common cause of acute intestinal ischemia and may result in the infarction of the midgut due to the absence of well-developed collaterals. Emboli are more likely to involve the SMA, presumably because its origin from the aorta is at a more acute angle than the celiac artery, IMA, or renal arteries.

6. What is the diagnostic triad of acute embolic intestinal ischemia?

Sudden onset of (1) severe abdominal pain, (2) bowel evacuation (vomiting or diarrhea), and (3) a history of cardiac disease (arterial emboli). An additional hallmark is pain out of proportion to the physical findings, which is found clinically because at the time of presentation the patient's abdomen is without acute signs of peritonitis (e.g., rigidity). If the patient is not treated, peritonitis eventually develops.

7. Which laboratory value is diagnostic of acute intestinal ischemia? Is acidosis?

None and no. Acidosis is a late finding in less than 25% of patients, but when present it is a poor prognostic indicator. Although leukocytosis is found in the majority of patients, no laboratory studies are specific. The diagnosis is pursued on clinical suspicion alone.

8. When acute intestinal ischemia is suspected, what study is diagnostic?

Emergent arteriography is diagnostic. It is important to obtain both anteroposterior and lateral views of the aorta to visualize the visceral vessels.

9. How is NOMI diagnosed and managed?

Angiography is required to document vasospasm in the absence of an organic occlusion. The right colon is most commonly affected because of its less consistent collateral blood flow. It is associated with and may be exacerbated by the concomitant use of digitalis in patients with systemic hypoperfusion. In severe cases associated with multisystem organ failure, the mortality rate approaches 70%. Treatment consists of infusing vasodilators (papaverine) through the angiogram catheter, but it is often less than effective. Of interest, the incidence is believed to be declining because of widespread use of calcium channel blockers and nitrates.

10. What is the primary cause of chronic mesenteric ischemia?

Atherosclerosis. Typically, atherosclerotic disease compromises flow to at least two of the three major arteries. Bowel infarction may be forestalled by development of collaterals.

11. What are the clinical features of patients with chronic mesenteric ischemia?

Weight loss is the most consistent sign of chronic mesenteric ischemia. Patients gradually and sometimes unknowingly become afraid to eat (food fear) because of postprandial pain (intestinal angina). In the absence of weight loss, the diagnosis of chronic intestinal ischemia is unlikely. Conversely, in patients with severe atherosclerosis and weight loss of unknown cause, mesenteric ischemia should be strongly considered. An epigastric bruit is an important sign suggestive of mesenteric occlusive disease.

12. How should patients with chronic mesenteric ischemia be evaluated?

Noninvasive ultrasound duplex scanning provides important physiologic information about the celiac axis and SMA. When surgery is planned or duplex scanning is equivocal (see Controversies), angiography is performed. The lateral view is the most informative.

13. If mesenteric vein thrombosis (MVT) is suspected, which test is best?

The signs and symptoms of MVT are similar to those of acute intestinal ischemia, but they often are more subtle. Delay in diagnosis is thought to contribute to the reported high mortality rate of 13–50%. Contrast-enhanced computed tomography (CT) scan has been considered the gold standard; however, recent evidence suggests that the sensitivity of magnetic resonance imaging (MRI) approaches 100%.

14. How do the operative findings differ in patients with atherosclerotic occlusion and patients with SMA embolism?

Because an SMA embolus usually lodges beyond the proximal jejunal and middle colic arteries, these bowel segments are usually spared. Thrombotic occlusion occurs at the ostia, where the atherosclerotic narrowing is most severe, causing ischemia of the entire midgut.

15. What is the appropriate surgical management of an SMA embolus?

Embolectomy, assessment of bowel viability 30 minutes after reperfusion, and resection of any infarcted bowel. Postoperative anticoagulation is essential to avoid further embolization.

16. How is visceral ischemia of thrombotic origin managed?

Mesenteric ischemia from thrombotic occlusion is the end-stage of progressive atherosclerotic occlusion. Thrombectomy alone is not sufficient; therefore, bypass or endarterectomy of the proximal diseased vessel(s) is necessary. Bowel viability is assessed after reperfusion.

17. What are the goals of arterial bypass?

Resolution of symptoms, improved nutrition, and prevention of visceral infarction are the primary goals of arterial bypass in chronic mesenteric ischemia. In some cases prophylactic arterial bypass may be done when collaterals have been compromised at the time of another operation (colon resection) and the bowel is believed to be in jeopardy.

18. Which intraoperative tests help the surgeon to determine bowel viability?

Both systemic intravenous infusion of fluorescein, which is evaluated using a Wood's lamp, and intraoperative Doppler examination of the bowel are helpful, but ultimately the decision is based on clinical judgment.

19. When the extent of bowel viability is in question, what should be done?

When massive resection would be required for all questionable bowel, the surgeon should schedule a second-look operation 12–24 hours later. Some segments that were initially questionable may become clearly viable during this period; salvaged small bowel may be critical in avoiding dependence on total parenteral nutrition (TPN).

20. How much small intestine is required to maintain adequate nutrition?

About 50–100 cm of small intestine is required to maintain adequate nutrition. The distal ileum and ileocecal valve are the most important segments to retain for vital bowel absorption and function.

21. Should a second-look operation be canceled because a patient improves?

Never. The decision is made in the operating room based on findings at the time of surgery. No clinical parameters within the ensuing 12–24 hours accurately indicate the status of the bowel in question.

22. What is the mortality rate of acute mesenteric ischemia?

Although the prognosis of embolic occlusion is somewhat better because of the dramatic presentation, the diagnosis of acute mesenteric ischemia is often made after infarction. The result is a high mortality rate (60–90%), regardless of cause.

23. What is ischemic colitis?

Ischemic colitis is circulatory insufficiency of the colon, which may result from occlusive, nonocclusive, and pharmacologic (cocaine and NSAIDs) causes. Seven percent of all patients having nonemergent abdominal aortic aneurysm surgery and nearly 60% of patients who survive a ruptured abdominal aortic aneurysm suffer from ischemic colitis. Most cases are mild, typically involving only the mucosa, abdominal pain, bloody diarrhea, and bloating. Severe disease (10–20% of cases) is characterized by transmural gangrenous infarction that presents with clear signs of peritonitis and bloody diarrhea.

24. How is ischemic colitis diagnosed and treated? What are its prognostic implications?

The diagnosis is made by endoscopy, which is prompted by bloody diarrhea. In idiopathic cases, angiography demonstrates patent large vessels because the responsible emboli/lesions are believed to involve peripheral, end-arterial vessels. Mild disease is typically treated conservatively with bowel rest, rehydration, and antibiotics. Severe disease requires surgical resection. Mortality rates, overall, are about 50%, but in patients requiring colon resection, the mortality rate may exceed 85%. The high mortality rate in the latter group is attributed to endotoxemic shock and multisystem organ failure.

CONTROVERSIES

25. What is celiac compression syndrome (Dunbar's syndrome)?

Celiac compression is a rare and controversial disorder most commonly described in women (female-to-male ratio = 4:1) between the ages of 20 and 50. Patients appear to suffer from chronic mesenteric ischemia without angiographic evidence of atherosclerotic disease. The mechanical compression is believed to be caused by the left crus of the diaphragm (marginal arcuate ligament), and diagnosis occasionally is confirmed by demonstrating transient celiac compression during expiration. The associated pain is the result of a complicated and still heavily debated redirection of flow (foregut steal) away from the SMA. Effective treatment has required not only release of the compression but also bypass to improve the likelihood of pain resolution.

26. Which is preferred for diagnosis of chronic mesenteric ischemia—fasting or postprandial duplex ultrasound?

Fasting peak systolic flow velocities (PSV) exceeding 275 cm/sec have been correlated with a 70% or greater stenosis in the corresponding artery. The sensitivity in such cases is 89%, and the specificity is 92%. Controversy exists as to whether it is necessary to determine postprandial flow velocities in patients who have already demonstrated occlusive criteria in the fasting state (> 275 cm/sec). Positive criteria for postprandial flow velocities stipulate that there must be less than a 20% increase in the PSV after a food challenge. The diagnostic advantage gained from a postprandial study appears minimal.

27. Which is the preferred treatment—antegrade or retrograde visceral artery bypass?

The terms antegrade and retrograde as they apply to intestinal bypass refer to the origin of the graft from the aorta as either proximal to the celiac axis or distal to the SMA, respectively. The stated advantages of antegrade bypass are less kinking of the graft and possibly better blood flow characteristics. The disadvantages are that supraceliac exposure is technically more difficult, and clamping may result in renal ischemia or spinal cord ischemia. Retrograde bypass grafts are more difficult to position to avoid kinking. The results for both are excellent.

28. What is the role percutaneous transluminal angioplasty (PTLA)?

The endovascular treatment of chronic mesenteric ischemia is a relatively new technique. The obvious avoidance of surgery is an important consideration, but the rare complications of dissection and embolus can be devastating in arterial beds without adequate collaterals. Success rates vary from 33% to 80%; restenosis and recurrent symptoms are reported in 30–50% of patients. No prospective trials have compared PTLA with conventional revascularization (arterial bypass).

BIBLIOGRAPHY

1. Allen R, Martin G, Rees C, et al: Mesenteric angioplasty in the treatment of chronic intestinal ischemia. J Vasc Surg 24:415–423, 1996.
2. Bradbury AW, Brittenden J, McBride K, Ruckely CV: Mesenteric ischemia: A multidisciplinary approach. Br J Surg 82:1446–1459, 1995.
3. Gewertz BL, Schwartz LB(eds): Mesenteric ischemia. Surg Clin North Am 77:275–502, 1997 [issue contains comprehensive reviews of the many areas related to mesenteric ischemia].
4. Gentile AT, Moneta GL, Lee RI, et al: Usefulness of fasting and post-prandial duplex ultrasound examinations for predicting high-grade superior mesenteric stenosis. Am J Surg 169:476–479, 1995.
5. Taylor LM: Management of visceral ischemic syndromes. In Rutherford RB (ed): Vascular Surgery, 4th ed. Philadelphia, W.B. Saunders, 1995.

48. DIVERTICULAR DISEASE OF THE COLON

Lawrence W. Norton, M.D.

1. What is a colonic diverticulum?

A colonic diverticulum is a protrusion of mucosa and submucosa through the muscular layers of the bowel wall. It has no muscular covering. Its formation may be related either to weakness of the bowel wall at the sites of vessel perforation or to increased intraluminal pressure caused by low dietary fiber and constipation.

2. What is the difference between diverticulosis and diverticulitis?

Diverticulosis refers to colonic diverticula without associated inflammation. Diverticulitis refers to diverticula associated with inflammation and infection. Only 15% of patients with diverticulosis develop diverticulitis.

3. How does a diverticulum cause pain?

Pain apparently results from perforation of the diverticulum The resulting leakage may be scant and contained within pericolic fat or extensive, involving the mesentery, other organs, or peritoneal cavity. Pain usually is located in the left lower quadrant—sigmoid diverticulitis.

4. Where in the colon are diverticula usually located?

In the United States, 95% of all diverticula occur in the left colon, primarily in the sigmoid colon. Diverticula, however, may occur anywhere in the colon. In Asia, right colon diverticula are more common.

5. At what age is diverticulitis most common?

Most patients with diverticulitis are in the sixth or seventh decade. Patients younger than 50 who develop diverticulitis tend to have more complications. Younger patients are more likely than older patients to have right colon diverticulitis.

6. What strategy may decrease diverticulitis in patients with diverticula?

A diet high in fiber appears to reduce the risk of diverticulitis. Large bulk in the colon decreases segmentation and intraluminal pressure.

7. What is the best imaging test for diagnosing acute diverticulitis?

Contrast enema was the diagnostic standard for many years, but computed tomography (CT) scan is now advocated by many as the best initial imaging study. CT scan can also diagnose local complications of diverticulitis.

8. What complications can result from perforation of a colonic diverticulum?

- Inflammatory phlegmon or abscessin the bowel mesentery
- Peritonitis
- Intraabdominal abscess
- Internal fistula
- Bosel obstruction

9. Can diverticular disease cause bleeding?

Yes. Diverticulosis is one of the most common causes of lower GI bleeding. Bleeding from diverticulitis is uncommon.

10. How can the site of diverticular bleeding be localized?

The most accurate means of localization is angiography performed via the inferior mesenteric artery and, if necessary, the superior mesenteric artery. Tagged red blood cell studies are less useful. Colonoscopy is rarely helpful.

11. When should an operation be performed for a bleeding colonic diverticulum?

Replacement of 5–6 units of blood (two-thirds of a patient's blood volume) within 24 hours and rebleeding during hospitalization are indications for emergency resection of the segment of colon containing a bleeding diverticulum.

12. If bleeding is life-threatening but cannot be localized within the colon, what treatment is required?

Subtotal colectomy with ileostomy and closure of the sigmoid colon at the peritoneal reflection (Hartmann's operation) or total abdominal colectomy with ileorectal anastomosis is required.

13. What three procedures may be used when perforation of the diverticulum results in an abscess? Which has the lowest operative mortality rate?

1. Diverting colostomy and abscess drainage (first of three stages)
2. Resection of involved colon with proximal colostomy and distal mucous fistula or closure by Hartmann's operation (first of two stages)
3. Resection with primary anastomosis (one stage)

Operative mortality is lowest after resection and proximal colostomy for fecal diversion. Despite reports of success with the one-stage procedure, most surgeons favor a safer two-stage approach for perforated diverticulitis (this strategy requires a second operation after 3 months for colostomy takedown).

14. What is the clinical evidence of a vesicocolic or ureterocolic fistula after diverticular perforation?

Pneumaturia, fecaluria, and chronic urinary tract infections (polymicrobial).

15. What procedure is required to repair a vesicocolic fistula?

A staged procedure was the standard until recently. Now most patients can be treated with a single procedure that includes sigmoid resection, colonic anastomosis, and primary repair of bladder defect with absorbable suture. A Foley catheter is usually left in place for 10 days after surgery.

BIBLIOGRAPHY

1. Birnbaum BA, Balthazar EJ: CT of appendicitis and diverticulitis. Radiol Clin North Am 32:855–898, 1994.
2. Cho KC, Morehouse HT, Alterman DD, et al: Sigmoid diverticulitis: Diagnostic role of CT—comparison with barium enema studies. Radiology 176:111–115, 1990.
3. Elfrink RJ, Miedema BW: Colonic diverticula. Postgrad Med 92:97–105, 1992.
4. Freeman SR, McNally PR: Diverticulitis. Med Clin North Am 77:1149–1167, 1993.
5. Konvolinka CW: Acute diverticulitis under age forty. Am J Surg 167:562, 1993.
6. Murray JJ, Schoetz DJ, Coller JA, et al: Intraoperative colonic lavage and primary anastomosis in non-elective colon resection. Dis Colon Rectum 34:527–531, 1991.
7. Roberts PL, Veidenheimer MC: Current management of diverticulitis. Adv Surg 27:"189–208, 1994.
8. Roberts PL, Abel M, et al: Practice parameters for sigmoid diverticulitis—supporting documentation. Dis Colon Rectum 38:126–132, 1995.
9. Rothenberger DA, Wiltz O: Surgery for complicated diverticulitis. Surg Clin North Am 73:975–992, 1993.
10. Schoetz DJ: Uncomplicated diverticulitis. Surg Clin North Am 73:965–974, 1993.

49. ACUTE LARGE BOWEL OBSTRUCTION

Elizabeth C. Brew, M.D.

1. What are the mechanical causes of large bowel obstruction?

The three most common mechanical causes are carcinoma (50%), volvulus (15%), and diverticular disease (10%). Extrinsic compression from metastatic carcinoma is another cause of obstruction. Less frequent causes include stricture, hernia, intussusception, benign tumor, and fecal impaction.

2. How is the diagnosis made?

1. The patient complains of crampy abdominal pain, distention, and obstipation. Nausea and vomiting occur later in large bowel obstruction and may be feculent. An acute onset of symptoms is more consistent with volvulus compared with the gradual development of obstructive complaints from patients with colon carcinoma.

2. Physical examination reveals abdominal distention and high-pitched bowel sounds with rushes. Rectal examination may reveal an obstructing rectal cancer or evidence of fecal impaction. Symptoms may progress to silence and localized tenderness, which may be signs of peritonitis or sepsis. This progression accompanied by a high fever or tachycardia requires immediate operative attention.

3. Flat and upright abdominal films reveal gas in the dilated colon with haustral markings proximal to the obstruction. If the patient has an incompetent ileocecal valve, it may be difficult to distinguish a large bowel from a small bowel obstruction. An upright chest film may show free air under the diaphragm if a perforation has occurred.

3. How is the diagnosis confirmed?

Plain abdominal films are usually sufficient to confirm a diagnosis. A contrast enema (barium or water-soluble contrast) is necessary to delineate the level and nature of an obstruction. A volvulus can be identified by a "bird's-beak" narrowing of the rectosigmoid at the neck of the volvulus. A stricture also can be demonstrated with the use of a contrast enema. Sigmoidoscopy or colonoscopy is an essential part of the evaluation, because it allows visualization of the colon and may be therapeutic in the case of a sigmoid volvulus.

4. Why is tenderness in the right lower quadrant important?

The cecum is the area that is most likely to perforate. When the cecum reaches 15 cm at its widest diameter, the tension on the wall is so great that decompression is essential to prevent perforation. The larger diameter of the cecum causes more tension of the cecal wall at the same intraluminal pressure (law of Laplace). The other area at risk for perforation is the site of a primary colon cancer.

5. Where is the obstructing cancer usually located?

Most obstructing colorectal carcinomas occur in the splenic flexure, descending colon, and hepatic flexure. In contrast, lesions of the right colon usually present with occult bleeding. Cecal and rectal cancers are uncommon causes of obstruction.

6. What is a volvulus? Where is it located?

A volvulus is an abnormal rotation of the colon on an axis formed by its mesentery and occurs either in the sigmoid colon (75%) or cecum (25%). **Sigmoid volvulus** occurs in an older population when chronic constipation causes the sigmoid colon to elongate and become redundant. **Cecal volvulus** requires a hypermobile cecum as a result of incomplete embryologic fixation of the ascending colon.

7. When is surgery indicated?

Surgery is performed early in colon obstruction. Urgent laparotomy is necessary in patients with suspected perforation or ischemia. Danger signs are quiet abdomen, right lower quadrant tenderness, and increasing pain. The patient's cardiopulmonary status should be assessed and optimized preoperatively. It is essential to correct dehydration and electrolyte imbalances with intravenous fluids. Nasogastric suction prevents further distention. Perioperative antibiotics, with both anaerobic and gram-negative coverage, are also necessary. Marking of possible stoma sites and deep venous thrombosis prophylaxis are other important preoperative considerations.

8. Which operation should be performed for a large bowel obstruction?

The traditional procedure for a large bowel obstruction has been a decompressing colostomy. However, careful assessment of the patient's condition, viability of the bowel, location of the obstruction, and absence of intraabdominal contamination often allows resection with or without a primary anastomosis. In fact, an initial diverting colostomy has not been shown to have any survival advantage and incurs the risk of further surgeries.

An **obstructing carcinoma** may be resected satisfactorily under emergency conditions in 90% of patients. Carcinomas of the right and transverse colon (proximal to the splenic flexure) are routinely treated with resection and primary anastomosis. Recently, obstructing cancers of the descending colon have been treated either with resection and colostomy or intraoperative lavage followed by resection and primary anastomosis. Techniques for nonoperative decompression of the colon, such as balloon dilation, laser therapy, and stent placement, are under study. Theoretically, these techniques will allow bowel perforation and elective colon resection.

A **volvulus** should be reduced and resected. Reduction of a sigmoid volvulus can be achieved nonoperatively by sigmoidoscopy or hydrostatic decompression with a contrast enema. The recurrence rate of volvulus after simple nonoperative reduction is 75%. Surgical therapy includes operative detorsion alone, detorsion with colopexy, sigmoid colectomy, or mesosigmoplasty. Cecal volvulus can be treated similarly with nonoperative decompression, cecopexy, or surgical resection.

The optimal treatment of **diverticular disease** is initial bowel rest, intravenous antibiotics, and percutaneous abscess drainage, if necessary. Colon resection and primary anastomosis can be performed after adequate bowel preparation.

9. What are the nonmechanical causes of large bowel obstruction?

Paralytic ileus (colonic pseudoobstruction) or toxic megacolon.

10. What is Ogilvie's syndrome?

Ogilvie's syndrome is an acute paralytic (adynamic) ileus or pseudoobstruction (i.e., enormous dilation of the colon without a mechanical distal obstructing lesion). Patients present with a massively dilated abdomen and a small amount of pain. Nonoperative management, including bowel rest, intravenous fluids, and gentle enemas, is the therapy of choice. Colonoscopy is both diagnostic and therapeutic in patients with colons larger than 10 cm in diameter. The risk of cecal perforation is high, and decompression of the colon should be attempted.

11. What is toxic megacolon?

Toxic megacolon is dilatation of the entire colon secondary to acute inflammatory bowel disease. The disease is manifested by acute onset of abdominal pain, distention, and sepsis. Initial therapy includes intravenous fluid resuscitation, nasogastric decompression, and broad-spectrum antibiotics. If symptoms do not resolve within a few hours, the patient requires an operation to avoid perforation. Surgical therapy most often consists of an emergency abdominal colectomy with formation of an ileostomy.

BIBLIOGRAPHY

1. Buechter KJ, Boustany C, Caillouette R, et al: Surgical management of the acutely obstructed colon: A review of 127 cases. Am J Surg 156:163, 1988.
2. Eckhauser MC, Mansour EG: Endoscopic laser therapy for obstructing and/or bleeding colorectal carcinoma. Am Surg 58:358, 1992.
3. Gosche JR, Sharpe JN, Larson GM: Colonoscopic decompression for pseudo-obstruction of the colon. Am Surg 55:111, 1989.
4. Lopez-Kostner F, Hool GR, Lavery IC: Management and causes of acute large-bowel obstruction. Surg Clin North Am 77:1265, 1997.
5. Murray JJ, Schoetz DJ, Coller JA, et al: Intraoperative colonic lavage and primary anastomosis in non-elective colon resection. Dis Colon Rectum 34:527, 1991.
6. Saida Y, Sumiyama Y, Nagao J, et al: Stent endoprosthesis of obstructing colorectal cancers. Dis Colon Rectum 39:552, 1996.
7. Tan SG, Nambiar R, Rauff A, et al: Primary resection and anastomosis in obstructed descending colon due to cancer. Arch Surg 126:748, 1991.

50. INFLAMMATORY BOWEL DISEASE

Gilbert Hermann, M.D.

1. What two clinical entities encompass the diagnosis of inflammatory bowel disease?

Crohn's disease and ulcerative colitis (acute or chronic).

2. Although the two diseases often overlap, they usually can be distinguished by clinical criteria. What are the major clinical differences?

Rectal bleeding is unusual in Crohn's disease but common in chronic ulcerative colitis. An abdominal mass and anal complications (fissure, fistula) are more common in Crohn's disease.

3. What are the major radiologic differences?

Terminal ileal involvement, skip areas, internal fistulas, and "thumb printing" are rare or absent in chronic ulcerative colitis but common in Crohn's disease.

4. What are the major histologic differences?

Granulomas in the intestinal wall and adjacent lymph nodes are absent in ulcerative colitis but occur in 60% of patients with Crohn's disease. The inflammatory process in Crohn's disease involves the entire bowel wall. In ulcerative colitis the inflammation usually is limited to the mucosa and submucosa.

5. Although Crohn's disease affects the gastrointestinal tract from the pharynx to the anus, what are the most common clinical patterns of gastrointestinal involvement?

Small bowel only, 28%; both ileum and colon (ileocolitis), 41%; and colon only, 27%. Crohn's involvement of the colon is also termed Crohn's colitis or granulomatous colitis.

6. Crohn's colitis and ulcerative colitis are often difficult to distinguish clinically. What are the major differences at colonoscopy?

Crohn's disease is focal and predominantly right-sided. The mucosa has a cobblestone appearance with transverse ulcerations in affected areas. Biopsies reveal transmural disease with possible focal granulomas. On colonoscopy, chronic ulcerative colitis may appear as a diffuse disease. However, if only a portion of the colon is involved, it is on the left side and almost always involves the rectum. Pathologic changes involve primarily the mucosa and submucosa.

7. What are the major indications for surgery in Crohn's disease?

It depends on the site of involvement. Enterocutaneous or enteroenteral fistulas (controversial), abscess, and intestinal obstruction are the most common surgical indications for small intestinal and ileocolic types. Perianal disease, medical failure, ileocolic fistulas, and abscess formation are the most common indicators for surgery in the colonic type.

8. What are the major indications for surgery in ulcerative colitis?

Medical intractability (including failure to thrive in children, diarrhea, weight loss, and abdominal pain), toxic megacolon with or without perforation, and concern about the development of colonic cancer (controversial) are the main indications.

9. What is the surgical procedure for treatment of ulcerative colitis?

Total colectomy with ileoanal pouch anastomosis is currently the standard procedure. A total colectomy with a Brooke ileostomy was the classic surgical approach and is still applicable in some situations. A Kock (continent) pouch can be used for younger (less than 55 years old) patients who do not wish to wear an ileostomy bag. Ileorectal anastomosis has been advocated by some (controversial).

10. What are the acceptable surgical procedures for the treatment of complications of Crohn's disease?

Complications requiring surgery are usually corrected by removing all areas of bowel involved in the complication. Experience with strictureplasty as opposed to resection has become more frequent in selected cases of small bowel obstruction (controversial). When resection is necessary, grossly clear margins are satisfactory. Skip areas are left alone unless they are directly adjacent to resected intestine.

11. What should the patient be told to expect about recurrence of the inflammatory bowel disease after surgery?

With chronic ulcerative colitis, surgery is definitive and curative. With Crohn's disease, however, the aim of surgery is to treat the complications (i.e., obstruction and sepsis). Recurrence of Crohn's disease can be expected in a high percentage of cases if the patient is followed long enough. Small bowel recurrence after total colectomy for Crohn's colitis does unfortunately occur.

CONTROVERSIES

12. Should all patients with enteroenteral fistulas secondary to Crohn's disease have surgery when the fistula is discovered?

For: Such patients do poorly, develop further intraperitoneal septic complications, and always eventually need surgery.

Against: Studies have indicated that many patients with enteroenteral fistulas do well without operative treatment as long as they remain asymptomatic.

13. Should all patients with documented chronic ulcerative colitis for over 10–15 years, whether active or not, have a colectomy to avoid the risk of carcinoma of the colon?

For: The risk of colon cancer in ulcerative colitis increases by approximately 0.5–1% per year 8–10 years after the diagnosis.

Against: Using surveillance colonoscopy and biopsy, only patients whose colons show dysplastic changes over time need a colectomy.

14. Is ileorectal anastomosis an acceptable operation after colectomy for ulcerative colitis?

For: The patients have reasonably normal bowel habits and avoid the problems and complications associated with other procedures.

Against: At least 50% of patients need reoperation for recurrence of disease. The remaining rectum also may be a site for the development of cancer.

15. Is standard (Brooke) ileostomy a good way to handle the terminal ileum after total colectomy for chronic ulcerative colitis?

For: The complication rate is very low. Over 90% of patients studied lead satisfactory lives.

Against: Psychosocial and sexual problems are associated with the use of external appliances, particularly in the teenage group, among whom chronic ulcerative colitis is quite common.

16. Is the continent Kock pouch a good procedure after colectomy for chronic ulcerative colitis?

For: It avoids use of an external appliance and is quite easy to manage.

Against: Approximately 20–30% of all patients who have a Kock pouch need to have a revision because slippage of the valve mechanism allows the pouch to become incontinent.

17. Is an ileoanal anastomosis with a surgically constructed ileoanal reservoir a good operation after colectomy for chronic ulcerative colitis?

For: It avoids external appliances or ostomies and thus is well accepted by patients. Currently this is probably the most commonly performed operation after colectomy.

Against: It is more difficult technically to construct; thus the complication rate is higher. The average number of bowel movements is 4–6/day, and there may be soilage at night. Pouchitis remains a problem.

18. Is strictureplasty an acceptable procedure for small bowel obstruction secondary to fibrotic stricture in Crohn's disease?

For: It preserves maximal length of small bowel in a disease prone to recurrence.

Against: Surgical morbidity may be higher, and stricture at the site of the strictureplasty may recur.

BIBLIOGRAPHY

1. Fazio V: Current status of surgery for inflammatory bowel disease. Digestion 59:470–480, 1998.
2. Holten L: Protocolectomy and ileostomy to pouch surgery for ulcerative colitis. World J Surg 22:378–341, 1998.
3. Hurst RD, Michelassi F: Strictureplasty for Crohn's disease: Techniques and long term results. World J Surg 22:359–363, 1998.
4. Rubenstein MC, Fisher RL: Pouchitis: Pathogenesis, diagnosis and management. Gastroenterologist 4:129–133, 1996.
5. Solomon MJ, Schmitz M: Cancer and inflammatory bowel disease: Bias, epidemiology, surveillance, and treatment. World J Surg 22:352–358, 1998.
6. Wolff BG: Factors determining recurrence following surgery for Crohn's disease. World J Surg 22:364–369, 1998.

51. UPPER GASTROINTESTINAL BLEEDING

G. Edward Kimm, Jr., M.D., and Allen T. Belshaw, M.D.

1. What is upper gastrointestinal (GI) bleeding?

Bleeding from a point in the digestive tract proximal to the ligament of Treitz (the transition point between duodenum and jejunum).

2. What are the most common causes of upper GI bleeding?

In descending order of frequency, duodenal ulcer, esophageal varices, gastritis, benign gastric ulcer, esophagitis, and Mallory-Weiss tear. All other causes account for less than 5% of cases.

3. What is the overall mortality rate of upper GI bleeding?

Approximately 10%. Mortality is usually associated with comorbid factors such as cardiac, pulmonary, hepatic and renal disease as well as advanced age (> 60) and large transfusion requirements (> 5 units of blood). Patients who rebleed during the same hospitalization have a mortality rate of 30%.

4. What is the most common presentation of upper GI bleeding?

Approximately 80% of patients present with melena (passage of black or tarry stools) or hematochezia (bright red blood per rectum). Hematemesis (bright red or coffee-ground emesis) is diagnostic of an upper source of GI bleeding. Occult bleeding may present only with guaiac-positive stool.

5. How much GI blood loss is necessary to cause melena?

As little as 50 ml. Occult bleeding (guaiac- or Hematest-positive) can be detected with as little as 10 ml of blood loss.

6. A 45-year-old man presents to the emergency department with massive hematemesis, tachycardia, and hypotension. What is your initial approach?

Acute gastrointestinal hemorrhage requires a prompt and systematic approach. As in all critically ill patients, initially assess the ABCs (airway, breathing, circulation). Start two large bore IV lines, and give one liter of Ringer's lactate while monitoring the patient. Nasogastric tube (NGT) and Foley catheter are placed, and the NGT is irrigated with saline. Laboratory testing includes type and crossmatch coagulation and liver function tests.

7. The above patient is hemodynamically stabilized after your interventions. What can be obtained from the history to determine a cause of the bleeding?

- Previous symptoms of peptic ulcer disease or NSAID use—bleeding duodenal or gastric ulcer
- History of gastroesophageal reflux disease—esophagitis
- Heavy alcohol use—gastritis or bleeding varices
- Recent retching or vomiting—Mallory-Weiss tear
- Weight loss—upper GI malignancy

8. What physical finding may be helpful in establishing the source of bleeding?

Physical exam is generally not helpful in determining the source of upper GI bleeding. The stigmata of liver disease (jaundice, caput medusa, ascites, muscle wasting) raise the suspicion of variceal bleeding.

9. What percentage of patients with known esophageal varices are bleeding from the varices on presentation?

Fifty percent.

10. Does bilious or clear NGT aspirate rule out an upper GI source of hemorrhage?

No. Although NGT aspiration can be useful in directing the search for a bleeding site, one should keep in mind that the false-negative rate may be as high as 20%.

11. What studies can be used to determine the source of bleeding?

Upper endoscopy (EGD) is the first and best test. Barium studies may miss a significant source of upper GI bleeding, such as erosive gastritis, and interfere with other more definitive tests, especially arteriography. Nuclear scans are of limited value in acute upper GI hemorrhage.

12. What is the sensitivity of EGD?

Endoscopy identifies the source of bleeding in up to 95% of cases of acute upper GI hemorrhage. Endoscopy has the advantage of directly visualizing the source of blood loss and provides the opportunity to biopsy a lesion and perform therapeutic maneuvers.

13. What amount of bleeding is required to see a "blush" on arteriography?

Two to 5 ml per minute. Although angiography is the most invasive of these tests, it can be useful in selected patients who are actively bleeding. In addition, the catheter can be left in place and used for delivery of vasopressin or embolization.

14. What treatment options are available to control variceal bleeding?

Upper endoscopy with sclerotherapy or band ligation. In experienced hands, placement of a Sengstaken-Blakemore tube (a double balloon tube permitting direct compression of both gastric and esophageal varices) controls bleeding in 90% of cases. Intravenous infusion of vasopressin or octreotide also may control bleeding but is less successful with more severe liver disease.

15. What are the indications for surgery in patients with upper gastrointestinal hemorrhage?

About 10% of patients eventually require surgery. Indications include:
• Persistent hypotension or shock
• Recurrent bleeding while on maximal medical therapy
• High-risk patients with significant comorbid disease
• Large transfusion requirements (transfusion of more than two-thirds of the patient's blood volume in 24 hours)

16. What is the surgical approach to an unstable patient with a nonlocalized upper GI bleed who does not respond to initial resuscitation?

Start with a generous gastroduodenostomy centered over the pylorus. If this does not reveal a source of bleeding, proceed with a proximal gastrotomy.

17. A patient presents with hematemesis and has a remote history of an abdominal aortic aneurysm repair. What uncommon cause of upper GI bleeding needs to be considered?

Aortoduodenal fistula. Any patient with a history of aortic surgery and evidence of GI bleeding should be aggressively worked up for aortoenteric fistula. The study of choice is endoscopy.

18. What is a Dieulafoy's ulcer?

Another uncommon cause of upper GI bleeding is Dieulafoy's lesion, which is a gastric vascular malformation with an exposed submucosal artery, usually within 2–5 cm of the gastroesophageal junction. It presents with painless hematemesis, often massive.

19. A patient recently admitted with a traumatic liver laceration for nonoperative treatment develops painless hematemesis. What do you suspect? How should you treat it?

Hemobilia, another rare cause of upper GI bleeding, usually occurs after liver trauma or hepatic resection. Treatment consists of angiographic embolization.

20. What are other rare causes of upper GI bleeding?

Watermelon stomach, portal hypertensive gastropathy, other vascular anomalies, upper GI neoplasm, duodenal diverticulum, and pancreatitis (resulting in erosion into the splenic artery or splenic vein thrombosis with sinistral portal hypertension).

BIBLIOGRAPHY

1. Abedi M, Haber GB: Watermelon stomach. Gastroenterologist 5:179, 1997.
2. Corley DA, Stefan AM, et al: Early indicators of prognosis in upper gastrointestinal hemorrhage. Am J Gastroenterol 93:336, 1998.
3. Gilbert DA: Epidemiology of upper gastrointestinal bleeding. Gastrointest Endosc 36:S8, 1990.
4. Katz PO, Salas L: Less frequent causes of upper gastrointestinal bleeding. Gastroenterol Clin North Am 22:875, 1993.
5. McGuirk TD, Coyle WJ: Upper gastrointestinal tract bleeding. Emerg Med Clin North Am 14:523, 1996.
6. Rikkers LF: The changing spectrum of treatment for variceal bleeding. Ann Surg 228:536, 1998.

7. Segal WN, Cello JP: Hemorrhage in the upper gastrointestinal tract in the older patient. Am J Gastroenterol 92:42, 1997.
8. Wilcox CM, Alexander LN, Cotsonis G: A prospective characterization of upper gastrointestinal hemorrhage presenting with hematochezia. Am J Gastroenterol 92:231, 1997.

52. LOWER GASTROINTESTINAL BLEEDING

Kathleen Liscum, M.D.

1. Describe the treatment of a patient who presents with lower gastrointestinal bleeding.

Treatment begins with the ABCs (airway, breathing, circulation). Venous access should be established immediately by placing two large-bore catheters in the upper extremities. Blood should be analyzed for hemoglobin, hematocrit, and type and cross-match. A Foley catheter should be placed to help monitor volume status.

2. What is the next step in evaluating the patient?

A nasogastric tube should be placed to rule out an upper gastrointestinal source. If the aspirate is bilious, the examiner can be fairly certain that the source is distal to the ligament of Treitz. However, if the aspirate reveals no bilious fluid, the patient may have a bleeding source in the duodenum with a competent pylorus.

3. What are the two most common causes of massive lower gastrointestinal bleeding?

Diverticular hemorrhage (diverticulosis) and bleeding vascular ectasias are the two most common causes. Historically diverticular disease was thought to be the most common cause of lower gastrointestinal bleeding, but vascular ectasias are now responsible for an increasing number of cases.

4. What other processes may be associated with passage of blood per rectum?

Colon cancer	Inflammatory bowel disease
Polyps	Anorectal disorders (hemorrhoids, fissure)
Ischemic colitis	Meckel's diverticulum
Infectious colitis	

5. After a good history and physical exam, what is the first step toward identifying the specific site of bleeding?

Anoscopy and rigid proctosigmoidoscopy should be done first to rule out anorectal fissures and an extraperitoneal source.

6. Name four options for localizing lower gastrointestinal bleeding.

Tagged red blood cell scan	Angiography
Sulfur colloid scan	Colonoscopy

7. Discuss the differences between sulfur colloid scan and tagged red blood cell scan.

The **sulfur colloid scan** can be accomplished quickly and detects bleeding as minimal as 0.1 ml/minute. The radiolabeled sulfur colloid is cleared quickly by the liver and spleen, which may obscure the bleeding site if it is located in the hepatic or splenic flexure. The test is complete within 20 minutes of administration of the radionuclide.

The **tagged red blood cell scan** requires a 30–60-minute delay while the red cells are labeled. The test detects bleeding as slow as 0.5 ml/minute. Because the tagged cells stay in the patient's system, it is also helpful in identifying the source when the patient is bleeding intermittently. The study takes at least 2 hours to complete.

8. What is the role of angiography in the evaluation?

Angiography detects bleeding rates of 0.5–1.0 ml/minute. When a bleeding site is identified, the angiographic appearance may provide further insight into the cause of the bleeding. Diverticular bleeding is often seen as extravasation of contrast, whereas vascular ectasias may be identified by a vascular tuft or early filling vein.

9. What therapeutic options are available with angiography?

Two options are available: (1) infusion of pitressin into a selected vessel and (2) embolization of the bleeding vessel.

10. Which patients should have angiographic embolization of the bleeding site?

Most surgeons believe that embolization should be reserved for patients who are poor operative risks. A 15% complication rate is associated with the procedure. Patients may perforate or develop a stricture as a result of bowel wall ischemia.

11. What is the role of vasopressin infusion?

Vasopressin should be used as a temporizing measure. Control of the bleeding with vasopressin allows time for resuscitation and essentially converts an emergent case into an urgent one. Vasopressin occasionally may be used as the only treatment for diverticular bleeding. If the patient has a repeated episode of bleeding after weaning from vasopressin, the surgeon must decide between embolization and surgery.

12. In what percentage of patients does lower gastrointestinal hemorrhage spontaneously resolve?

Spontaneous resolution occurs in 75% of patients with vascular ectasias and 90% of patients with diverticular bleeding.

13. What are the generally accepted indications for operative intervention?

Most surgeons believe that an operation is indicated if the patient has received 6 units of blood (two-thirds of the patient's blood volume in 24 hours) without resolution of bleeding. Any patient who continues to bleed or has recurrent bleeding after vasopressin or embolization should undergo resection.

14. What is the role of blind subtotal colectomy in the management of patients with massive lower gastrointestinal bleeding?

Blind subtotal colectomy is limited to the small group of patients in whom a specific bleeding source cannot be identified. The procedure is associated with a 16% mortality rate. Younger patients tend to tolerate the procedure better than elderly patients. Older patients often suffer with severe diarrhea, urgency, and incontinence. However, blind segmental colectomy is associated with an even higher mortality rate (39%) and a 54% rebleeding rate.

15. What is the most common cause of lower gastrointestinal hemorrhage in the pediatric population?

Meckel's diverticulum.

BIBLIOGRAPHY

1. American Society for Gastrointestinal Endoscopy: The role of endoscopy in the patient with lower gastrointestinal bleeding. Gastrointest Endosc 48:685–688, 1998.
2. Belaiche J, D'Heans G, Cabooter M, et al: Acute lower gastrointestinal bleeding in Crohn's disease: Characteristics of a unique series of 34 patients. Belgian IBD Research Group.
3. Gunderman R, Leef JA, Lipton MJ, Reba RC: Diagnostic imaging and the outcome of acute lower gastrointestinal bleeding. Acad Radiol Suppl 2:S303–S305, 1998.
4. So JB, Kok K, Hgoi SS: Right-diverticular disease as a source of lower gastrointestinal bleeding. Am Surg 65:299–302, 1999.
5. Wilcox CM, Clark WS: Causes and outcome of upper and lower gastrointestinal bleeding: The Grady Hospital experience. South Med J 92:44–50, 1999.

53. COLORECTAL POLYPS

Carlton C. Barnett, Jr., M.D.

1. What are polyps?

A polyp is an elevation of the mucosal surface, consisting of a rounded projection into the alimentary lumen. Polyps occur throughout the gastrointestinal tract but are most common in the colon and rectum. Two-thirds of colorectal polyps occur in the rectum and sigmoid and descending colon. The remainder are distributed between the right and transverse colon.

2. What are the major types of polyps?

Polyps are classified by their morphologic features as either pedunculated or sessile. Pedunculated polyps have a head attached by a stalk to the mucosa of the colon or rectum. The stalk usually is covered with normal mucosa. Sessile polyps rest on a broad base. In either type the muscularis mucosa is an important landmark for differentiating invasive from noninvasive lesions. Lymphatics and veins do not extend across the muscularis mucosa. Submucosal lesions such as carcinoid and lipomas also may appear to be colorectal polyps.

3. At what age do polyps occur?

Adenomatous colorectal polyps occur infrequently under the age of 30. The incidence increases with age; autopsy series report an incidence as high as 70% in patients over 45. This figure is generated from postmortem examination with high-power microscopic techniques. The clinical incidence is 25% for persons over age 60.

4. Which polyps have malignant potential?

Adenomatous polyps may be precursors for cancer. Three histologic types of adenomatous polyps are recognized. Polyps containing more than 75% tubular (glandular) elements are called **tubular.** Polyps containing more than 75% villous elements are called **villous,** and those containing greater than 25% of both glandular and villous elements are called **villotubular.**

5. What are the four histologic types of adenomatous polyps?

1. **Carcinoma in situ** is a lesion solely above the muscularis mucosa.
2. **Pseudocarinomatous polyps** have displaced benign adenomatous epithelium with a normal histologic lamina propria surrounding the epithelium.
3. **Invasive carcinoma** penetrates the muscularis mucosa. The incidence of invasive carcinoma is about 2.7–5% in large series based on endoscopic polypectomy.
4. **Polypoid carcinoma** occurs when the entire polyp degenerates into adenocarcinoma. Because the carcinoma is above the muscularis mucosa, this type of polyp is not necessarily associated with adverse outcome.

6. Does polyp type increase the likelihood of finding adenocarcinoma?

Yes. Adenocarcinoma is more likely with villous polyps than with tubular polyps of similar size. Wolff and Shinya showed 3.3% vs. 12.6% for tubular compared with villous adenomas. Coutsoftides et al. showed 5.6%, 16%, and 41% incidences of adenocarcinoma for tubular, villotubular, and villous adenomas, respectively.

7. What is the relationship between polyp size and risk of adenocarcinoma?

Polyps < 2 cm have a 1–10% risk of containing cancer, 1–2-cm polyps have a 7–10% risk, and polyps > 2 cm have a cancer risk between 35% and 53%. Sixty percent of villous polyps are > 2 cm, whereas 77% of tubular polyps are < 1 cm at the time of discovery.

8. Does the size of an adenomatous polyp correlate with adverse outcome?

No. Although the chances that a polyp contains cancer increase with an increase in polyp size, there is no direct correlation with adverse outcome. Stryker et al. found that most polyps associated with invasive adenocarcinoma were 1.0–1.4 cm. Cranley et al. found that 45% of invasive cancers were associated with polyps < 2.0 cm.

9. What classification system for adenomatous polyps correlates with long-term outcome?

The Haggit classification system correlates the level of invasion into the polyp with long-term outcome:

0—adenocarcinoma confined to the mucosa
1—confined to the head of the polyp
2—confined to the neck of the polyp
3—confined to the stalk of the polyp
4—invasive into the submucosa underlying the polyp

Level 4 invasion has been shown in multiple studies to correlate with adverse outcome (death due to colorectal carcinoma or nodal disease).

10. Which polyps have no malignant potential?

Hyperplastic (metaplastic) polyps are the most common polyps in the colon and rectum. They generally are small (1–5 cm) and constitute over 90% of the polyps in the colon and rectum that are smaller than 3 mm. Unlike adenomatous polyps, hyperplastic polyps are caused by failure of normally matured mucosal cells to spread over the mucosal lumen. These cells then accumulate on the luminal surface, forming a polyp.

Hamartomas are collections of normal tissue in abnormal places (e.g., within the colonic mucosa).

Inflammatory polyps are commonly seen in diseases such as ulcerative colitis, Crohn's disease, and schistosomiasis. They represent islands of healed or healing mucosal epithelium and are not permanent. The appearance of inflammatory polyps reflects the severity of the underlying disease. Lipomas may occur in polypoid form with head and stalk.

11. What is a juvenile polyp?

Juvenile polyps occur in the colon and rectum of infants, children, and adolescents. Histologically they consist of large mucus-filled glands with excessive connective tissue. The etiology of these polyps is unclear. They may represent a response to inflammation, or they may be hamartomas. Juvenile polyps are symptomatic for rectal bleeding and as lead points for intussusception. Conservative treatment via polypectomy is sufficient.

12. How are colorectal polyps diagnosed?

Polyps are usually asymptomatic unless they enlarge. The most common symptom is occult bleeding. Screening for colorectal polyps with fecal occult blood tests has 40% specificity and only 30% sensitivity. Colonoscopy is the preferred test when polyps are suspected because it allows identification as well as diagnostic and therapeutic biopsies. Barium enema is also effective in diagnosing polyps > 5 mm if double-contrast techniques are used; however, it does not allow therapeutic intervention if polyps are discovered.

13. What are the risks of colonoscopy?

The major risks of colonoscopy are bleeding and perforation. For diagnostic colonoscopy these risks are extremely low—0.2% and 1.0%, respectively. Both risks are still less than 1% for therapeutic colonoscopy. Bleeding is usually self-limited and rarely necessitates laparotomy.

14. How can one determine whether endoscopic polypectomy is adequate treatment?

The patient's overall health must be strongly considered in deciding between surgical and endoscopic treatment. Obviously patients in poor health are preferentially treated with polypectomy. In general, if a margin > 1 mm can be obtained, there is no invasion of the muscularis mucosa, and the histologic grade of the lesion is I or II (well to moderately differentiated), the patient is amenable to endoscopic polypectomy. Patients with margins < 1 mm, invasion into vessels or lymphatics, and histologic grade III (poorly differentiated) lesions should undergo colon resection if medically feasible.

15. What is the proper treatment of a villous adenocarcinoma of the rectum?

Villous adenomas of the middle and upper rectum are often large and involve a substantial portion of the circumference of the bowel. Such lesions are best treated by low anterior resection. Lesions in the lower rectum may be excised locally if clear mucosal margins can be obtained. Large lesions low in the rectum with invasion may have to be treated by abdominoperineal resection. In selected lesions a posterior approach in which the rectum is entered after resection of the coccyx may allow adequate margins as well as spare rectal function. Patients with prohibitive operative risk may undergo treatment via fulgation or laser ablation.

16. What are the screening recommendations for patients with polyps?

Adenomatous polyps. Full colonoscopy should be performed, because patients with a polyp have a 30–50% risk of synchronous lesions. If a single lesion is discovered and removed, patients should have repeat screening at 3 years. If patients are found to have multiple polyps, they should undergo screening at 1 and 4 years. If patients are found to have no new lesions after one 3-year screening cycle, screening can be performed every 5 years.

Malignant polyps should be removed based on the criteria discussed in question 14. Follow-up endoscopy should be performed at 3 months to ensure that no residual tumor is present at the polypectomy site. After this, follow-up should be the same as for multiple adenomatous lesions. The relative risks of segmental colectomy in individual patients should be considered.

17. Which clinical syndromes are associated with colorectal polyps?

Familial polyposis coli (FPC) or **adenomatous polyposis coli** (APC) is inherited as an autosomal dominant trait characterized by multiple adenomatous polyps throughout the gastrointestinal tract. Diagnosis is made clinically by observing at least 100 adenomatous polyps in the colon; over 1000 are found in many cases. FPC appears to be caused by the loss of tumor suppressor genes on the long arm of chromosome 5. Multiple family members often are diagnosed with colorectal cancer, generally at a younger age than in sporadic cases. Bleeding, diarrhea, and abdominal pain are common presenting symptoms. FPC is associated with nearly a 100% risk of cancer.

Gardner syndrome also is inherited as an autosomal dominant trait. Patients have polyposis, as do patients with FPC, but in addition they have osteomas of the skull, epidermoid cysts, and multiple soft tissue tumors.

Turcot syndrome is a rare autosomal recessive trait consisting of central nervous system tumors and multiple adenomatous polyps.

Peutz-Jehgers syndrome consists of multiple hamartomatous polyps throughout the alimentary tract. These polyps are associated with cutaneous melanotic spots on the lips, within the oropharynx, and on the dorsum of the fingers and toes. The malignant potential is very low.

18. What is the natural history of FPC?

In a review of over 1000 cases of FPC, the mean age at diagnosis of polyps was 34, and the mean age at diagnosis of colorectal cancers was 40. The mean age of death was 43. It is now recommended that patients with FPC undergo colectomy at age 25. Patients also are at risk for the late development of foregut adenocarcinoma.

19. What are the surgical treatment options for FPC?

Treatment options include total proctocolectomy with permanent ileostomy, proctocolectomy with continent (Kock pouch), abdominal colectomy with rectal preservation, abdominal colectomy with ileorectal anastomosis, and ileal pouch-anal anastomosis. In patients in whom the rectum is preserved, continued endoscopic surveillance is necessary.

20. What role do genetic defects play in the progression of colorectal polyps to adenocarcinoma?

The progression of adenomatous polyps to colorectal cancer is believed to involve an accumulation of genetic defects via the activation of protooncogenes or the inactivation of tumor suppressor genes. The p53 gene is normally responsible for tumor suppression. Using immunohistochemical techniques to examine colorectal polyps, it has been shown that 65% of adenocarcinomatous polyps have abnormal p53 gene expression compared with only 24% of adenomatous polyps. Overexpression of abnormal p53 is more common in villous than tubular polyps. Of interest, the degree of abnormal p53 expression does not correlate with tumor differentiation.

21. Does the activation of protooncogenes play a role in the development of adenocarcinoma from adenomatous polyps?

Yes. Activation of the *c-K-ras* gene by a point mutation has been found in more than 50% of colon carcinomas. In addition, activation of the tyrosine kinase of the *c-src* gene product pp60[s-src] has been demonstrated in polyps of high malignant potential; the activity of tyrosine kinase is significantly elevated above the level of primary tumors in liver metastases.

BIBLIOGRAPHY

1. Bond JH: Polyp guideline: Diagnosis, treatment and surveillance for patients with nonfamilial colorectal polyps. Ann Intern Med 119:836–843, 1993.
2. Cooper HS, Deppisch LM, Gourley WK, et al: Endoscopically removed malignant colorectal polyps: Clinicopathologic correlations. Gastroenterology 198:1657–1665, 1995.
3. Darmon E, Cleary KR, Wargovich MJ: Immunohistochemical analysis of p53 overexpression in human colonic tumors. Cancer Detect Prevent 18:187–195, 1994.
4. Haggitt RC, Glotzbach RE, Soffer EE, Wruble CD: Prognostic factors in colorectal carcinoma arising in adenomas: Implications for lesion removal by endoscopic polypectomy. Gastroenterology 89:328–336, 1985.
5. Iwama T: The impact of familial adenomatous polyposis coli (FAP) on the tumorigenesis and mortality: Its rational treatment. Ann Surg 217:101, 1993.
6. Kohler LW, Pemberton JH, et al: Quality of life after proctocolectomy: A comparison of Brooke ileostomy, Kock pouch and ileal pouch-anal anastomosis. Gastroenterology 101:679–684, 1991.
7. Macrae FA, St. John DJB: Relationship between patterns of bleeding and Hemoccult sensitivity in patients with colorectal cancers or adenomas. Gastroenterology 82:891–898, 1982.
8. Nivatvongs S, Rojanasakul A, Reimann HM, et al: The risk of lymph node metastasis in colorectal polyps with invasive adenocarcinoma. Dis Colon Rectum 34:323–328, 1991.
9. Stein BL, Coller JA: Management of malignant colorectal polyps. Surg Clin North Am 73:47–66, 1993.
10. Talamonti MS, Roh MS, Curley SA, Gallick GE: Increase in activity and level of pp60[c-src] in progressive stages of human colorectal cancer. J Clin Invest 91:53–60, 1993.

54. COLORECTAL CARCINOMA

Kathleen Liscum, M.D.

1. What are the top three causes of cancer deaths in the United States?

Lung, breast or prostate, and colon cancer.

2. List the common presenting symptoms of a patient with colorectal cancer.

Intermittent rectal bleeding	Constipation
Vague abdominal pain	Tenesmus
Fatigue secondary to anemia	Perineal pain
Change in bowel habits	

3. What options are available to evaluate patients with guaiac-positive stool?

To evaluate the entire colon and rectum one may perform a barium enema and proctoscopy or colonoscopy. Colonoscopy is approximately 10 times more expensive, but it is also more sensitive for lesions < 1 cm.

4. List the major risk factors for colorectal cancer.

Adenomatous polyps
Family history of colorectal cancer
Age over 40
Chronic ulcerative colitis
Crohn's colitis
Personal history of colon cancer
Exposure to pelvic radiation for prostate or cervical cancer
Familial polyposis
Hamartomatous polyps (Peutz-Jeghers syndrome), inflammatory polyps, and hyperplastic polyps are not considered premalignant.

5. What are the current screening recommendations of the American Cancer Society for colorectal cancers?

A yearly digital rectal exam is recommended for all patients 40 and older. For patients over 50 a yearly digital rectal exam with occult blood testing is suggested. In addition, patients over 50 should have flexible sigmoidoscopy every 3–5 years.

6. In what part of the colon and rectum are most cancers found?

Historically a higher incidence of cancers has been found in the rectum and left colon. However, over the past 50 years there has been a gradual shift toward an increased incidence of right colon cancers. This change in patterns may reflect improvement in early detection.

7. Surgical options for colorectal cancer depend on tumor location. What operation should be performed for a lesion 25 cm from the anal verge?

Sigmoid colectomy.

8. What operation should be performed for a lesion 9 cm from the anal verge?

Low anterior resection (LAR).

9. What operation should be performed for a lesion 4 cm from the anal verge?

Abdominoperineal resection (APR).

10. What is the significance of adenomatous polyps in the colon?

Patients with adenomatous polyps are 6 times more likely to develop colorectal cancer than patients without polyps. Evidence suggests that all colon cancers arise from adenomatous polyps. The adneoma-carcinoma sequence describes this transformational process. Patients with familial adenomatous polyps (FAP) have > 100 polyps that cover the colonic wall. If such patients go untreated, without exception they develop adenocarcinoma of the colon by the age of 40.

11. How does the surgeon prepare the colon for operation?

Bowel preparation includes both mechanical cleansing and appropriate antimicrobial prophylaxis. This combination has resulted in significant decreases in morbidity and mortality from colon surgery. Mechanical cleansing is accomplished by lavage with polyethylene glycol (Go-Lytely) or a combination of cathartics and enemas (Fleet's Prep).

Antimicrobial prophylaxis should cover the expected aerobic and anaerobic flora of the gut. Significant controversy exists over whether the antibiotics should be given enterally (e.g., neomycin, 1 gm, and metronidazole, 1 gm, 3 times orally at 4-hour intervals on the evening before surgery) or parenterally (e.g., cefotetan, 2gm intravenously within 1 hour before surgery). Many clinicians give both to obtain intraluminal and systemic effects.

12. What is Dukes' staging system?
In 1932 Dukes described a staging system for rectal cancer:
Dukes A: Tumor confined to bowel wall
Dukes B: Tumor invading through the bowel wall
Dukes C: Tumor cells found in the regional lymph nodes
Since his original article this classification has been modified several times. One of the most commonly used modifications is the inclusion of Dukes D stage, which correlates with distant metastases.

13. Which patients with colorectal cancer require postoperative adjuvant therapy?
Patients with colon cancer and lymph node involvement (Dukes C) should receive chemotherapy postoperatively to treat micrometastases. Two large studies have documented a survival advantage for such patients. However, no studies have documented a survival advantage for patients with Dukes B disease who are treated with chemotherapy.
Patients with rectal cancer and a significant chance of local recurrence (Dukes B and C) should be treated with radiation therapy, which may be given preoperatively, postoperatively, or with a combined "sandwich" technique.

BIBLIOGRAPHY

1. Breivik J, Gaudernack G: Genomic instability, DNA methylation, and natural selection in colorectal carcinogenesis. Semin Cancer Biol 9:245–254, 1999.
2. Douek M, Wickramasinghe M, Clifton MA: Does isolated rectal bleeding suggest colorectal cancer? Lancet 354:393, 1999.
3. European Group for Colorectal Cancer Screening: Recommendations to include colorectal screening in public health policy. J Med Screen 6:80–81, 1999.
4. Ilyas M, Straub J, Tomlinson IP, Bodmer WF: Genetic pathways in colorectal and other cancers. Eur J Cancer 35:335–351, 1999.
5. Jadallah F, McCall JL, van Rij AM: Recurrence and survival after potentially curative surgery for colorectal cancer. N Z Med J 112:248–250, 1999.
6. Lipkin M, Reddy B, Newmark H, Lamprecht SA: Dietary factors in human colorectal cancer. Annu Rev Nutr 19:545–586, 1999.
7. Roberts-Thomson IC, Butler WJ, Ryan P: Meat, metabolic genotypes and risk for colorectal cancer. Eur J Cancer Prev 8:207–211, 1999.
8. Tilsed JV: Recent advances in surgery for colorectal surgery. Crit Rev Oncol Hematol 30:201–205, 1999.

55. ANORECTAL DISEASE

John B. Moore, M.D., F.A.C.S.

1. What aspect of the initial patient encounter is most important in the diagnosis of anorectal disease?
Clinical history, including duration of complaints, exacerbating or alleviating issues, precipitating events, dietary and bowel habits, and current or previous treatments.

2. What is the most common cause of painless bright red blood per rectum?
Internal hemorrhoids.

3. What are the proximal and distal anatomic landmarks of the anal canal? What is its average length?

The anal canal starts at the anorectal junction (which is the upper border of the internal sphincter muscle/puborectalis muscle) and ends at the anal verge. The average length is only 3–4 cm. The midpoint of the anal canal is called the dentate line.

4. What is the anatomic and surgical significance of the dentate line?

The dentate line is the location of the anal crypts that drain the intramuscular and intersphincteric anal glands, which are the site of anorectal abscesses and fistulas in ano. Above the dentate line, the anal canal receives visceral innervation (involuntary control), is covered by columnar epithelium, and is the origin of internal hemorrhoids. Below the dentate line, the anal canal receives somatic innervation (voluntary control), is lined with squamous epithelium, and is the location of external hemorrhoids.

ANORECTAL ABSCESS/FISTULA IN ANO

5. What is the most common cause of anorectal abscess?

Ninety percent result from cryptoglandular infection.

6. What are the four potential anorectal spaces used to classify anorectal abscesses?

1. Perianal (area of the anal verge)

2. Ischiorectal (area lateral to the external sphincter muscles, extending from the levator ani muscles to the perineum)

3. Intersphincteric (area between the internal and external sphincter muscles, continuous inferiorly with the perianal space and superiorly with the rectal wall)

4. Supralevator (area superior to the levator ani muscles, inferior to the peritoneum, and lateral to the rectal wall)

7. Define fistula in ano.

A fistula is an abnormal communication between any two epithelial-lined surfaces. The internal opening of the fistula in ano involves the anoderm at the dentate line, whereas the external orifice is located at the anal margin.

8. What is the incidence of fistula in ano after appropriate surgical incision and drainage of acute anorectal abscesses?

50%.

9. What is the most important factor leading to the successful surgical eradication of anorectal abscesses and/or fistulas?

You must know anorectal anatomy, including the potential spaces.

10. What is Goodsall's rule?

The location of the internal opening of an anorectal fistula is based on the position of the external opening. An external opening posterior to a line drawn transversely across the perineum originates from an internal opening in the posterior midline. An external opening, anterior to this line, originates from the nearest anal crypt in a radial direction.

11. What is the most important determinant of successful surgical treatment of fistula in ano?

Identification of the internal opening.

ANAL FISSURE

12. What is the most common location for idiopathic anal fissure?

90% are posterior, and 10% are anterior.

13. What are the most common symptoms of anal fissure?
Tearing anal pain and bleeding with bowel movements.

14. What is the underlying pathophysiology of fissure in ano?
Local trauma, anatomy of the anal canal, internal anal sphincter dysfunction, and ischemia.

15. What is the differential diagnosis for anal fissure, especially if atypical in location?
Anorectal abscess, thrombosed hemorrhoid, inflammatory bowel disease, or malignancy.

16. How do you best diagnose anal fissure?
By clinical history and visual inspection—*not* by digital examination or anoscopy.

17. What are the nonoperative treatment options?
High-fiber diet, stool-bulking agents, increased hydration, frequent warm sitz baths, and topical agents containing antiinflammatories, local anesthetics, and vasodilators (nitroglycerin).

18. What is the most common operation performed to treat intractable fissure in ano?
Fissurotomy with lateral internal anal sphincterotomy.

HEMORRHOIDS

19. What are hemorrhoidal tissues and their normal functions?
Hemorrhoids are cushions of vascular tissue that contribute to anal continence and protect the sphincter mechanism during defecation. Hemorrhoids are not veins, but sinusoids. Bleeding originates from presinusoidal arterioles, thus explaining the bright red arterial color.

20. What are the most common causes of pathologic hemorrhoids?
Constipation, prolonged straining, pregnancy, and internal sphincter dysfunction.

21. What is the most important difference between internal and external hemorrhoids?
Internal hemorrhoids are located above the dentate line with visceral innervation, whereas external hemorrhoids are located below the dentate line with somatic innervation. Ablation of internal hemorrhoids causes a pressure sensation with an urge to defecate, whereas a similar approach to external hemorrhoids causes the usual acute pain.

22. What are the most common complaints associated with pathologic internal hemorrhoids?
Bleeding, mucous discharge, and prolapsing tissue.

23. What are the most common complaints associated with external hemorrhoids?
Pain, inflammation, thrombosis, and difficulty with anal hygiene.

24. Are treatment options for symptomatic internal hemorrhoids based on a gradation system of physical characteristics?
Yes. Treatment is based on degree of prolapse:
Grade 1: none
Grade 2: spontaneous reduction
Grade 3: manual reduction
Grade 4: unreducible

25. How can you treat symptomatic grades 2 and 3 and occasionally grade 4 internal hemorrhoids?
Diet and stool-bulking, rubber band ligation, injection sclerotherapy, cryotherapy, infrared photocoagulation, anal dilatation, or electrocautery.

26. What is the last-resort treatment for recalcitrant symptomatic internal hemorrhoids or combined internal and external hemorrhoids?

Operative hemorrhoidectomy.

PILONIDAL SINUS DISEASE

27. What is the most common clinical presentation of a pilonidal sinus?

Pain and swelling in the sacrococcygeal region, which typically are associated with a chronic draining sinus tract.

28. Is pilonidal disease acquired or congenital?

Acquired. Hair follicles in the midline sacrococcygeal area enlarge and become infected, resulting in an abscess.

29. How is acute pilonidal abscess treated?

Incision and drainage.

30. What is the definitive therapy for pilonidal disease?

Excision of the entire pilonidal cavity and associated sinus tracts down to the fascia with primary or delayed closure.

31. What theory explains the rarity of pilonidal disease after the age of 40?

Changes in body habitus.

BIBLIOGRAPHY

1. Beck DE: Handbook of Colorectal Surgery. St. Louis, Quality Medical Publishing, 1997.
2. Beck DE, Wexner SD (eds): Fundamentals of Anorectal Surgery. Philadelphia, W.B. Saunders, 1998.
3. Cameron JL: Current Surgical Therapy, 6th ed. St. Louis, Mosby, 1998.
4. Cho DV: Endosonographic criteria for an internal opening of fistula-in-ano. Dis Colon Rectum 42:515–518, 1999.
5. Hodgkin W: Pilonidal sinus disease. J Wound Care 7:481–483, 1998.
6. Law WL, Chu KW: Triple rubber band ligation for hemorrhoids: Prospective randomized trial of local anesthetic injection. Dis Colon Rectum 42:363–366, 1999.

55. INGUINAL HERNIA

James Bascom, M.D.

1. "Groin" hernia refers to what three hernias?

Direct and indirect inguinal hernias and femoral hernias.

2. Francois Poupart, a French surgeon and anatomist (1616–1708), described a ligament that bears his name. What is the anatomic name of the Poupart ligament?

Inguinal ligament, which is a key element in most groin hernia repair.

3. Franz K. Hesselbach, a German surgeon and anatomist (1759–1816), described a triangle that is the common site of direct hernias. What are the anatomic margins of Hesselbach's triangle?

The triangle is defined inferiorly by the inguinal ligament, superiorly by the inferior epigastric vessels, and medially by the rectus fascia. The floor of the triangle is formed by the transversalis fascia. The original description used Cooper's ligament as the inferior limit, but because of the common use of the anterior approach to hernias the more apparent inguinal ligament was substituted as the inferior limit of the triangle. With the increasing use of preperitoneal approaches to hernia repair, Cooper's ligament is again much more apparent and useful as an anatomic touchstone.

4. Sir Astley Paston Cooper, an English surgeon and anatomist (1768–1841), described a ligament bearing his name. What is the anatomic name for the ligament and the proper name of Cooper's ligament repair?

The anatomic name of Cooper's ligament is iliopectineal ligament. The McVay repair was popularized by Chester McVay (1911–1987). With Barry Aston, professor of anatomy at Northwestern University, McVay provided the modern description of the groin anatomy.

5. Antonio de Gimbernat, a Spanish surgeon and anatomist (1734–1816), had his interesting name attached to the lacunar ligament, which marks the medial margin of a groin area opening. What is the opening? What hernia protrudes into this opening?

The femoral hernia protrudes into the femoral canal.

6. Indirect inguinal hernia (particularly in children) and hydrocele are associated with what congenital abnormality?

Persistence of an open processus vaginalis, in the case of a hernia, allows descent of bowel into the inguinal canal. With fluid accumulation, partial obstruction presents as a hydrocele of the spermatic cord.

7. What are the diagnostic criteria for hernia in an infant or child?

1. Inguinal, scrotal, or labial lump that may or may not be reducible.
2. History of a lump seen by a health care provider.
3. History of a lump seen by the mother.
4. The "silk sign" (the feeling of rubbing together two surfaces of silk cloth when gently rubbing together the two surfaces of a hernia sac).
5. An incarceration sometimes felt on rectal exam.

8. What can be done to reduce an incarcerated hernia in an infant or child?

The four-point program is easier said than done, but worth the effort:

1. Sedate the patient.
2. Place the patient in the Trendelenburg position.
3. Apply a cold pack (over petroleum gauze to avoid skin injury) in inguinal area.
4. In the absence of spontaneous reduction—and if the patient is quiet—use gentle manipulation.

9. How often can incarceration be successfully reduced? What next?

About 80% of incarcerated hernias can be reduced in children; in adults, the percentage is lower. Despite the fact that 80–90% of inguinal hernias occur in boys, most incarcerations occur in girls. The hernia should be repaired electively within a few days after incarceration. The 20% of hernias that are still incarcerated are operated immediately.

10. What is a Bassini repair?

The Bassini repair sutures together the conjoined tendon and the inguinal ligament up to the internal ring. This classic procedure, introduced in 1887 at the Italian Society of Surgery in Genoa, revolutionized hernia repair. Until recently, it has been the standard of repair. After graduation from medical school and while fighting for Italian independence, Edoardo Bassini (1844–1924) was bayoneted in the groin and as a prisoner was hospitalized for months with a fecal fistula.

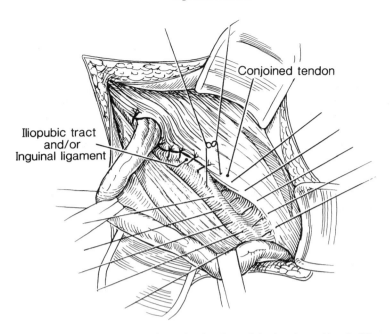

The standard right inguinal hernia repair using the conjoined tendon and inguinal ligament.

11. What is the recurrence rate with indirect and direct hernias that have been repaired with classic Bassini repair technique?

Over a follow-up period of 50 years, the recurrence rate of adult indirect hernias is 5–10%; of direct hernias, 15–30%.

12. Describe a McVay hernia repair.

The line of interrupted sutures starts at a the pubic tubercle and joins the tendinous arch of the transversus abdominis muscle to Cooper's ligament up to the femoral canal. At this point 2 or 3 transitional sutures are placed from Cooper's ligament to the anterior femoral fascia, effectively closing the medial extreme of the femoral canal. The final set of sutures joins the transversus abdominis arch and the anterior femoral fascia. The stitches usually incorporate the inguinal ligament at the upper limit of the repair, the site of the new internal inguinal ring and cord structures. About 15 years ago, McVay described laying in a mesh patch and stitching it, at its periphery, to the same anatomic structures. This application of mesh closely resembles the Lichtenstein repair (see question 17), except that it uses Cooper's ligament.

13. For what type of hernia is the McVay Cooper's ligament repair most useful?

Femoral and direct hernias.

14. What is the Shouldice repair?

The Shouldice repair, popularized at the Shouldice Clinic near Toronto, imbricates or overlays the transversalis fascia and conjoined tendon with 4 continuous lines, using 2 fine-wire sutures. The suture tract runs from the pubic tubercle to a new internal ring. Care is taken with the inferior epigastric vessels. The result is layered approximation of the conjoined tendon to the inguinal ligament tract.

15. What is the reported recurrence rate for the Shouldice repair?

1%—the lowest reported rate for nonmesh repairs of inguinal hernias in adults.

16. For what type of groin hernia is the Shouldice repair not appropriate?
Femoral hernia.

17. Describe the Lichtenstein repair.
The Lichtenstein repair consists of a sutured patch of polypropylene mesh (Marlex, C.R. Bard, Inc., Covington, GA) that covers Hesselbach's triangle and the indirect hernia area. It is considered a tension-free repair because the mesh is sutured in place without pulling ligaments or tissues together as in all other repairs. The mesh is divided at its upper end to wrap closely around the spermatic cord and its associated structures in the normal position of the internal inguinal canal. The Lichtenstein procedure is rapidly becoming the most widely used repair of adult inguinal hernia. The reported recurrence rate is < 1%.

18. What are the advantages of using the Marlex mesh?
Central to acceptance and success of the Lichtenstein hernia repair has been the development of and experience with the Marlex mesh. The monofilament mesh is strong, inert, and resistant to infection. The interstices are rapidly and completely infiltrated with fibroblasts, and the mesh is not subject to deterioration, rejection, or fragmentation.

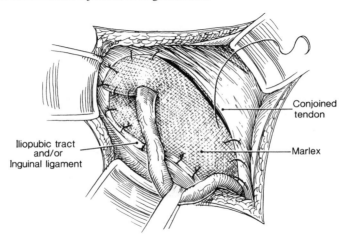

The Marlex mesh repair of a right inguinal hernia. Note that the same structures are used but not brought together; thus, the name of the "tension-free" repair.

19. For what groin area is the Lichtenstein repair not appropriate?
Femoral hernia.

20. What repair is acceptable for the femoral hernia?
Several different repairs can be used. Mesh in the form of a plug can be inserted and fixed in place. A McVay Cooper's ligament repair can be done. A preperitoneal approach to the hernia can be used to suture or plug the defect. A suture repair or a sartorius facial flap applied from below the inguinal ligament in a femoral approach also may be used. The preperitoneal approach is increasingly used for complicated inguinal and femoral hernias.

21. What is the preperitoneal or Stoppa procedure?
The preperitoneal or Stoppa procedure is a groin hernia repair on the internal side of the abdominal wall between the peritoneum and fascial surfaces that do not open into the peritoneal cavity. The anatomic landmarks are very different and initially quite challenging to the surgeon accustomed to the external abdominal wall approach. The technique is suited for recurrent hernias in

which scarring and obliterated anatomy increase the risk of cord injury and recurrence. Other problems such as large hernias and femoral hernias are corrected with this approach. Conceptually the laparoscopic hernia repair uses the same approach.

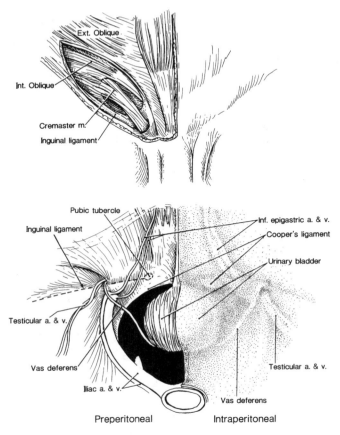

The different appearance and landmarks are seen in the anterior view (above) and the posterior view (below) of the inguinal/femoral area. In the posterior view the importance of the inferior epigastric vessels, bladder, and Cooper's ligament as anatomic landmarks is apparent.

22. Where are the spaces of Retzius and Bogros? Why are they increasingly important?

Retzius' space is between the pubis and the urinary bladder. **Bogros' space** is between the peritoneum and the fascias and muscle planes on the posterior aspect of the abdominal wall below the umbilicus and down to Cooper's ligaments. Laterally the space goes to the iliac spines. In either the open Stoppa procedure or the laparoscopic preperitoneal repair, the spaces of Retzius and Bogros are developed for mesh placement and surgical exposure.

23. How tight around the spermatic cord should a surgically fashioned, internal inguinal ring be?

About 5 mm, which is less than a fingertip and more than a forceps tip.

24. What is the common fascial defect of larger indirect and all direct inguinal hernias?

Weakness or attenuation of the transversalis fascia.

25. On examination the femoral hernia may be confused with what other inguinal hernia?
The femoral hernia may be confused with a direct inguinal hernia because of the tendency of the femoral hernia to present at the lateral edge of the inguinal ligament.

26. What is the difference between an incarcerated and a strangulated hernia?
Incarcerated: structures in the hernia sac still have a good blood supply but are stuck in the sac because of adhesions or a narrow neck of the hernia sac.
Strangulated: herniated structures, such as bowel or omentum, have lost their blood supply because of anatomic constriction at the neck of the hernia. The herniated, ischemic tissue is therefore in various stages of gangrenous changes. Strangulated hernias are surgical emergencies.

27. What is the operation for an uncomplicated indirect infant hernia?
High ligation of the sac.

28. What is the operation for an uncomplicated indirect hernia in young adults?
The appropriate operation consists of high ligation and possibly 1 or 2 stitches in the transversalis fascia to tighten the internal ring. This is the basic Marcy technique, developed by Henry Orlando Marcy (1837–1924); it is smaller and more anatomically focused than the Bassini repair.

29. What is the operation for an uncomplicated but sizable direct hernia in elderly adults?
Traditionally, the Bassini or McVay repair was chosen. More recently, because of the low recurrence rate, the Shouldice or Lichtenstein repair is favored.

30. What organ systems should be reviewed with particular care in the work-up of patients with hernia (especially elderly patients with recent onset of hernia)?
The gastrointestinal, urinary, and pulmonary systems should be reviewed with particular care. One is looking for causes of chronic strain or sudden forces that may have induced the hernia. Straining at stooling or urinating, unusual coughing, or difficulty with breathing, if corrected, may be of great value to the patient and reduce the chance of recurrent hernia.

31. What is a sliding hernia?
A sliding hernia is formed when a retroperitoneal organ protrudes (herniates) outside the abdominal cavity in such a manner that the organ itself and a peritoneal surface constitute the hernia sac.

32. What organs can be found in sliding hernias?

Colon	Bladder
Cecum	Fallopian tubes
Appendix	Uterus (rare)
Ovary	

33. What are common operative and postoperative complications of hernia repairs?
Intraoperative complications
- Injury to spermatic cord, especially in children
- Injury to spermatic vessels, resulting in atrophy or acute necrosis of testes
- Injury to ilioinguinal nerve, genitofemoral nerve, and lateral femoral cutaneous nerve. (The lateral femoral cutaneous nerve is uniquely vulnerable in laparoscopic and properitoneal procedures.)
- Injury to the femoral vessels

Postoperative complications
- Infection—high risk in children with diaper rash and patients with bowel injury or necrosis
- Hematoma—should resolve in time
- Nerve injury—the nerve is not always divided and with time may improve. If pain persists, try xylocaine block for both diagnosis and treatment. If a nerve block is not successful, one may consider reexploration to free the nerve from scar or to excise a postsurgical neuroma.

34. What are the common sites of hernia recurrence?

Direct hernias often recur at the pubic tubercle. Indirect hernias recur at the internal ring. The cause is usually related to poorly placed or insufficient stitches. Other possible causes include infection, poor tissue, poor collagen formation, or too much tension at the surgical suture line. A single line of repair under moderate tension probably will fail in a significant number of patients, regardless of adequacy of repair or healing process. Tension is almost always bad in surgery.

35. How long should the patient avoid heavy lifting after a hernia repair?

The standard advice for decades has been 6 weeks. The current advice varies from no limitation with the Lichtenstein or preperitoneal repairs to 6 weeks for a Bassini repair. The self-limitation of pain is an excellent guide.

CONTROVERSIES

36. Anatomic issues.

At issue is the **iliopubic tract**, which is central to the Anson/McVay anatomic description of the inguinal area and featured in the McVay Cooper's ligament repair. Although the McVay repair is used in England, the iliopubic tract is not referred to or described in English anatomic texts.

The term **conjoined tendon**, although commonly used, is considered by many to be anatomically inaccurate and misleading. The internal oblique and transversus abdominis muscles that make up the conjoined tendon are obvious and can be used surgically either alone or together. The tendinous edge of the transversus abdominis muscle and the tendinous edge of the internal oblique muscle start at their insertion on the pubic tubercle and course laterally and superiorly to the medial edge of the internal ring. At this point the tendinous elements diminish, leaving only muscle tissues, and continue laterally and superiorly to their origins.

Whether the lacunar ligament or the iliopubic tract defines the medial border of the femoral canal is controversial. The compromise position is that in the normal unstretched state the iliopubic tract is the border, whereas in the presence of hernia (stretched state) the lacunar ligament (Gimbernat's ligament) is the border. At surgery it is enough to say that a palpable, visible curved ligament is present and used in some femoral repairs.

37. Surgical issues.

The controversy over implanting mesh, as in the Lichtenstein repair, has been resolved in favor of mesh. Another controversy concerns the use of the laparoscope for hernia repair. A further issue is intraabdominal or preperitoneal placement of mesh. At present, most surgeons accept laparoscopic repair as an alternative for preperitoneal hernia repair. The indications for a preperitoneal approach to hernia repair are still being defined, although the preperitoneal approach is acceptable for repair of recurrent hernia and unusually large or difficult hernias. The preperitoneal approach is used with increasing frequency for repair of femoral hernias.

The repair should be appropriate to the circumstance of the hernia. Thus, hernia location and size as well as the patient's age, general condition, and recurrence status should be factored into the strategy of repair.

BIBLIOGRAPHY

1. Frankum CE, Renshaw BJ, White J, et al: Laparoscopic repair of bilateral and recurrent hernia. Am Surg 65:839–842, 1999.
2. Johansson B, Hallerback B, Glise H, et al: Laparoscopic mesh versus open perperitoneal mesh versus conventional technique for inguinal hernia repair: A randomized, multi-center trial (SCUR Hernia Repair Study). Ann Surg 230:225–231, 1999.
3. MRC Laparoscopic Groin Hernia Trial Group: Laparoscopic versus open repair of groin hernia: A randomised comparison. Lancet 354:185–190, 1999.
4. Smith AI, Royston CM, Sedman PC: Stapled and nonstapled laparoscopic transabdominal preperitoneal (TAPP) inguinal hernia repair: A prospective randomized trial. Surg Endosc 13:804–806, 1999.

IV. Endocrine Surgery

57. HYPERPARATHYROIDISM

Robert C. McIntyre, Jr., M.D.

1. What is the prevalence of hyperparathyroidism?

There are approximately 100,000 new cases of hyperparathyroidism (HPT) annually in the United States. Primary HPT occurs in 1 in 500 women over 40 years old and in 1 in 2000 men. Approximately 10% of patients with primary HPT are referred for surgery.

2. What are the symptoms of hyperparathyroidism?

Primary HPT is associated with "painful bones, renal stones, abdominal groans, and psychic moans." The three most common symptoms are fatigue, depression, and constipation. The classical symptoms and signs are listed below.

Bones: arthralgia, osteoporosis, pathologic fractures

Stones: renal stones, renal insufficiency, polyuria, polydipsia

Abdominal groans: pancreatitis, peptic ulcer disease, constipation

Psychic moans: fatigue, weakness, depression

3. What are the leading causes of hypercalcemia?

HPT is the most common cause of hypercalcemia among outpatients and the second most common cause in the hospital setting. The most common cause of hypercalcemia in hospitalized patients is malignancy. Primary HPT and malignancy account for 90% of cases of hypercalcemia.

4. What is the differential diagnosis of hypercalcemia?

Endocrine
    Hyperparathyroidism
    Hyperthyroidism
    Addison's disease
Malignancy
    Bone metastasis
    Paraneoplastic syndrome
      Solid tumors (squamous or small cell lung carcinoma)
    Hematologic malignancy (myeloma, leukemia, lymphoma)
Increased intake
    Milk alkali syndrome
    Vitamin D intoxication
Granulomatous disease
    Sarcoidosis
    Tuberculosis
Miscellaneous
    Familial hypocalciuric hypercalcemia
    Thiazides
    Lithium

5. What is the essential laboratory evaluation for hyperparathyroidism?

Elevated serum calcium (> 10.3 mg/dl) should be assessed at least twice. Hypercalcemia must be associated with elevation of parathyroid hormone (intact). Serum phosphate levels are low in nearly 80% of patients. Serum chloride is increased in 40% of patients. A chloride-to-phosphate ratio greater than 33 suggests primary HPT. Increased alkaline phosphatase levels are uncommon and occur only in the setting of advanced bone disease. A 24-hour urine collection for calcium excretion should be done to exclude benign familial hypocalciuric hypercalcemia (FHH). In patients with primary HPT, the 24-hour urine calcium is > 200 mg/day vs. < 100 mg/day in FHH.

6. Describe the anatomy of the parathyroid glands.

The upper parathyroid glands arise from the dorsal part of the fourth brachial pouch along with the lateral lobes of the thyroid. The lower parathyroid glands arise from the dorsal part of the third brachial pouch along with the thymus.

The average weight of a normal parathyroid gland is 35–50 mg. In most cases, the upper parathyroid gland lies on the posterior portion of the upper one-half of the thyroid, cephalad to the inferior thyroid artery and posterior to the recurrent laryngeal nerve. The normal lower parathyroid gland is found on the lateral or posterior surface of the lower pole of the thyroid gland.

Four glands are present in 89% of patients, 5 in 8%, 6 in 3%, and less than 4 in 0%.

Because the upper parathyroid glands, unlike the lower glands, do not migrate a great distance during development, their location is more constant. The most common ectopic sites of the upper glands are posterior to the esophagus or in the posterior superior mediastinum. The lower parathyroid glands are more commonly ectopic and may lie within the thyrothymic ligament, thymus, mediastinum (but outside the thymus), carotid sheath, thyroid, and upper neck in the undescended position.

7. What are the indications for parathyroidectomy?

All patients with symptomatic HPT or with serum calcium 1 mg/dl above normal should undergo parathyroidectomy. The treatment of asymptomatic patients with minimal elevation (10.3–11.0 mg/dl) of serum calcium is controversial. However, at least three factors favor operation in the majority of patients:

1. Patients with untreated primary HPT have an increased death rate due to cardiovascular disease.

2. The cost of parathyroidectomy is equivalent to medical follow-up at 5–6 years.

3. Experienced endocrine surgeons have a high success rate (95%) with very low morbidity and mortality rates.

Most experts recommend parathyroidectomy for all patients who do not have an absolute contraindication to surgery.

8. What localization studies are available and when are they indicated?

Experienced radiologists may localize parathyroid tumors in as many as 90% of cases. The single best localization study is the sestamibi scan. Other noninvasive localization studies include ultrasound, computed tomography, or magnetic resonance imaging. Invasive localization procedures include arteriography and venous sampling. The tests are most accurate with a single abnormal parathyroid gland. Localization procedures in cases of hyperplasia may be misleading.

Localization studies are not routinely indicated before an initial operation, but they are mandatory before all reoperative parathyroidectomies for persistent or recurrent HPT and in patients with previous thyroid surgery.

Preoperative sestamibi scintigraphy is used by some surgeons for the initial operation to allow unilateral neck exploration or minimally invasive radioguided parathyroidectomy.

9. What is the pathology of primary HPT?

Primary HPT is due to a single adenoma in 87% of cases, hyperplasia in 9%, double adenoma in 3%, and carcinoma in 1%. In familial HPT, multiple endocrine neoplasia syndromes (MEN I and MEN II), and HPT due to end-stage renal disease, hyperplasia is the rule.

10. Outline the surgical strategy of an initial exploration for primary HPT.

A meticulously dry, blood-free operative field must be maintained at all times. Tissue in the region of the recurrent laryngeal nerve should not be clamped or divided until the nerve is definitively identified. A bilateral operation is the standard approach. If a solitary adenoma and three normal glands are found, the adenoma is removed and one of the normal glands biopsied. Frozen section examination confirms that the tissue is parathyroid. Four-gland enlargement (hyperplasia) indicates either subtotal parathyroidectomy (leaving approximately 50 mg of well-vascularized parathyroid tissue in the neck) or total parathyroidectomy with autotransplantation to the forearm of 50 mg of parathyroid tissue. If a remnant is left in the neck, it should be marked with a nonabsorbable suture or staple. In the setting of hyperplasia, a thymectomy eliminates the possibility of thymic supernumerary glands. If more than one enlarged gland is found in association with normal-appearing glands (double adenoma), all abnormal glands should be removed, with frozen section confirmation of parathyroid tissue. The glands left in situ should be marked as above.

Newer operative techniques include endoscopic neck exploration, minimally invasive radioguided parathyroidectomy, and intraoperative "rapid" parathyroid hormone assays.

11. What should one do if an adenoma is not found in the usual locations?

If an adenoma cannot be found in the usual locations, each normal gland should be biopsied for confirmation and marked. Do not remove normal parathyroid glands. If three normal glands are identified and the fourth cannot be located, the surgeon should assess whether the missing gland is an upper or lower parathyroid. A missing upper gland often lies in the tracheo-esophageal groove, posterior to the esophagus or in the posterior superior mediastinum. The common mistake in this situation is that the dissection is not carried posterior enough to the prevertebral fascia. The location of a missing lower gland is more varied. First, the thyrothymic ligament should be inspected for ectopic parathyroid glands. The thymus then can be resected through the neck incision. If the adenoma is still not found, the surgeon should search for an undescended parathyroid. Next, the carotid sheath should be opened. In addition, the area lateral to the jugular vein should be explored. Finally, the thyroid lobe on the side of the missing parathyroid should be palpated for nodules. If a nodule is palpated, it should be excised and examined by frozen section; it may be an intrathyroidal parathyroid. If no nodule is palpated, a blind thyroid lobectomy should be performed.

A sternotomy should not be done as part of an initial exploration. If the above maneuvers are unsuccessful in revealing a parathyroid adenoma, the surgeon should stop. A diagram of the location of the identified glands should be made for future reference. Persistent hypercalcemia indicates the need for localization procedures.

12. What is the outcome of surgery for primary HPT?

The expected cure rate should be 95% for patients undergoing an initial exploration for primary HPT. After parathyroidectomy, 80% of symptomatic patients have improvement in bone density and renal function. Even in asymptomatic patients urinary calcium and deoxypyridinoline levels decrease. Patients have fewer episodes of nephrolithiasis, gout, and peptic ulcer disease. Parathyroidectomy also appears to improve longevity in patients with primary HPT.

13. What are the complications of parathyroidectomy?

Permanent recurrent laryngeal nerve injury occurs in < 1% of patients; however, a temporary nerve paresis occurs in 3%. Hungry bone syndrome may lead to temporary hypocalcemia in up to 20% of patients, but permanent hypoparathyroidism occurs in only 2% of cases. An elevated preoperative alkaline phosphatase level may predict which patients are likely to experience postoperative hypocalcemia.

14. What are the physical signs of hypocalcemia after surgery?

Chvostek's sign is spasm of the facial muscles due to tapping of the facial nerve trunk. Trousseau's sign is carpal spasm elicited by occlusion of the brachial artery for 3 minutes with a blood pressure cuff.

15. How should patients with hypocalcemia be treated?

Patients with tetany due to hypoparathyroidism require emergency treatment with intravenous calcium to prevent laryngeal stridor and convulsions. Ten ml of 10% calcium gluconate (90 mg elemental calcium per 10 ml) should be given in 100 ml saline over 20 min. followed by an infusion of calcium (4 ampules of calcium gluconate in a liter of saline) at 50 ml/hr. Maintaining calcium levels of 7.5–9 mg/dl is adequate. Oral calcium should be started as soon as possible in the form of calcium carbonate (Tums or Oscal) at 2–3 gm daily in divided doses (3–4 times/day). Calcium citrate is preferred for patients with renal lithiasis because the citrate may be prophylactic against renal lithiasis. In most patients, vitamin D preparations increase intestinal absorption and can be given as calcitriol (Rocaltrol), 0.25–0.75 µg per day.

16. Define persistent and recurrent hyperparathyroidism.

Operative success is defined by long-term normocalcemia. Persistent HPT is defined as hypercalcemia within 6 months of surgery; recurrent HPT is defined as hypercalcemia after 6 months.

17. What is the strategy for management of the patient with persistent or recurrent hyperparathyroidism?

First, the patient should be reevaluated to ensure that the hypercalcemia is due to primary HPT and not some other cause. Patients should be evaluated for familial hypocalciuric hypercalcemia, which does not warrant reoperation. Previous operative notes and pathology reports should be reviewed to assist in planning repeat therapy. Localization studies should be used extensively. Before reexploration, vocal cord function should be assessed in all patients.

Repeat cervical exploration is done through the previous incision. Because the strap muscles are usually adherent to the thyroid, a lateral approach through the plane between the sternocleidomastoid and strap muscles may be used instead of the usual medial approach. With positive localization studies or retrospective determination of the side of the missing adenoma, the dissection may be limited if an adenoma is found.

An alternative to repeat exploration is angiographic ablation of parathyroid tissue, which is especially useful for mediastinal adenomas because it avoids a median sternotomy. It is done by delivering ionic contrast through an arterial catheter wedged into the feeding vessel.

18. Who performed the first parathyroidectomy?

In 1925, Felix Mendl performed the first successful parathyroidectomy at the Hochenegg Clinic in Vienna. His patient was Albert, a 34-year-old tram car conductor who could not work because of severe osteitis fibrosa cystica.

19. Who was Captain Martell?

An officer in the U.S. Merchant Marine, Captain Martell was the first patient in the U.S. to undergo surgery for primary HPT. Captain Martell had progressive HPT that reduced his height from 6 feet to a kyphotic 5 feet 6 inches. After seven operations the adenoma was finally removed from the mediastinum; however, the captain died in chronic renal failure.

BIBLIOGRAPHY

1. Boggs JE, Irvin GL III, Molinari AS, Deriso GT: Intraoperative parathyroid hormone monitoring as an adjunct to parathyroidectomy. Surgery 120:954–958, 1996.
2. Burney RE, Jones KR, Christy B, Thompson NW: Health status improvement after surgical correction of primary hyperparathyroidism in patients with high and low preoperative calcium levels. Surgery 1125:608–614, 1999.
3. Chan AK, Duh QY, Katz MH, et al: Clinical manifestations of primary hyperparathyroidism before and after parathyroidectomy. A case-control study. Ann Surg 222:402–412; discussion, 412–414, 1995.
4. Clark OH: Asymptomatic hyperparathyroidism: Is parathyroidectomy indicated? Surgery 116:947–953, 1994.
5. Denham DW, Norman J: Cost-effectiveness of preoperative sestamibi scan for primary hyperparathyroidism is dependent solely upon the surgeon's choice of operative procedure. J Am Coll Surg 186:293–305, 1998.

6. Hedback G, Oden A, Tisell LE: The influence of surgery on the risk of death in patients with primary hyperparathyroidism. World J Surg 15:399–405; discussion, 406–407, 1991.
7. Kaplan EL, Yashiro T, Salti G: Primary hyperparathyroidism in the 1990's. Choice of surgical procedures for this disease. Ann Surg 215:300–317, 1992.
8. Liechty RD, Weil R: Parathyroid anatomy in hyperplasia. Arch Surg 127:813–816, 1992.
9. McIntyre RC, Kumpe DA, Leichty RD: Re-exploration and angiographic ablation for persistent and recurrent hyperparathyroidism. Arch Surg 129:499–505, 1994.
10. Norman J, Chheda H: Minimally invasive parathyroidectomy facilitated by intraoperative nuclear mapping. Surgery 122:998–1003; discussion, 1003–1004, 1997.
11. Palmer M, Adami HO, Bergstrom R, et al: Survival and renal function in untreated hypercalcemia. Population-based cohort study with 14 years of follow-up. Lancet 1:59–62, 1987.

58. HYPERTHYROIDISM

Robert C. McIntyre, Jr., M.D.

1. What are the symptoms and signs of hyperthyroidism?

General:	Heat intolerance, perspiration, flushing, tremor, sleep disturbance
Psychological:	Nervousness, emotional lability, anxiety, aggressiveness, delusions
Cardiovascular:	Palpitations, tachycardia, supraventricular dysrhythmias
Respiratory:	Breathlessness, hoarseness
Gastrointestinal:	Increased appetite, weight loss, increased frequency of bowel movements
Reproductive:	Gynecomastia, irregular menses
Bone:	Osteoporosis
Other:	Ophthalmopathy, dermopathy

2. What causes hyperthyroidism?

The most common form of hyperthyroidism is Graves' disease (90%), which is due to production of thyrotropin receptor-stimulating antibodies. Ten percent of hyperthyroidism among middle-aged and elderly patients is due to Plummer's disease (toxic nodular goiter), which is characterized by nodules that function independently of the normal feedback regulation.

Less common forms of hyperthyroidism include thyroiditis (subacute, silent, postpartum), in which inflammation leads to an increase in the release of thyroxine and triiodothyronine. Iatrogenic hyperthyroidism is due to excessive administration of thyroxine or triiodothyronine.

Rare causes of hyperthyroidism include neonatal hyperthyroidism, pituitary thyrotropin-secreting tumor, exogenous iodine, and factitious disease. Very rare causes are thyroid cancer, choriocarcinoma, hydatidiform mole, embryonal testicular carcinoma, and struma ovarii.

3. How should hyperthyroidism be investigated?

Hyperthyroidism is confirmed by low serum levels of thyrotropin and high serum levels of thyroxine. If the serum thyroxine level is normal, a high serum level of triiodothyronine indicates triiodothyronine toxicosis; a normal triiodothyronine level excludes hyperthyroidism. A normal serum thyrotropin level almost always excludes hyperthyroidism. A high thyrotropin level with an increase in free thyroxine indicates the rare patient with a thyrotropin-producing pituitary tumor.

Serum total thyroxine may be increased in the setting of increased serum thyroid-binding globulin. This finding occurs in pregnancy, patients taking estrogen therapy, and patients with an inherited increase in thyroid binding globulin.

Toxic nodular goiter is confirmed by a radionuclide scan that shows uptake into a single thyroid nodule or patchy uptake into more than one hyperfunctioning nodule. Scintigraphy reveals low or absent uptake of radioiodine in thyroiditis.

4. What are the three treatment options?

Antithyroid drugs, radioiodine, and surgery.

5. Which drugs are useful for the treatment of hyperthyroidism? What are their mechanisms of action?

Methimazole (the active metabolite of carbimazole) and propylthiouracil (PTU) are the mainstays of treatment. The goal of treatment is remission of Graves' disease during therapy or euthyroidism before treatment with radioiodine or surgery. Both drugs inhibit the organification of iodine and coupling of iodothyronines. PTU also inhibits the peripheral monodeiodination of thyroxine (T_4) to triiodothyronine (T_3). Both drugs also reduce the serum concentration of thyrotropin receptor antibodies and increase suppressor T-cell activity. Thus, they may have an immunosuppressive action. Treatment is started with 20 mg/day of methimazole or 100 mg of PTU 3 times/day. The dose may be reduced after 6 weeks of treatment as the patient shows clinical and biochemical improvement. Therapy is usually maintained for 2 years. Patients must be monitored for side effects, which include rash, pruritus, agranulocytosis, hepatitis, cholestatic jaundice, and lupus-like syndrome.

Beta-adrenergic antagonists ameliorate the signs and symptoms of disease. They should not be used alone except for short periods prior to radioiodine or surgical therapy. Nadolol (80 mg/day) and atenolol (100 mg/day) are the most common agents.

Iodine given as Lugol's solution (5% iodine and 10% potassium iodide in water, 0.3 ml/day) or potassium iodide (60 mg 3 times/day) inhibits the release of thyroid hormone. It is useful for short-term therapy in preparation for surgery, after radioiodine therapy to hasten the fall in hormone levels, and for treatment of thyroid storm.

6. What is the outcome of drug treatment?

Long-term remission of Graves' hyperthyroidism during antithyroid drug therapy occurs in 50% of patients. Relapse is most common in the first 6 months after cessation of treatment.

7. What are the indications and objectives for radioiodine therapy?

Radioiodine therapy is the treatment of choice for recurrence after antithyroid drug therapy. The objective of radioiodine therapy is to destroy enough thyroid tissue to cure hyperthyroidism, yet to preserve enough tissue to avoid hypothyroidism.

8. What is the regimen of radioiodine treatment?

The usual dose of radioiodine is 10 mCi. If hyperthyroidism is not cured, the dose should be repeated in 6 months. Pretreatment with antithyroid drug therapy should achieve a euthyroid state. The drugs should be discontinued 4 days before radioiodine therapy and resumed 4 days after therapy. Steroids prevent progression of ophthalmopathy. Prednisone is used at a dose of 0.5 mg/kg body weight, starting 3 days after radioiodine therapy and continuing for 1 month. The dose is tapered over 2 months.

Pregnancy is an absolute contraindication. Women of childbearing age should be evaluated with a pregnancy test before treatment and should avoid pregnancy for 6 months after treatment. Evidence indicates that radioiodine may exacerbate ophthalmopathy.

9. What is the outcome of radioiodine treatment?

Euthyroidism is not achieved for months after treatment. Once euthyroidism is achieved, recurrence of hyperthyroidism is rare. Hypothyroidism, the only serious side effect, is dose-dependent. It occurs at a rate of 3% per year, affecting 50% of patients at 10 years, and nearly 100% at 25 years.

10. What are the indications for thyroidectomy for hyperthyroidism?

1. Pregnant patients who are difficult to treat medically
2. Patients with large goiter and low radioiodine uptake
3. Children
4. Noncompliant patients

5. Patients with nodules suspected to be cancer
6. Patients with compression of the trachea or esophagus
7. Patients with cosmetic concerns
8. Patients with ophthalmopathy

11. How should patients be prepared for surgery?

Any patient with hyperthyroidism should be rendered euthyroid before surgery. Patients may be treated with antithyroid medication plus potassium iodine. Beta-adrenergic antagonists also may be used alone or in combination with the above regimen.

12. What is the extent of thyroidectomy?

The two surgical options for Graves' disease are subtotal thyroidectomy or near-total thyroidectomy. The goals of subtotal thyroidectomy are to preserve 4–8 gm of well-vascularized thyroid tissue and to avoid hypothyroidism. Because of the small risk of recurrence (10%), however, some surgeons prefer near-total thyroidectomy. In Plummer's disease, lobectomy or partial thyroidectomy for unilateral lesions and contralateral subtotal thyroidectomy for multiple lesions render the patient euthyroid.

13. What is the incidence of hypothyroidism after surgery?

All patients having a near-total thyroidectomy become hypothyroid and need thyroxine replacement. Hypothyroidism occurs in 50% of patients with subtotal thyroidectomy.

14. What is the appropriate treatment for toxic nodular goiter?

Hyperthyroidism due to toxic nodular goiter is permanent and without spontaneous remission; antithyroid drugs are not appropriate long-term therapy. Radioiodine is the most common form of therapy. Larger doses (50 mCi) minimize the risk of persistent hyperthyroidism in such patients, who tend to be older and to have prominent cardiovascular symptoms of hyperthyroidism.

15. What is the appropriate treatment for hyperthyroidism due to thyroiditis?

Subacute thyroiditis should be suspected if the patient has pain and tenderness in the thyroid region. The hyperthyroidism is usually mild and of short duration (weeks). Patients are treated with a β-adrenergic antagonist and salicylate or glucocorticoid. Hypothyroidism may occur but usually is not permanent.

16. What is the appropriate treatment for thyroid storm?

Thyrotoxic crisis should be treated in the intensive care unit. General measures include hydration, antipyresis (acetaminophen), and nutrition. Specific measures include inhibition of T_4 synthesis and conversion to T_3 with PTU at a dose of 100 mg orally, via nasogastric tube, or rectally every 6 hours. Iodides inhibit T_4 release (saturated solution of potassium iodide, 5 drops by mouth or nasogastric tube every 6 hr). Steroids (dexamethasone, 2 mg every 6 hr) also inhibit T_4 release and conversion to T_3. Beta-adrenergic antagonists (propranolol or esmolol) may control cardiovascular manifestations. The last management option is T_4 removal by plasmapherisis, hemoperfusion, or dialysis.

17. Who performed the first thyroidectomy?

Johann von Mikulicz-Radecki performed the first thyroidectomy in 1885.

18. What surgeon won the Nobel prize for his work with thyroid disease?

Theodor Kocher won the Nobel prize in medicine in 1909. He was successful in reducing the high mortality rate of thyroidectomy to less than 1%. His most significant achievement was in describing postoperative hypothyroidism as *cachexia strumipriva*.

BIBLIOGRAPHY

1. Bartalena L, Marcocci C, Bogazzi F, et al: Relation between therapy for hyperthyroidism and the course of Graves' ophthalmopathy. N Engl J Med 338:73–78, 1998.
2. David E, Rosen IB, Bain J, et al: Management of the hot thyroid nodule. Am J Surg 170:481–483, 1995.
3. Franklin JA, Daykin J, Drolc Z, et al: Long term follow-up of treatment of thyrotoxicosis by three different methods. Clin Endocrinol 34:71–76, 1991.
4. Franklyn JA: The management of hyperthyroidism. N Engl J Med 330:1731–1737, 1994.
5. Patwardhan NA, Moroni M, Rao S, et al: Surgery still has a role in Graves' hyperthyroidism. Surgery 114:1108–1113, 1993.
6. Singer PA, Cooper, D S, Levy EG, Ladenson PW, et al: Treatment guidelines for patients with hyperthyroidism and hypothyroidism. JAMA 27:808–812, 1995.
7. Surks MI, Chopra IJ, Mariash CN, et al: American Thyroid Association guidelines for use of laboratory tests in thyroid disorders. JAMA 263:1529–1532, 1990.

59. THYROID NODULES AND CANCER

Robert C. McIntyre, Jr., M.D.

1. What is the prevalence of thyroid nodules and cancer?

The prevalence of thyroid nodules increases throughout life. Approximately 10% of 50-year-old women have a palpable nodule. Nodules are about 4 times more common in females than in males. After exposure to radiation, nodules develop at approximately 2% annually, reaching a peak at 25 years. Nodules are 10 times more frequent in glands examined by ultrasound, at surgery, or at autopsy. Less than 50% of thyroid nodules that appear solitary on physical exam are truly solitary.

Each year in the United States, there are approximately 12,000 new cases and 1,000 deaths due to thyroid cancer. Up to 35% of thyroid glands examined at autopsy contain occult papillary cancer (<1.0 cm.).

2. What is the importance of the distinction between solitary and multiple thyroid nodules?

Traditionally multiple thyroid nodules were considered benign and solitary thyroid nodules malignant. However, multiple series suggest that a dominant nodule in a multinodular gland carries the same risk of cancer as a solitary nodule (5%).

3. What is the differential diagnosis of thyroid nodules?

Adenoma
    Macrofollicular (colloid)   Embryonal
    Microfollicular   Hurthle cell
Carcinoma
    Papillary   Anaplastic
    Follicular   Lymphoma
    Medullary   Metastatic
Cyst
Nodular goiter with a dominant nodule
Other
    Inflammatory diseases (e.g., Hashimoto's thyroiditis)
    Developmental abnormalities

4. What features of the history and physical exam indicate a higher risk of cancer?

Nodules occurring at the extremes of age are more likely to be cancerous, particularly in males. Rapid growth and local invasion raise the possibility of malignancy, but associated symptoms (hoarseness, dysphagia) are rare. A history of radiation exposure increases the frequency of both benign and malignant nodules. A family history of medullary or papillary thyroid cancer or Gardner's syndrome (familial polyposis) increases the risk of cancer.

Cancer is more often found in patients with firm, solitary nodules. Fixation to adjacent structures, vocal cord paralysis, and enlarged lymph nodes also are associated with an increased risk of malignancy.

5. What is the proper laboratory evaluation of a patient with a thyroid nodule?

The only biochemical test that is routinely needed is a serum thyroid-stimulating hormone concentration to identify patients with unsuspected hyperthyroidism. In patients with suspected medullary thyroid carcinoma, basal serum calcitonin and calcium/pentagastrin-stimulated calcitonin should be measured. In patients with known medullary carcinoma, serum calcium levels and 24-hour urine collection for assessment of catecholamines and their metabolic products should be done to exclude multiple endocrine neoplasia (MEN) before thyroidectomy. A further option to evaluate for MEN is lymphocyte-derived DNA analysis for *ret* protooncogene mutations.

6. Which single test best predicts the need for surgical intervention?

The single best test to predict the need for surgery is fine-needle aspiration (FNA). If an adequate specimen is obtained, there are three possible results: benign (70%), suspicious (10%), and malignant (5%). FNA is most reliable for the diagnosis of papillary carcinoma and in patients with medullary and anaplastic cancer. It is least reliable in distinguishing benign from malignant follicular and Hurthle cell neoplasms. The overall accuracy exceeds 95% in experienced hands. When FNA reveals cancer, it is 97% correct (3% false-positive rate); when it indicates a benign nodule, cancer is present in 4% of cases (4% false-negative rate). On the other hand, when the FNA is suspicious, 20–30% of nodules are malignant.

7. What other tests may be useful in the evaluation of a thyroid nodule?

Thyroid radionuclide studies with isotopes of either iodine (most common) or technetium often are performed but cannot reliably differentiate malignant from benign nodules. Scans may be useful in patients with indeterminate FNA results, because hyperfunctioning nodules are almost always benign.

Ultrasound categorizes nodules as cystic, solid, or mixed and is the best measure of the size of a nodule. Ultrasound can be used to determine the presence of other nodules in a patient with a solitary nodule on physical exam. It is particularly useful to follow the size of a nodule. Like radionuclide scans, ultrasound cannot distinguish malignant from benign nodules; thus, it is not routinely used in the evaluation of a nodule.

8. Should a solitary thyroid nodule be suppressed with thyroxine for 3–6 months to determine whether it is benign or malignant?

Most nodules change very little over the short term. In one series of 74 patients with colloid nodules, 13% of nodules decreased in size, 22% disappeared, 46% did not change, and 19% enlarged. Studies of thyroxine therapy suggest that treatment is not superior to placebo in patients with solitary nodules. Most nodules do not change in size, 30% decrease in size, and a few increase in size. On the other hand, there are reports of decreased size in malignant nodules. FNA remains the single best test to determine the need for surgery.

9. What are the types and distribution of thyroid cancer?

Papillary	70%	Medullary	5%
Follicular	20%	Anaplastic and lymphoma	5%

10. What are the axioms of thyroid surgery, as noted by Clark?

1. A meticulously dry operative field must be maintained.

2. Tissue in the region of the recurrent laryngeal nerve should not be cut or clamped until the nerve is definitively identified.

3. Every parathyroid gland should be treated as if it were the last functioning gland.

4. If malignancy is suspected, the entire operation should be done as if the lesion were cancer.

11. What is the minimal extent of thyroidectomy for a solitary thyroid nodule?

The goal of surgery is to remove all foci of neoplastic tissue and any palpable cervical adenopathy. With the exception of small lesions in the thyroid isthmus, the minimal procedure for suspected malignancy should be lobectomy, including the isthmus. Enucleation is to be avoided. Frozen section is accurate for papillary, medullary, and anaplastic carcinoma. Frozen section is no more accurate than FNA for follicular and Hurthle cell carcinoma. Functioning "toxic" nodules may be resected by a partial lobectomy because they are usually benign. If the lesion is large, a lobectomy is preferred.

12. What is the most common form of thyroiditis in nodules?

The most common inflammatory disorders of the thyroid presenting as nodules are Hashimoto's thyroiditis, subacute thyroiditis, and Reidel struma (rare). These conditions usually do not require surgery. Thyroidectomy is indicated for compressive symptoms or when cancer cannot be excluded.

13. What is the surgical therapy for thyroid carcinoma?

Thyroid carcinoma should be treated by near-total or total thyroidectomy except in young patients with small, well-differentiated tumors (≤ 1 cm) and no evidence of lymph node or extrathyroidal disease. In such cases, lobectomy with resection of the isthmus is adequate therapy. Near-total thyroidectomy eliminates multifocal cancer in the thyroid, allows postoperative radioiodine for the diagnosis and therapy of metastatic disease, decreases risk of local-regional recurrence, and improves the accuracy of serum thyroglobulin as a marker for persistent or recurrent disease. Enlarged cervical lymph nodes should be removed and examined by frozen section. If metastatic cancer is identified, a neck dissection is performed by extending the Kocher collar incision laterally to the anterior border of the trapezius muscle (McFee extension). "Berry picking" results in an increased rate of regional recurrence and should be avoided in favor of anatomic dissections.

Because medullary thyroid cancer is not responsive to radioiodine or levothyroxine, a total thyroidectomy should be performed. A central neck dissection is mandatory to evaluate metastatic disease. If the central nodes are positive for cancer on frozen section, a modified neck dissection is performed.

Surgery for anaplastic carcinoma is palliative and usually is limited to debulking and tracheostomy for relief of compressive symptoms.

14. Describe the arterial supply and venous drainage of the thyroid.

The blood supply to the thyroid gland comes from the superior and inferior thyroid arteries. Occasionally, a midline thyroid internal mammary artery arises from the aortic arch. The superior thyroid artery is the first branch of the external carotid artery. The inferior thyroid artery arises from the thyrocervical trunk.

There are three major veins: superior, middle, and inferior thyroid veins. The superior and middle thyroid veins drain into the internal jugular vein, and the inferior vein drains into the innominate vein.

15. Describe the anatomy of the recurrent laryngeal nerves.

The right recurrent laryngeal nerve (RLN) arises from the vagus and loops around the right subclavian artery. The left vagus nerve gives off the left RLN, looping around the aorta. The RLNs run obliquely through the neck, usually in the tracheoesophageal groove. Low in the neck the nerves are more lateral and course medially as they ascend. The right nerve runs more obliquely than the left. Occasionally the RLN may branch before entering the larynx, usually on the left side. The motor fibers are usually in the most medial branch. In 1% of cases the right RLN is not recurrent and enters the neck from a lateral and superior direction.

16. What defect results from injury to the RLN?

Injury to a single RLN results in a paralyzed vocal cord, which causes a weak, hoarse voice. Patients also have abnormal swallowing and problems with aspiration. Injury to both nerves causes paralysis of both cords and obstruction of airflow. This situation necessitates a tracheostomy. RLN injury occurs in 1% of thyroidectomies.

17. Describe the anatomy of the superior laryngeal nerve and the defect that occurs with its injury.

The superior laryngeal nerve gives off the external laryngeal nerve, which runs medial to the superior pole vessels to enter the cricothyroid muscle. This motor nerve increases tension of the vocal cords allowing for high notes (Amelita Galli-Curci nerve). The internal laryngeal nerve provides the sensory innervation to the posterior pharynx. It lies superior to the thyroid cartilage. Injury to the nerve leads to a weak, low voice that lacks resonance. Patients also may have problems with aspiration.

18. What is the other major complication of thyroidectomy?

Permanent hypoparathyroidism occurs in 1% of thyroidectomies.

19. What is the postoperative therapy for well-differentiated thyroid carcinoma?

Patients with risk factors should be treated with postoperative radioiodine (I-131). Risk factors include older age (> 45 years old), male gender, direct local invasion, nodal spread, and distant disease. All patients with well-differentiated thyroid cancer should be treated with levothyroxine (Synthroid) to suppress serum levels of thyroid-stimulating hormone (0.2-0.5 µU/ml). This three-component therapy (surgery, I-131, levothyroxine) results in the lowest recurrence rate.

20. How should a patient be followed after therapy for well-differentiated thyroid carcinoma?

In young, low-risk patients, physical examination of the neck is done every 6 months for 2 years and then yearly thereafter. In high-risk patients, close follow-up includes repeat neck examination in addition to assessment of serum thyroglobulin levels and diagnostic radioiodine scans.

Patients with recurrent cervical disease by palpation or ultrasound should have repeat surgery if the procedure can be performed with low morbidity. After removal of gross disease, patients should be treated with radioiodine. Distant disease should be treated with radioiodine if the metastases take up iodine.

BIBLIOGRAPHY

1. Cady B: Presidential address: Beyond risk groups—a new look at differentiated thyroid cancer. Surgery 124:947–957, 1998.
2. Chen H, Nicol TL, Udelsman R: Follicular lesions of the thyroid. Does frozen section evaluation alter operative management? Ann Surg 222:101–106, 1995.
3. Chen H, Zeiger MA, Clark DP, et al: Papillary carcinoma of the thyroid: Can operative management be based solely on fine-needle aspiration? J Am Coll Surg 184:605–610, 1997.
4. Gharib H, Goellner JR: Fine-needle aspiration biopsy of the thyroid: An appraisal. Ann Intern Med 118:282–289, 1993.
5. Hay ID, Grant CS, Bergstralh EJ, et al: Unilateral total lobectomy: Is it sufficient surgical treatment for patients with AMES low-risk papillary thyroid carcinoma? Surgery 124:958–964; discussion 964–966, 1998.
6. Ladenson PW, Braverman LE, Mazzaferri EL, et al: Comparison of administration of recombinant human thyrotropin with withdrawal of thyroid hormone for radioactive iodine scanning in patients with thyroid carcinoma. N Engl J Med 337:888–896, 1997.
7. Maxon HR, Smith HS: Radioiodine 131 in the diagnosis and treatment of metastatic well differentiated thyroid cancer. Endocrinol Metab Clin North Am 19:685–718, 1990.

8. Mazzaferri EL: Management of solitary thyroid nodule. N Engl J Med 328:553–559, 1993.
9. McHenry CR, Sandoval BA: Management of follicular and Hurthle cell neoplasms of the thyroid gland. Surg Oncol Clin North Am 7:893–910, 1998.
10. Moley JF, DeBenedetti MK: Patterns of nodal metastases in palpable medullary thyroid carcinoma: Recommendations for extent of node dissection. Ann Surg 229:880–887; discussion 887–888, 1999.
11. Ridgway EC: Clinical review 30: Clinician's evaluation of a solitary thyroid nodule. J Clin Endocrinol Metab 74:231–235, 1992.
12. Wells SA Jr, Chi DD, Toshima K, et al: Predictive DNA testing and prophylactic thyroidectomy in patients at risk for multiple endocrine neoplasia type 2A. Ann Surg 220:237–247; discussion, 247–250, 1994.

60. SURGICAL HYPERTENSION

Thomas A. Whitehill, M.D.

1. What are the surgically correctable causes of hypertension?

Renovascular hypertension, pheochromocytoma, Cushing's syndrome, primary hyperaldosteronism (Conn's syndrome), coarctation of the aorta, and unilateral renal parenchymal disease. Surgical hypertension accounts for 5% of all hypertensive patients.

2. Which form of surgical hypertension is most common?

Renovascular hypertension. Although the overall frequency of renovascular hypertension among patients with elevated diastolic blood pressure is less than 1%, moderate or severe diastolic hypertension may be caused by renal artery occlusive disease in as many as 25% of cases. Pheochromocytoma, hyperaldosteronism, Cushing's disease, and coarctation of the aorta each are found in only 0.1% of all hypertensive patients.

3. What are the most common causes of renovascular hypertension?

Atherosclerosis is the most common cause (70%); it affects men twice as often as women. The second most common cause is fibromuscular dysplasia (25%). Of the many pathologic subtypes, the most common is medial fibrodysplasia (85%); it invariably affects women. Last is development renal artery stenosis (10%); it often is associated with neurofibromatosis and abdominal aortic coarctation.

4. What clinical criteria support the pursuit of investigative studies for suspected renovascular hypertension?

Although no clinical characteristics are pathognomonic of renovascular hypertension, the following findings strongly suggest the presence of an underlying renal artery stenotic lesion:

1. Hypertension in the very young or in a woman less than 50 years of age
2. Rapid onset of severe hypertension after age 50
3. Hypertension refractory to three-drug regimens
4. Initial presentation with diastolic blood pressure greater than 115 mmHg or sudden worsening of presumed preexisting hypertension
5. Accelerated or malignant hypertension
6. Deterioration of renal function after the initiation of antihypertensive agents, especially angiotensin-converting enzyme (ACE]) inhibitors
7. Systolic/diastolic upper abdominal/flank bruits

5. What is the renin-angiotensin-aldosterone axis?

Renin is released from the juxtaglomerular apparatus of the kidney in response to changes in renal cortical afferent arteriolar perfusion pressure. Renin acts locally and in the systemic circulation on renin substrate (angiotensinogen), a nonvasoactive alpha$_2$ globulin produced in the liver, to form angiotensin I. Angiotensin I undergoes enzymatic cleavage by ACE in the pulmonary circulation to produce angiotensin II, a potent vasopressor responsible for the vasoconstrictive element of renovascular hypertension. Angiotensin II increases adrenal gland production of aldosterone with subsequent retention of sodium and water; this process establishes the volume element of renovascular hypertension.

6. How do ACE inhibitors work?

Direct inhibition of ACE decreases concentrations of angiotensin II, which leads to decreased vasopressor activity and decreased aldosterone secretion. Removal of angiotensin II negative feedback on renin secretion leads to increased plasma renin activity.

7. Should renovascular hypertension be treated medically or surgically?

Although prospective randomized studies comparing drug and interventional therapy have not been published, surgical treatment and percutaneous transluminal renal angioplasty (PTRA) have been favored over drug therapy by most clinicians. The key is timely recognition and acknowledgement of the problem.

8. When should renovascular hypertension be treated with PTRA?

Clear indications for PTRA include nonorificial atherosclerotic lesions and medial fibrodysplastic lesions limited to the main renal artery.

9. What findings on history and physical examination should lead to a suspicion of pheochromocytoma?

Pheochromocytomas are tumors primarily of the adrenal medulla. Approximately 90% are found within the adrenal gland, and the remaining 10% are scattered along the abdominal paravertebral sympathetic chain or in ganglia located remotely (e.g., urinary bladder, pelvic nerves). Tumors are classified as functioning when they produce catecholamines, always autonomously and usually in great excess. The predictable clinical effects of increased endogenous cathecholamine outpouring is sustained hypertension; sustained hypertension with episodes of increased blood pressure, tachycardia, or flushing; or, rarely, normotension with infrequent and unpredictable episodes of hypertension.

10. How is pheochromocytoma diagnosed?

Diagnosis is best confirmed by 24-hour urine collection for excreted catecholamines, metanephrines, and vanillylmandelic acid. The best single test to confirm the diagnosis of pheochromocytoma is still debated; some believe that the metanephrine level is the most precise (85%). It also has been argued that plasma catecholamines are the most precise and specific test, but given the variability of results in individual patients and in many assays, the current approach should continue to emphasize the use of urinary catecholamines. Eighty percent of patients with pheochromocytoma have at least one urinary metabolite greater than twice the normal value. The diagnosis of pheochromocytoma should be followed by studies to localize the tumor.

11. What is the best test to localize pheochromocytoma?

For most patients with sporadic (nonfamilial) pheochromocytoma, computed tomography (CT) identifies the lesion in the adrenal gland, especially if it is larger than 1 cm. Extraadrenal lesions should be sought only if a lesion is not found on CT scan. Magnetic resonance imaging (MRI) is complementary to CT: CT better detects the lesion, whereas MRI distinguishes one type of lesion from another.

The most appropriate test to localize solitary lesions or multiple lesions or metastases is ^{131}I-metaiodobenzylguanidine (MIBG), a norepinephrine analog. MIBG labels catecholamine precursors and is taken up and concentrated in adrenergic storage vesicles. The false-negative rate is less than 5%, and the false-positive rate is 1–2%. Another scintigraphic radiopharmaceutical,

^{131}I-6$_\beta$-iodomethyl-19-norcholesterol (NP-59), a cholesterol analog, can distinguish adrenocortical hyperplasia from functioning adenomas or carcinomas. It accurately localizes the adrenal cortex and any functioning tumors.

12. Describe the acute antihypertensive treatment in patients with pheochromocytoma.

Hypertension from pheochromocytoma is caused by activation of vascular smooth muscle alpha$_1$ receptors, which results in vasoconstriction. Thus, the best acute treatment is intravenous administration of the alpha$_1$ antagonist, phenoxybenzamine. Sodium nitroprusside is also a reasonable choice. Beta blockers should be avoided initially because they cause both unopposed peripheral alpha$_1$-receptor stimulation and decreased cardiac output. Congestive heart failure may be precipitated by blocking the heart (β) before lowering the blood pressure (α).

13. How is primary hyperaldosteronism (Conn's syndrome) diagnosed?

Conn's syndrome, which results from autonomous mineralocorticoid hypersecretion, is characterized by hypertension, hypokalemia, hypernatremia, metabolic alkalosis, and periodic muscle weakness and paralysis, often due to an aldosterone-secreting adenoma. The syndrome is now identified by the combined findings of hypokalemia, suppressed plasma renin activity despite sodium restriction, and high urinary and plasma aldosterone levels after sodium repletion in hypertensive patients.

14. Why does Cushing's syndrome or Cushing's disease cause hypertension?

Patients with Cushing's syndrome or disease have hypercortisolism or excessive amounts of glucocorticoids. In the cardiovascular system, glucocorticoids appear to produce an increased chronotropic and inotropic effect on the heart, along with an increased peripheral vascular resistance. Receptors in the distal renal tubules respond to glucocorticoids by inducing increased tubular resorption of sodium. These receptors belong to a different class from receptors mediating the more potent actions of aldosterone.

15. What findings suggest aortic coarctation?

Coarctation of the aorta is suggested in patients who have a lower blood pressure in the legs than in the arms; they also have notably diminished or absent femoral pulses. Rib notching may be evident on chest radiograph in patients with long-standing, hemodynamically significant coarctation. Bruits may be heard over the chest or abdominal wall. Adults may have an ongoing history of congestive heart failure or mild renal failure.

16. How does aortic coarctation cause hypertension?

No single cause has been identified. Mechanical obstruction to ventricular ejection is one component leading to elevation of arterial pressure. Hypoperfusion of the kidneys with resulting activation of the renin-angiotensin-aldosterone axis probably contributes to some degree. Abnormal aortic compliance, variable capacity of collateral vessels, and abnormal setting of baroreceptors also have been implicated in the pathogenesis of hypertension.

BIBLIOGRAPHY

1. Blumenfeld JD, Sealey JE, Schlussel Y, et al: Diagnosis and therapy of primary hyperaldosteronism. Ann Intern Med 121:877–885, 1994.
2. Bonelli FS, McKusick M, Textor SC, et al: Renal artery angioplasty: Technical results and outcome in 320 patients. Mayo Clin Proc 70:1041–1052, 1995.
3. Gagner M, Breton G, Pharland D, et al: Is laparoscopic adrenalectomy indicated for pheochromocytoma? Surgery 120:1076–1080, 1996.
4. Lairmore TC, Ball DW, Baylin SB, et al: Management of pheochromocytomas in patients with multiple endocrine neoplasia type 2 syndromes. Ann Surg 217:595–603, 1993.
5. Lamki LH, Haynie TP: Role of adrenal imaging in surgical management. J Surg Oncol 43:139–147, 1990.
6. Stanley JC: The evolution of surgery for renovascular disease. Cardiovasc Surg 2:195–202, 1994.
7. Tullis MJ, Zierler RE, Glickmore OP, et al: Results of percutaneous transluminal angioplasty for atherosclerotic renal artery stenosis: A follow up study with duplex ultrasound. J Vasc Surg 25:46–54, 1997.

V. Breast Surgery

61. BREAST MASSES

Christina A. Finlayson, M.D.

1. What are the three parts of breast screening that assist in the early diagnosis of breast cancer?

Breast self-examination (BSE) should begin at age 20 and be performed monthly. The breast is usually easiest to examine on the days immediately following the menstrual cycle. BSE can be frustrating to patients, particularly when they have fibrocystic change, because they are not certain what they are feeling or supposed to feel. The technique of BSE should be taught early and reinforced regularly. If a palpable tumor develops, women who regularly perform BSE present with tumors 1 cm or smaller more frequently than women who do not perform BSE.

Clinical or physician breast examination (CBE) also should begin at age 20 and be performed annually for women at average risk for breast cancer. Although tumors between 0.5 cm and 1.0 cm occasionally can be detected by an experienced clinician, tumors between 1.0 and 1.5 cm can detected 60% of the time. As the tumor grows, 96% of tumors larger than 2.0 cm can be identified on clinician physical examination.

Screening mammography has had the most substantial impact on the early diagnosis of, and subsequent decrease in mortality from, breast cancer.

2. When should routine mammography begin?

When mammography screening begins at age 40, a 30% decrease in death from breast cancer can be realized. Mammography should be performed annually.

3. Does a normal or negative mammogram guarantee that no cancer is present?

No. Mammography has a false-negative rate of at least 15%. For a breast cancer to be detected on mammography, it must have tissue characteristics that are different from the surrounding tissue. Some tumors, particularly lobular carcinoma, invade the surrounding breast tissue in a way that does not alter the characteristics of the breast tissue. Such tumors are often not visible on mammogram.

4. What is the difference between a screening and a diagnostic mammogram?

Screening mammography is done in asymptomatic women to look for clinically occult breast cancer. Two views of each breast are obtained. When a woman has a breast complaint such as a mass or an abnormal screening mammogram, diagnostic mammography is performed. A diagnostic mammogram pays particular attention to the area of clinical concern. Additional views taken at multiple angles or compression views taken with increased magnification of the abnormality help to distinguish between benign and malignant changes.

5. How are mammographic abnormalities characterized?

The American College of Radiography has developed a standard interpretation score to decrease ambiguity in mammographic reporting:

Bi-Rads	0	Requires further evaluation
	1	Negative (normal exam without any findings)
	2	Benign (normal exam with a definitely benign finding)

3   Probably benign (< 3% chance of malignancy)
4   Suspicious (30% chance of malignancy)
5   Highly suspicious or malignant

- **Category 0** is a temporary designation that requires further diagnostic imaging by either ultrasound or compression (magnification) views of the abnormality. After further evaluation, such mammograms are reclassified into one of the other categories.
- **Categories 1 and 2** require no further evaluation; the usual mammographic schedule is not altered.
- For **category 3**, a short-interval (6-month) diagnostic mammogram of the affected breast is recommended. Alternatively, a biopsy may be performed.
- **Categories 4 and 5** require a biopsy.

6. Which biopsy techniques aid in the diagnosis of mammographic abnormalities?

Several image-guided biopsy techniques maximize diagnostic yield while minimizing patient discomfort and loss of normal tissue:

Tru-cut core biopsy is performed with a 14–18-gauge coring needle. Several tissue samples (at least seven) are obtained.

Mammotome biopsy is performed with an 11-gauge vacuum-assisted biopsy needle. Mammotome can remove an entire lesion or area of calcification. A marking clip can be left in the breast at the site of the abnormality. Core biopsy and mammotome can be performed with local anesthesia alone.

The **advanced breast biopsy instrument** (ABBI) removes up to a 2-cm core of breast tissue. It usually requires local anesthesia and mild sedation and usually is performed in the operating room.

Needle localization breast biopsy is a surgical procedure is a surgical procedure requiring the radiologist to place a thin wire into the breast at the site of the abnormality. In the operating room, the wire and the breast tissue surrounding the wire are removed. This procedure can be done with local anesthesia with or without sedation.

Although **fine-needle aspiration** (FNA) is excellent for evaluation of palpable abnormalities, its sensitivity and specificity for image-guided biopsy are not acceptable.

With the exception of FNA, each of these techniques has an equivalent success rate in identifying the pathology associated with the mammographic abnormality. A 5% false-negative rate is associated with each of these techniques.

7. What are the characteristics of a dominant breast mass?

Identification of a dominant mass, especially in premenopausal women, can be challenging. Typically, a dominant mass can be palpated in three dimensions, and its density is distinct from surrounding breast tissue. Symptoms of equal importance are nodule, lump, thickening, and asymmetry. Breast cancer cannot be excluded by physical examination alone. "Failure to be impressed by physical exam findings" is the most common reason cited for a delay in the diagnosis of breast cancer.

8. What are the four most important palpable breast masses?

Most dominant masses are benign. Examples include cysts, fibroadenomas, and fibrocystic masses. Carcinoma, although not the most common form of breast mass, is the reason that all persistent, dominant masses require a tissue diagnosis. Other less common causes of palpable breast masses are lipomas, granulomas, fat necrosis, epidermal inclusion cysts, and lactational adenomas.

9. What are the differential characteristics of the most common palpable masses?

A **cyst** is a regular, mobile mass that may be tender. It may be quite firm or fluctuant. A **fibroadenoma** is usually smooth, firm, elongated (longer than it is wide), and mobile with discrete borders. **Fibrocystic changes** often are described as "lumpy-bumpy" breast tissue. There may be a discrete focal area of fibrosis that is more dominant than the background irregular tissue.

Carcinoma is an irregular, hard, painless mass. In advanced stages it may become fixed to the chest wall or be associated with overlying skin changes. Although this is the classic presentation, carcinoma may present in a form similar to benign lesions. Lobular carcinoma often appears as a soft mass or area of thickening. Because physical examination alone is unreliable in definitively excluding breast cancer, a biopsy must be obtained for all persistent, dominant masses.

10. A 32-year-old woman presents with the complaint of a breast slump. Which questions about the patient's history are important in the evaluation of the mass?

The size of the mass, whether it has changed in size, how long it has been present, whether it is painful, skin changes, nipple discharge, or changes in relation to the menstrual cycle may be helpful. Evaluation of any breast condition includes an assessment of risk factors for breast cancer, including personal or family history of breast, ovarian, or other cancers; age at menarche; age at first full-term pregnancy; age at menopause, if applicable; birth control or hormone replacement use; and history of previous breast biopsy.

11. The mass identified in question 10 is discrete, not tender, and easily palpable and has gradually increased in size. What is the most appropriate next step?

Breast imaging can be useful in further defining the characteristics of a breast mass. Ultrasound of a discrete mass can determine if it is cystic or solid. There are specific ultrasound criteria for defining a simple cyst. A simple cyst can be aspirated or observed. A complex cyst must be further evaluated by aspiration (to see if it completely resolves) or by excisional biopsy. With a complex cyst, FNA or core biopsy has a higher risk of sampling error of the solid component. A solid mass requires a tissue diagnosis.

12. How is a cyst aspiration performed?

A 22-gauge needle is inserted into the cyst, and fluid is withdrawn. Generally, a 10-ml syringe is adequate, although occasionally cysts contain larger amounts of fluid. If the cyst is quite deep and difficult to fix between the clinician's fingers, the aspiration can be performed under ultrasound guidance. Aspiration of a cyst is both diagnostic and therapeutic. After aspiration, the mass should resolve completely. If a mass persists or recurs after two aspirations, it should be excised. Cyst fluid may be clear or cloudy yellow, green, gray, or brown. A purely blood aspirate or an aspirate of what appears to be old blood should be sent for cytology, and excision of the lesion should be considered.

13. What techniques are available for diagnosis of a palpable, solid breast mass?

FNA, core biopsy, incisional biopsy, and excisional biopsy have a role in diagnosing palpable breast masses. Which technique is used depends on the nature of the lesions and available technical support.

FNA recovers cells from the mass and requires a dedicated cytopathologist for accurate interpretation. Several benign and malignant lesions can be characterized accurately by FNA, but FNA cannot discriminate between invasive and in situ carcinoma. To be used effectively, it must be correlated with physical examination and breast imaging.

Core biopsy is also a sampling technique that removes 14–18-gauge pieces of tissue for histologic evaluation by the pathologist. Because it is a sampling, there is a risk of missing the lesion and obtaining a false-negative result. Again, correlation with physical examination and imaging is important to avoid failure to diagnose a breast cancer.

Incisional biopsy is rarely used today. It has a role when a highly suspicious lesion that is a candidate for neoadjuvant treatment fails to be definitively diagnosed on core biopsy.

Excisional biopsy completely removes the target lesion. It provides the most tissue for pathologic evaluation and, in benign disease, is both diagnostic and therapeutic.

14. What is the role for breast imaging in the evaluation of a palpable breast mass?

Breast imaging helps to define the lesion as well as screens the remainder of the breast for secondary lesions. In general, breast imaging is done before biopsy because the artifact from the biopsy can interfere with the interpretation of the study.

In women younger than 30, in whom the risk of malignancy is low, mammography should be reserved for the most suspicious lesions. For women over 30, evaluation of a mass suspicious for malignancy includes mammography to characterize the mass as well as evaluate the remainder of the breast. For masses that have a low suspicion for malignancy, ultrasound can reliably differentiate between cystic and solid masses. A cyst aspiration or biopsy can be performed accordingly.

15. What is the "triple negative test" or "diagnostic triad"?

There are three components to diagnosing a palpable breast abnormality: physical examination, breast imaging, and biopsy. Benign lesions do not have to be removed, but the difficulty is in differentiating between a benign and a malignant lesion. When the characteristics of a mass on physical examination indicate low suspicion for malignancy, the mammogram is benign, and FNA recovers benign cells, the likelihood that the lesion is benign is 98%. Treatment options include excision for definitive diagnosis or observation. If observation is elected, the abnormality should be reexamined within 3 months to confirm that it is stable. If any component of the diagnostic triad is worrisome, definitive diagnosis, usually with excisional biopsy, is necessary.

BIBLIOGRAPHY

1. Bjurstam N, Bjorneld L, Duffy SW, et al: The Gothenburg breast screening trial: First results on mortality, incidence, and mode of detection for women ages 39–49 years at randomization. Cancer 80:2091–2099, 1997.
2. Cady B, Steele GD, Morrow M, et al: Evaluation of common breast problems: Guidance for primary care providers. Cancer 48:49–63, 1998.
3. Farwell MF, Foster RS Jr, Costanza M: Breast cancer and earlier detection efforts: Realized and unrealized impact on state. Arch Surg 128:510–513, 1993.
4. Harris JR, Lippmann ME, Morrow M, et al (eds): Diseases of the Breast. Philadelphia, Lippincott-Raven, 1996.
5. Morris A, Pommier RF, Schmidt WA, et al: Accurate evaluation of palpable breast masses by the triple test score. Arch Surg 133:930–934, 1998.
6. Singletary SE, Bevers T, Dempsey P, et al: Screening for and evaluation of suspicious breast lesions: NCCN practice guidelines. Oncology 12:89–138, 1998.

62. PRIMARY THERAPY FOR BREAST CANCER

Benjamin O. Anderson, M.D., F.A.C.S.

1. How is breast cancer diagnosed?

A diagnosis of cancer requires tissue confirmation. A diagnosis of breast cancer usually is made by **excisional biopsy** (removal of the entire mass) performed under local anesthesia. Needle biopsies are helpful in selected patients, as long as the limitations of sampling techniques are understood. **Fine-needle aspiration** (FNA) is useful for verifying a clinical impression of malignancy but requires formal histologic (as opposed to cytologic) confirmation at some point, because false-positive cytologies occasionally occur. **Core-needle biopsy**, if positive for cancer, may be considered a definitive diagnosis of cancer (see chapter 61). However, a negative core-needle biopsy may represent sampling error and therefore can be difficult to interpret. Core-needle biopsies can distinguish invasive from noninvasive (in situ) cancers (see question 4), whereas FNA cytology cannot.

2. What is the role of mammography after biopsy of a cancer?

Mammography after diagnosis is most valuable for identifying additional cancers in the same breast or opposite breast. Mammography also may be useful in counseling patients who must choose between breast conservation (lumpectomy and radiation) and mastectomy (see question 8). Women with highly dense or cystic breasts often have mammograms that defy accurate interpretation. Such women may consider mastectomy instead of breast conservation, because local cancer recurrence in the conserved breast is difficult to detect promptly.

3. Does a delay between biopsy and definitive treatment adversely affect cure?

Probably not—if the delay is only for a few days or weeks. Delays of more than 3–4 weeks should be avoided. A possible exception is the pregnant patient, in whom tumor growth may be quite rapid; prompt treatment appears to be particularly important.

4. What is the difference between noninvasive (in situ) and invasive breast cancers?

Noninvasive (in situ) cancers are malignant cells that remain confined to the duct or lobule in which they originated. In situ cancers have minimal chance of spreading to nodes or distant sites, because they have contacted neither lymphatic nor vascular channels through which they metastasize. Invasive cancers have traversed the basement membrane of their originating duct or lobule and, therefore, have metastatic potential. With little chance for spread, in situ cancers without invasion do not warrant lymph node dissection as part of definitive surgery.

5. How is breast cancer staged?

	HISTOLOGY	TUMOR SIZE	NODAL METASTASES	DISTANT METASTASES
Stage 0	Noninvasive	Any	—	—
Stage I	Invasive	< 2 cm	No	No
Stage II	Invasive	2–5 cm < 5 cm > 5 cm	No Yes No	No
Stage III	Invasive	> 5 cm Any size Skin or chest wall invasion	Yes Fixed nodes Yes or no	No
Stage IV	Invasive	Any size	Yes or no	Yes

6. Why is staging of breast cancer important?

Cancer staging is important because (1) it defines a common descriptive vocabulary and (2) the stages correlate with likelihood of relapse and fatality. The TNM (tumor, node, metastasis) staging summarizes data about tumor size, axillary node metastases, and distant metastases. In general, stage I breast cancers are small cancers without nodal metastases; stage II cancers are intermediate-sized cancers with or without axillary nodal metastases; stage III cancers are locally advanced cancers, usually with axillary nodal metastases; and stage IV cancers already have metastasized to distant sites.

7. Where does breast cancer spread (other than to lymph nodes)? Which diagnostic tests are useful for identifying such metastases?

Breast cancers most commonly metastasize to bone, lung, liver, and brain. Screening for bone metastases begins with whole-body radionuclide bone scanning. Bone scans are quite sensitive but less specific for metastases. Lesions seen on bone scan are further studied by standard radiographic techniques to distinguish metastases from benign inflammatory conditions. Lung metastases are identified by chest radiograph or CT scan. Liver function tests (LFTs) are commonly used to screen for liver metastases. Unfortunately, LFTs are neither specific nor sensitive for this purpose. LFTs are most commonly elevated because of benign hepatic pathology rather than metastases, and 25% of breast cancer patients with known liver metastases have normal LFTs. Liver imaging tests (ultrasound or abdominal CT), although more expensive, are more reliable for the diagnosis of liver metastases. Brain metastases are generally imaged by CT or MRI scanning.

8. Which preoperative studies should be done before mastectomy or lumpectomy to identify metastases?

Identification of stage IV (metastatic) cancers at first presentation is infrequent, because they represent 5% or fewer of all initially diagnosed breast cancers. Metastatic studies, therefore, should be used selectively at first diagnosis. All patients with symptoms suggesting metastatic disease (bone pain, pulmonary symptoms, jaundice, seizures) should be evaluated by appropriate preoperative testing once invasive breast cancer has been diagnosed. The asymptomatic patient, by comparison, warrants a limited evaluation. The standard minimal preoperative work-up for invasive disease consists of a chest radiograph and LFTs. In reality, the utility of these tests among early-stage cancers is quite low. Routine chest radiography identifies unsuspected lung metastases in fewer than 1% of patients. Chest radiography often is justified for other reasons and is useful as a baseline test for future comparison. LFTs, on the other hand, may become eliminated from the standard preoperative breast cancer work-up because of their limited sensitivity and specificity for metastatic disease (see question 7).

9. What are the alternatives for primary treatment of invasive breast cancer?

1. **Modified radical mastectomy.** Removal of the breast, including the nipple-areolar complex, and removal (dissection) of axillary lymph nodes have survival benefit equivalent to radical mastectomy, which also removes the pectoralis major muscle. The true radical mastectomy is rarely performed today. The pectoralis major muscle may be removed, with minimal morbidity, in a modified radical mastectomy to facilitate dissection of the highest (level III) lymph nodes.

2. **Partial mastectomy (lumpectomy or quadrantectomy).** Breast conservation therapy includes resection limited to removal of the breast tumor with a margin of normal breast tissue (negative margins), axillary dissection, and postoperative adjuvant breast irradiation. Breast conservation therapy has been shown in retrospective and prospective randomized studies to have survival rates equivalent to those for modified radical mastectomy among defined patient subgroups (see question 13). Although some surgeons reserved breast-conserving therapy for patients without axillary node metastases, this restriction is no longer thought to be correct. Treatment of the breast tumor and treatment of axillary nodes appear to be independent issues, according to current data.

3. **Primary irradiation to the breast.** Primary breast irradiation without surgery—not to be confused with postoperative adjuvant irradiation—is under evaluation in European cancer centers. Primary breast irradiation is not accepted currently as standard treatment in the United States, because it has not been shown to have curative potential equivalent to that of surgically based approaches with proved efficacy.

10. What is the overall survival rate after definitive treatment?

Stage I: 70–90% 10-year survival rate

Stage II: 50–70% 10-year survival rate

Stage III: 20–50% 10-year survival rate

Adjuvant (postoperative) chemotherapy and/or hormonal therapy increases these survival rates by 40–50%, based on many prospective randomized trials.

11. What is the National Surgical Adjuvant Breast Project B-06 (NSABP B-06)? What is its significance?

The NSABP B-06 is a multicenter study that randomized nearly 2,000 women with stages I and II tumors (< 4 cm) to three treatment modalities: segmental mastectomy (SM) alone, SM with radiation, and total mastectomy (TM). All patients underwent axillary dissection, and patients with positive nodes received adjuvant chemotherapy. At least two significant conclusions were reached. Patients who underwent SM without radiation therapy had lower rates of disease-free survival than patients who underwent SM with radiation therapy. There was **no difference in overall survival rates** between the two groups, but radiation therapy was of benefit in control of local tumor (i.e., decreased recurrence in the breast). In patients who underwent SM (with or without radiation), there was **no difference in disease-free survival or overall survival rates**, indicating that breast conservation surgery is an effective treatment in the appropriate setting.

12. What is a quadrantectomy (as opposed to lumpectomy or SM)?

A quadrantectomy is resection of the tumor along with the involved quadrant of the breast, including the skin. Quadrantectomy, lumpectomy, and SM are clinically the same procedure, differing primarily in the amount of breast tissue that is removed.

13. Are some patients poor candidates for breast conservation therapy?

Patients should be counseled against lumpectomy and irradiation in certain circumstances. Contraindications (relative or absolute) to breast conservation include (1) cancers that cannot be excised with negative margins without mastectomy, (2) cancers that are too large relative to the breast to obtain acceptable cosmetic results, (3) multicentric cancers (i.e,. multiple cancers in the same breast), and (4) patients who do not desire or who have a specific contraindication to adjuvant radiation therapy (e.g., pregnancy).

14. Which patients who have undergone radical mastectomy may undergo immediate breast reconstruction (i.e., at the same operation)?

Controversy surrounds patient selection for immediate reconstruction. Most agree that patients with noninvasive (in situ) or early invasive (stage I and selected stage II) breast cancers may be offered immediate reconstruction with either a myocutaneous flap or a breast implant. It is disadvantageous to perform immediate reconstruction in patients with locally advanced (stage III) breast cancer because (1) the patient may require chest wall irradiation and (2) a subsequent chest wall recurrence, which is more likely with advanced cancers, may be potentially difficult to detect with an overlying flap of tissue.

15. Which studies should be obtained after definitive surgery to screen for metastases and as baseline studies for future comparison?

The utility of metastatic screening tests correlates with the locoregional tumor and nodal (TN) staging determined at surgery. Patients with locally advanced (stage III and some stage II) cancers are at high risk for developing cancer recurrence with metastases. Bone scan and liver imaging (CT or ultrasound) are generally helpful as baseline studies. These tests occasionally reveal previously unappreciated metastatic disease. Conversely, such baseline studies are best avoided in asymptomatic patients with stage I (small, node-negative) cancers, because the chance of cure is high and the likelihood of finding metastases is remote. With stage I breast cancer, for example, the likelihood of a false-positive result on bone exceeds the likelihood of a true positive result by 250%. Brain imaging (CT or MRI), because of low yield in asymptomatic patients, usually is reserved for patients with neurologic symptoms.

16. What is the treatment of ductal carcinoma in situ (DCIS)?

In the past DCIS—also known as intraductal carcinoma—was thought to be a multicentric disease demanding mastectomy. This belief led to the paradoxical conclusion that a noninvasive cancer (DCIS) without the potential for metastatic spread required a more aggressive surgical approach than an invasive cancer of similar dimensions. As widespread screening mammography resulted in the detection of more cases of smaller, nonpalpable DCIS, this approach was reevaluated. Data from the NSABP B-17 trial (randomized excision vs. excision with radiation therapy) suggest that DCIS can be safely treated by breast conservation therapy (lumpectomy plus adjuvant radiation), provided that it can be excised with negative margins and that the remainder of the breast can be adequately evaluated and followed for development of subsequent malignancy.

17. Can some cases of DCIS be treated by lumpectomy without radiotherapy?

Using carefully collected retrospective data, Silverstein, Lagios, and colleagues developed a prognostic index (scoring system) for DCIS based on histologic grade, tumor size, and margin width. Their data suggest that small (< 1 cm), non–high-grade DCIS lesions resected with wide surgical margins do not require radiation therapy in addition to lumpectomy. However, forgoing radiation treatment after lumpectomy for DCIS remains controversial. Recent reports suggest that late local recurrence rates (15–25 years) for non–high-grade DCIS may exceed 25%.

18. What should be the treatment of lobular carcinoma in situ (LCIS)?

LCIS behaves differently from its ductal counterpart. LCIS may not invariably degenerate into invasive cancer, but women with proven LCIS have a 20–25% chance of developing breast cancer during their lifetime. Unfortunately, the cancer may be ductal or lobular in origin and may develop with equal likelihood in the ipsilateral or contralateral breast. Most authorities interpret the histologic finding of LCIS as a significant marker for high risk of breast cancer and suggest careful surveillance with serial mammography and physical examination. Bilateral mastectomy, the only logical surgical procedure for this condition, is extreme and has not been shown to improve overall survival rates for LCIS.

In the NSABP P-01 Tamoxifen Prevention Trial, women at heightened risk for the development of breast cancer (> 1.66% risk over the next 5 years) were shown to develop fewer breast canceres when given tamoxifen rather than placebo. For women with LCIS, the 5-year breast cancer incidence was 6.8% in the placebo group and 2.5% in the tamoxifen group, representing a 56% reduction in breast cancers. However, the number of breast cancers that were prevented rivaled the number of tamoxifen-associated complications, including endometrial cancers and thrombotic events. No survival benefit to tamoxifen prophylaxis has yet been observed. At this time, women with LCIS should be offered tamoxifen as an option for treatment and cancer prevention, although they may reasonably decline when presented with the complete data.

19. What is inoperable breast cancer?

Inoperable breast cancer has advanced beyond the boundaries of surgical resection. The spread may be regional (internal mammary lymph nodes, stage IIIB) or distant (distant metastases, stage IV). Supraclavicular lymph node metastases, which are beyond the margins of surgical resection, convey the same unfortunate prognosis as metastasis to distant solid organs and currently are staged as such. Primary therapy with such advanced cancers is systemic treatment (chemotherapy or hormonal therapy) rather than surgery. Surgery combined with radiation therapy becomes an adjuvant therapy for local control of disease after a good response to systemic treatment.

20. What is neoadjuvant therapy for breast cancer?

Locally advanced but operable (stage IIIA and some stage II) cancers have a high likelihood of recurrence after surgery. Neoadjuvant therapy is induction chemotherapy before surgery to decrease the local tumor burden and to begin treatment of micrometastatic disease at the earliest possible time. It is not yet known whether the timing of chemotherapy relative to surgery influences survival time from diagnosis. The role of neoadjuvant therapy is under evaluation in prospective and randomized trials. If a cancer is so locally advanced that negative margins are likely to be unobtainable even by mastectomy, neoadjuvant chemotherapy should be considered. In addition, preliminary data suggest that neoadjuvant therapy may convert some cancers that otherwise would require mastectomy into potential candidates for breast conservation surgery, although the safety of this approach warrants careful scrutiny.

21. What is sentinel lymph node mapping for breast cancer?

Removing normal lymph nodes in a standard node dissection provides important staging information, but at significant risk for later complications, the most notable of which is lymphedema of the arm. Sentinel lymph node mapping is a technique by which a radioactive tracer (Tc-labeled sulfur colloid) and/or a blue dye (lymphazurin) is injected in the breast to find the first upstream node to which a cancer would spread. If the sentinel lymph node or nodes are found to be negative for cancer, the remaining node dissection may potentially be avoided. Sentinel node mapping for breast cancer is not yet the standard of care in the U.S., but it is rapidly becoming a part of surgical practice. Mapping appears to be most appropriate for small breast cancers with clinically normal axillae. The technique may be less reliable with larger cancers, when the primary cancers have been previously excised from the breast for diagnosis, and/or when the patient was treated with neoadjuvant chemotherapy (see question 20). The risk of sentinel node mapping is that it may understage a patient by suggesting that the cancer is node-negative when in fact nodal metastases are present in other "nonsentinel" lymph nodes. As a result, the patient may be treated with less systemic chemotherapy than is appropriate and necessary to minimize cancer mortality.

BIBLIOGRAPHY

1. Anderson BO, Petrck JA, Byrd DR, et al: Pregnancy influences breast cancer stage at diagnosis in women 30 years of age and younger. Ann Surg Oncol 3:204–211, 1996.
2. Colleoni M, Orvieto E, Nole F, Orlando L, et al: Prediction of response to primary chemotherapy for operable breast cancer. Eur J Cancer 35:574–579, 1999.
3. Fisher B, Bryant J, Wolmark N, et al: Effect of preoperative chemotherapy on the outcome of women with operable breast cancer. J Clin Oncol 16:2672–2685, 1998.
4. Fisher B, Costantino JP, Wickerham DL, et al: Tamoxifen for prevention of breast cancer: Report of the National Surgical Adjuvant Breast and Bowel Project P-1 study. J Natl Cancer Inst 90:1371–1388, 1998.
5. Fisher B, Redmond C, Fisher ER, et al: Ten-year results of a randomized clinical trial comparing radical mastectomy and total mastectomy with or without radiation. N Engl J Med 312:674–681, 1985.
6. Fisher R, Redmond C, Poisson R, et al: Eight year results of a randomized clinical trial comparing total mastectomy and lumpectomy with or without irradiation in the treatment of breast cancer. N Engl J Med 320:822–828, 1989.
7. Giess CS, Keathing DM, Osborne MP, Rosenblatt R: Local tumor recurrence following breast-conservation therapy: Correlation of histopathologic findings with detection method and mammographic findings. Radiology 212:829-35, 1999.
8. Harlow SP, Krag DN, Ames SE, Weaver DL: Intraoperative ultrasound localization to guide surgical excision of nonpalpable breast carcinoma. J Am Coll Surg 189:241–246, 1999.
9. Heimann R, Karrison T, Hellman S: Treatment of ductal carcinoma in situ. N Engl J Med 341:999–1000, 1999.
10. Kaufman CS, Delbecq R, Jacobson L: Preoperative needle biopsy is helpful to the breast surgeon. J Am Coll Surg 189:335–336, 1999.
11. Silverstein MJ, Lagios MD, Craig PH, et al: A prognostic index for ductal carcinoma in situ of the breast. Cancer 77:2267–2274, 1996.
12. Singer A: Accuracy of intraoperative frozen-section analysis of axillary nodes. Br J Surg 86:1092–1093, 1999.

VI. *Other Cancers*

63. WHAT IS CANCER?

John Ridge, M.D., Ph.D.

1. What is a neoplasm?

A neoplasm is a new growth of tissue (tumor) in which cells grow progressively under conditions that do not prompt the growth of normal cells. A malignant neoplasm (cancer) is composed of cells that invade other tissues and spread.

2. What kinds of cancers are there?

Malignant tumors of epithelial (surface tissue) cells are **carcinomas**. Malignant tumors of mesenchymal (connective tissue) cells are **sarcomas.** Carcinomas and sarcomas are **solid** tumors. Hematologic malignancies, such as leukemia, are **liquid** tumors of mesenchymal origin.

3. What about skin cancers?

Most basal cell and squamous skin cancers are life-threatening only if neglected. They occur in tremendous numbers and are seldom fatal with proper treatment. Although the general principles of cancer management apply to skin cancers, they usually are not considered in the same class with other solid tumors.

4. Why is cancer bad for you?

Simple replacement of normal tissue by tumor eventually causes organ dysfunction. If a tumor outgrows its blood supply and becomes necrotic, local inflammation may ensue. Often obstruction develops as the tumor grows. Hence, the cancer may block the gastrointestinal tract, bile ducts, or airway. Sometimes the cancer bleeds. Nerve invasion or inflammation may cause pain. Cancers also may elaborate humoral factors that cause symptoms.

5. Are all cancers life-threatening?

Cancer is a fatal disease. Currently more than one-half of patients with cancer are cured in the United States. It is uncommon for a patient with an untreated cancer to die of something else.

6. How do cancers start?

No one knows, but abnormal cells begin dividing under circumstances when normal cells would not. Many steps are involved, with effects on the control of cell differentiation, division, and growth. The abnormal cells must then infiltrate through surrounding normal tissues. Most cancers eventually spread to distant sites as well.

7. What do oncogenes have to do with this process?

The genes involved with the transformation of normal cells into malignant cells are termed **oncogenes**. They add functions to normal cells, leading to more aggressive behavior. Tumor suppressor genes inhibit growth, and their loss also may result in cancer.

8. How does cancer spread?

Patients die of cancers because the tumors invade normal tissues and then spread. Cancer cells escape control mechanisms and promote self-feeding blood vessel formation. This angiogenesis precedes invasion of normal tissues. Cancer cells then infiltrate locally and make their way into blood and lymph. Circulating cancer cells may come to rest in lymph nodes or distant tissues, where metastatic foci form and begin to recruit additional blood supplies in their new environment.

9. Do all cancers spread?

About one-fourth of patients with solid tumors have detectable metastases at the time of diagnosis. Less than one-half of the remainder will develop metastases during the course of treatment. At diagnosis a cancer is usually at least one centimeter in diameter (and often much larger), containing millions of cells. It is surprising that metastases have not occurred in all patients at the time of diagnosis.

10. Does this process have an effect on how surgeons treat cancers?

Operations to treat benign conditions are designed to remove as little tissue as possible while creating a new and desirable physiologic or anatomic state. Cancer operations, on the other hand, are designed to remove as much tissue as possible while leaving the patient with acceptable function. Cancer operations are designed to remove the primary tumors as well as the lymph nodes draining the primary site.

11. Why are lymph nodes removed during cancer operations?

More than 100 years ago William S. Halsted appreciated that tumor recurrence in the area of the scar after mastectomy was related to tumor in remaining lymph nodes when only the breast was removed. Halsted believed that cancer of the breast spread in an orderly fashion (or perhaps even contiguously) from the primary tumor to regional lymph nodes and eventually to distant sites. He popularized en bloc dissection of the breast with axillary lymph nodes for treatment of breast cancer. Conceptually, this approach was adopted for surgical treatment of solid tumors.

12. What is a sentinel lymph node?

Sentinel lymph nodes are the first stop for tumor cells metastasizing through lymphatics from the primary tumor. Often there is more than one sentinel node, even for a small tumor. If no tumor is present in a sentinel lymph node, it is unlikely that tumor is present in any of the other nodes. Sentinel lymph nodes have been identified for many organs (including the skin, breast, colon, and thyroid). Sentinel node evaluation to select patients for full lymph node dissection has become the standard of care for melanoma and seems promising for cancer of the breast.

13. Do solid tumors spread in an orderly way?

Not necessarily. Another view of breast cancer behavior became popular by the 1970s. Bernard Fisher postulated that cancer is widespread at its inception. He stated that "breast cancer is a systemic disease . . . and that variations in effective local regional treatment are unlikely to effect survival substantially."

14. How do these different models of cancer affect treatment?

Surgeons who believe that tumors spread in an orderly way tend to perform aggressive lymph node dissections in concert with resection of the primary tumor. They generally believe that lymphadenectomy will cure some patients who have lymph node involvement without distant metastases and that local recurrence is a preventable cause of death. Surgeons who believe that lymph node metastases are markers for systemic disease are usually far less aggressive in performing lymph node dissections, because (in their eyes) removal of lymph nodes that contain tumor will not cure patients who probably already have metastatic disease.

15. Do we know which model is correct?

Both are probably inadequate. Some solid tumors (such as squamous cancer of the head and neck and colon cancer) often have no distant disease, even when they have lymph node metastases. Their spread seems to be an orderly process. Other solid tumors seem to metastasize widely even when they are very small. For such cancers lymph node involvement is a reliable sign of metastases. Sarcomas seldom metastasize to lymph nodes, but patients may develop metastases limited to the lungs alone; such patients sometimes are cured by resection.

16. How else can solid tumors be treated with curative intent?

Instead of surgical removal of the primary tumor and appropriate lymph nodes, the entire area may be treated with curative radiation. Some types of cancer are more responsive to radiation than others. The side effects of curative radiation treatment are formidable and cannot be ignored. When radiation kills cancer cells, it injures adjacent normal tissues. The damage to normal tissues worsens over the course of the patient's life. The tolerance of nearby tissues to radiation is the limiting factor in treatment of cancers with radiation alone.

17. What is adjuvant therapy?

Adjuvant means "assisting or aiding." Adjuvant chemotherapy is of proven benefit in the treatment of breast cancer, colorectal cancer, and ovarian and testicular tumors. Adjuvant radiation therapy may be used after operations to reduce the risk of tumor recurrence about the surgical site. It is often used in treating rectal cancer, breast cancer, head and neck cancer, and sarcomas.

18. What cancer treatments are available in addition to surgery, radiation therapy, and cytotoxic chemotherapy?

Hormonal manipulation has been used for decades to slow growth of some tumors. Stimulation of the patient's immune system to combat cancer is potentially promising. This approach may involve vaccines, training of T cells, or enhancement of the immune response. New types of anticancer agents include drugs that interfere with tumor angiogenesis, monoclonal antibodies against growth factor receptors, drugs that alter intracellular signaling pathways, and drugs that restore cell cycle control.

19. Does the body fight cancer on its own?

Certainly. Some scientists believe that early cancers are regularly extirpated by the immune system (as we "catch" cancer every day) and that clinical cancers reflect a breakdown in immune surveillance. Immunosuppressed people are susceptible to some kinds of cancers. Regression of primary melanoma is well described. "Spontaneous remissions" of melanoma and renal cell carcinoma have interested oncologists for decades. Indeed, these are the tumors that initially seemed to respond well to adoptive immunotherapy and treatment with interleukin-2.

20. What is a tumor-infiltrating lymphocyte (TIL)?

TILs are lymphoid cells that infiltrate solid tumors and appear sensitized against autologous tumor antigens. Compared with circulating lymphocytes, TILs are far more reactive to cancer.

21. What are palliative treatments?

Palliative means "affording relief but not curing."

22. Give examples of palliative procedures.

Resection of the primary tumor in the face of distant metastases may be performed to treat bleeding or obstruction. Procedures to bypass intestinal or biliary obstruction in patients with unresectable cancer are common. Tracheotomies are created for patients who are unable to breathe because of upper airway obstruction, and feeding tubes may permit enteral nutrition in patients who cannot eat. Removal of isolated brain metastases often improves the patient's quality of life. Many patients with functioning endocrine tumors benefit from reduction in tumor mass.

23. What is cytoreductive surgery?

Cytoreductive ("debulking") procedures are designed to decrease tumor burden. Simply reducing tumor bulk is seldom sufficient to prolong survival. For cytoreductive surgery to be beneficial, the nonsurgical (adjunctive) therapy must be highly effective—such as radiation for glioblastoma.

CONTROVERSY

24. Is lymph node dissection for breast cancer of therapeutic value, or does it merely help select patients who should receive chemotherapy?

Those who believe that axillary lymph node dissection confers only information about tumor behavior rather than a therapeutic benefit usually cite the NSABP B-04 trial. This multicenter study randomized 1665 patients to receive (1) radical mastectomy, (2) total mastectomy with radiation, or (3) mastectomy followed by axillary dissection if tumor developed in the axilla. There was no statistically significant difference in survival curves between patients whose axilla was treated initially and patients who received delayed treatment to the axilla. In addition to other problems, however, the study lacked the power to prove the point. To have a 90% chance of detecting a 7% survival difference between the treatment groups the NSABP should have enrolled 2000 patients (not just 550) in each arm. Hence, a substantial survival advantage due to axillary dissection might not have been recognized. Indeed, subsequent randomized trials in the management of breast cancer, as well as evaluation of patterns of care, demonstrate a survival advantage conferred by axillary dissection.

BIBLIOGRAPHY

1. Bilchik, AJ, Guiliano A, Essner R, et al: Universal application of intraoperative lymphatic mapping and sentinel lymphadenectomy in solid neoplasms. Cancer J Sci Am 4:351–358., 1998.
2. Bland KI, Scott-Conner CEH, Menck H, et al: Axillary dissection in breast-conserving surgery for stage I and II breast cancer: A National Cancer Data Base study of patterns of omission and implications for survival. J Am Coll Surg 188:586–596, 1999.
3. Cabanes PA, Salmon RJ, Vilcoq JR, et al: Value of axillary dissection in addition to lumpectomy and radiotherapy in early breast cancer. Lancet 339:1245–1248., 1992
4. Fisher B, Redmond C, Fisher ER, et al: Ten-year results of a randomized clinical trial comparing radical mastectomy and total mastectomy with or without radiation. N Engl J Med 312:674–681, 1985.
5. Harris JR, Osteen RT: Patients with early breast cancer benefit from effective axillary treatment. Breast Cancer Res Treat 5:17–21, 1985.
6. Hellman S: Natural history of small breast cancers. J Clin Oncol 12:2229–2234., 1994
7. McKinnell RG, Parchment RE. Perantoni AO, Pierce GB: The Biological Basis of Cancer. Cambridge, Cambridge University Press, 1998.
8. Rosenberg SA: New Opportunities for the development of cancer immunotherapies. Cancer J Sci Am 4(Suppl 1):S1–S4, 1998.

64. MELANOMA

William R. Nelson, M.D.

1. What is *melanoma?*

The term *melanoma* implies a malignant tumor; malignant melanoma is redundant. The most malignant of all skin cancers, melanoma usually forms from a preexisting nevus or mole but may develop de novo.

2. What are the types of moles? Which are most prone to malignant change?

Intradermal: the most benign form.

Junctional: the junctional component may be the site of melanoma formation.

Compound: intradermal and junctional together; intermediate activity.

Spitz: once called juvenile melanoma, it is actually a spindle cell epithelioid nevus, quite benign.

Dysplastic: the most likely to turn malignant (especially in dysplastic nevus syndrome).

3. What are the risk factors in melanoma formation?
- Large number of moles (over 50 moles over 2 mm in diameter)
- Changing nevi
- Family history of melanoma
- Light, poorly tanning skin; blonde or reddish brown hair
- History of episodic, acute, severe sunburns
- Dysplastic nevus syndrome
- History of prior melanoma

Immunosuppression also can increase the risk. Congenital nevi are certainly more likely to turn malignant than the usual benign variety.

4. What is the familial melanoma syndrome?
The inherited familial mole and melanoma syndrome (FAM-M) has been defined as the occurrence of melanoma in one or more first- or second-degree relatives and the presence of over 50 moles of variable size, some of which are atypical histologically. The risk of melanoma in this syndrome runs as high as 100% in the person's lifetime.

5. Is a specific gene involved in melanoma development in the FAM-M syndrome?
Genetic studies have revealed a specific gene (p16) in many people with the FAM-M syndrome.

6. Which people are at low risk for melanoma formation?
Children under 10 years of age, black, Asian, native American, dark-complected whites, and, of course, people without any other risk factors.

7. What are common sites of melanoma development?
Posterior trunk in men and lower extremities in women. All sun-exposed areas are possible sites. Uncommon sites for melanoma formation are the soles of the feet, palms, and genitalia; these areas, however, are sites for melanoma formation in black patients. Unusual noncutaneous sites for melanoma formation are the eye, anus, and oral mucosa.

8. Where is melanoma most common?
Melanoma is most common in Australia, especially the northern part of the continent where light skin descendants of the original settlers are exposed to tropical sun.

9. What are the warning signs of melanoma?
- **A** = **A**symmetry
- **B** = Irregular **b**order
- **C** = **C**olor: variable; spotted; often very black with irregular tan areas; red or pink spots; ulcerated when advanced (bleeds easily)
- **D** = **D**iameter (> 5–6 mm)

10. What are the types of melanoma and their incidence?
Superficial spreading: 75% of all cases
Nodular: 15% of cases; most malignant; well circumscribed, deeply invasive
Lentigo maligna melanoma: 5% of cases; relatively good prognosis
Acral lentiginous: 5% of cases; often in people of color; soles, palms, subungual sites

11. Which moles should be considered for removal?
Growing and darkening nevi should be considered for removal, especially in sun-sensitive patients. Itching is a sign of early malignant change. Ulceration is a late sign. Because melanoma may be familial in origin, children of patients with melanomas should be carefully screened for very dark nevi.

12. How should suspicious nevi be biopsied?

It was once believed that incisional biopsy was contraindicated in all lesions suspected of being melanomas. Currently wedge biopsy is believed to be safe for any large lesion requiring complex repair if excised. The best method, however, is total excision of the lesion with a narrow (1-mm) margin of normal skin plus primary repair. Thorough pathologic study is essential.

13. Do melanomas spontaneously regress or even disappear?

Rarely melanomas can regress or even disappear. Remarkably, such patients have a poor prognosis despite the fact that the primary lesion has regressed or even sloughed off, because metastatic disease to nodes and viscera then is quite common.

14. What are the Breslow and Clark classifications of melanoma invasion?

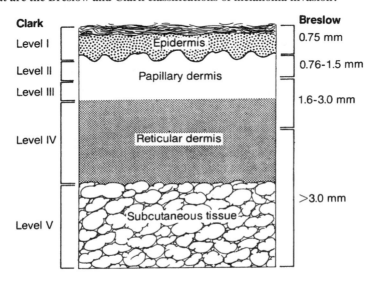

The Clark and Breslow classifications of melanoma invasion. (From Young OM, Mathes ST: In Schwartz SI (ed): Principles of Surgery, 6th ed. New York, McGraw-Hill, 1994, with permission.)

Clark selected five levels of melanoma thickness in the skin:

Level I: intradermal melanoma that does not metastasize; may be better termed atypical melanotic hyperplasia, a benign lesion.
Level II: melanoma that penetrates the basement membrane into the papillary dermis.
Level III: melanoma that fills the papillary dermis and encroaches on the reticular dermis in a pushing fashion.
Level IV: melanoma that invades the reticular dermis.
Level V: melanoma that works its way into the subcutaneous fat.

The **Breslow method** requires an optical micrometer fitted to the ocular position of a standard microscope. This technique is a more exact determination of tumor invasion. Lesions are classified as follows: 0.75 mm, 0.76–1.5 mm, 1.51–3.99 mm, and 4.0 mm. Lesions less than 1 mm include melanoma in situ and thin invasive tumors. The cure rate in the latter is over 95% with excision. Tumors of 1.0–4.0 mm are called intermediate but involve risk of metastasis. Lesions over 4.0 mm are high-risk lesions with a poor cure rate.

All melanomas should be checked by both methods, because some tumors may show a low Breslow measurement with a deeper Clark level, indicating a great risk of recurrence and spread. Measurement of thickness is all important, and the tumor should be measured from the total height of the lesion vertically at the point of maximal thickness. In addition, if ulceration is present, the measurement should be from the bottom of the ulcer crater down to the deepest margin of the lesion.

15. What are the chances of nodal and systemic spread of the various degrees of melanoma invasion?

Regional node metastases occur in about 2% of melanomas less than 0.76 mm in depth; the distant spread is almost 0%. In tumors of 0.76–1.5 mm thickness, nodes are positive in 25%, and distant spread is 8%. In tumors of 1.5–4.0 mm thickness, node metastasis occurs in 57% and distant spread is 15%. In tumors over 4 mm, node metastasis occurs in up to 62%, and distant spread is about 72%.

16. What are the characteristics of a subungual melanoma?

Subungual lesions are often mistaken for a chronic inflammatory process; therefore, most patients present quite late. They are usually older than patients with other forms of cutaneous melanoma. The great toe is most common site of origin. Amputation at or proximal to the metatarsal phalangeal joint and regional sentinel lymph node biopsy are advised by most authors. The primary lesions are usually deeply invasive, and lymph nodes are positive in the great majority of cases either at the time of the original diagnosis or at subsequent follow-up.

17. Which skin lesions often mimic a primary melanoma?
- Spitz nevus (spindle cell epithelioid nevus)
- Atypical benign nevus
- Halo nevus
- Recurrent benign nevus after inadequate excision
- Metastatic melanoma to skin
- Mycosis fungoides
- Extramammary Paget's disease
- Bowen's disease
- Dark sebaceous keratoses
- Kaposi's sarcoma
- Pigmented basal cell carcinoma

18. Does elective node dissection improve cure rates in melanoma?

Data by Balch from American and Australian studies indicate that selective node dissection significantly increased actuarial survival rates for patients with primary melanomas of depths between 1.50 and 3.99 mm (intermediate tumors in the level III range). However, a report from the Sydney Australia Unit demonstrates no benefit with elective lymph node dissection in truncal and limb melanomas over 1.5 mm in depth. Recently, beginning with the work of Morton, who used lymphoscintigraphy to identify routes of lymph drainage and sentinel lymph node (SLN) identification, SLN biopsy has come to the fore. In this approach, the first-echelon node is removed. If negative for metastasis, further node dissection is not performed. (If the SLN is positive, lymph node dissection is completed.)

19. How is SLN biopsy changing the treatment of melanoma?

Rather than perform elective dissections, surgeons can determine by SLN biopsy whether nodal spread has occurred and then carry out a therapeutic procedure.

20. Describe the technique of SLN biopsy.

The SLN identification technique requires the cooperation of surgeon, radiologist, and pathologist. Lymphoscintigraphy with the injection of radioactive technetium sulfur colloid (99mTeSC) is performed around the site of the primary melanoma. Scans are then performed in about 15 minutes. The SLN is then located and the overlying skin is marked with an intradermal tattoo. In approximately 4 hours, the patient is taken to the operating room for injection of blue dye around the primary site (lymphazurin 1%). In 10 minutes a hand-held gamma probe identifies the hot spot, and a small incision is made over this area for removal of the SLN. The node is then examined histologically.

21. Do routine histologic studies miss micrometastases? What newer methods help to identify such spread?

It has been estimated that a routine sectioning and study of a lymph node expose only 1% of the total volume of tissue. Cell cultures were originally used to identify micrometastases. This technique has been abandoned in favor of an assay with a combination of reverse transcriptase (RT) plus polymerase chain reaction (PCR). In one study, histologically RT-PCR-positive patients had a recurrence rate of 60%. If both assays were negative, the rate was 2%; 47% of patients were histologically negative and RT/PCR positive. The recurrence rate was 10%.

22. What are the results of lymph node studies in patients undergoing SLN biopsy and node dissection?

Brobeil and associates found 13.9% micrometastases in SLNs. In lesions over 4.0 mm 30% of nodes were positive. From 1.5–4 mm, 18% of nodes were positive, and in lesions of 1.0–1.5 mm 7% of nodes contained melanoma. In lesions less than 0.76 mm no positive nodes were found. In patients who underwent node dissection after the SLN-positive report, 8% had further positive nodes. All patients with positive lymph nodes in the dissections had tumors over 3.0 mm.

23. How important is anatomic site in the prognosis of melanoma patients?

Patients with melanomas of the trunk have a poorer prognosis than patients with lesions of the extremities.

24. Do women have a better prognosis with melanoma?

For unexplained reasons, survival rates are definitely higher in female patients, as substantiated in series controlled for variables of age, site, Clark's level, histology, and Breslow's thickness.

25. Does ulceration of a melanoma make a difference in outcome?

According to the Alabama and Sydney studies, patients with ulcerated stage I and II melanomas have a 10-year survival rate of 50%, whereas patients with nonulcerated lesions of the same stages have a 10-year survival rate of 75%. Tumor thickness and ulceration are the two most dominant features of aggressive primary melanomas.

26. If indicated, which types of node dissection should be performed?

If there is no evidence of gross involvement of nodes except for the histologically positive SLN, a functional type dissection is preferred by most authorities because it preserves vital nerves and vessels.

27. Is in-continuity removal of primary site and nodes ever indicated?

In-continuity removal of primary site and nodes is carried out if the primary lesions are near lymph node areas and if the SLNs are positive.

28. How much normal skin should be removed around a melanoma?

Melanoma in situ can be cured with an excisional margin of 0.5 mm, whereas a thin melanoma of less than 0.75 mm can be excised with a 1.0 cm margin of normal skin and underlying subcutaneous tissue (down to the fascia). For thicker lesions, a 2-cm margin is now advised.

29. Does pregnancy worsen the prognosis of melanoma?

In the past it was believed that pregnancy decreased survival rates in patients with melanoma, but more recent studies have indicated no significant alterations in rates of cure.

30. Does melanoma respond to chemotherapy or immunotherapy?

Various chemotherapy regimens are used, some in combination with cytokines such as interferon (IFN) and interleukin. Much work continues on these helpful approaches. A significant impact on survival in the relapse-free interval has been obtained with adjuvant IFN-alpha 2B in patients at risk for recurrence. This treatment has been applied especially to patients with microscopic positive nodes, including the SLN.

31. Can radiotherapy be of help in melanoma treatment?
Radiotherapy, once believed to be ineffective in melanoma, has been shown recently to be quite helpful as palliative treatment of metastatic disease.

32. Can amputation be used in the management of locally advanced melanoma?
In selected cases, amputations may be palliative. This approach applies to huge fungating masses or cases with extensive satellites.

33. What is isolation perfusion? How is it used in melanoma?
This technique is often used in the treatment of local spread of melanoma in an extremity (in-transit spread). Chemotherapy drugs or biologic preparations (such as interferon or tumor necrosis factor) are circulated through an isolated extremity using a pump oxygenator. This method is highly effective in some cases, although recurrence may develop.

34. What is the treatment of a patient with metastatic nodes confined to a single area when the primary site is unknown?
If careful studies show no other foci of melanoma, radical lymph node dissection should be carried out. Cure rates as high as 15% have been reported in these unusual situations.

35. How do you manage postlymphadenectomy edema of an extremity, especially the leg?
Edema of the lower extremity can be kept to a minimum with the use of tailor-made support stockings placed immediately after surgery.

36. What procedures should be used in the follow-up care of patients undergoing curative surgery for melanoma?
Besides frequent physical examinations, chest radiographs and liver function tests are important.

37. Is cure possible in a patient with a single, isolated distant metastasis of melanoma?
In a series reported by Overett and Shiu, a survival rate of 33% was achieved in a large series of patients undergoing resection of single isolated distant metastases. Such patients, of course, must be carefully studied to rule out other evidence of spread.

BIBLIOGRAPHY

1. Alpertini JJ, Cruse CW, et al: Intraoperative radiolymphoscintigraphy improves sentinel lymph node identification for patients with melanoma. Ann Surg 223:217–224, 1996.
2. Balch CM, Houghton AN, Sober AJ, Soong S: Cutaneous Melanoma. St. Louis, Quality Medical Publishing, 1998.
3. Brobel TE, Glass F: Results of complete lymph node dissection in 83 melanoma patients with positive sentinel nodes. Ann Surg Oncol 5:119–125, 1998.
4. Gershenwald JE, Colome MI, et al: Patterns of recurrence following negative sentinel lymph node biopsy in 243 patients with stage I or II melanoma. J Clin Oncol 16:2253–2260, 1998.
5. Rineborg U, Anderson R, et al: Resection margins of 2 versus 5 cm for cutaneous malignant melanoma with a tumor thickness of 0.8 to 2.0 mm—Swedish Melanoma Study Group. Cancer 77:1809–1814, 1996.
6. Morton DL, Wen DR, Wong JH, et al: Technical details of intraoperative lymphatic mapping for early stage melanoma. Arch Surg 127:392–399, 1992.
7. Reintgen D, Balch CM, Kirkwood J, Ross M: Recent advances in the care of the patient with malignant melanoma. Ann Surg 225:1–14, 1997.
8. Sharpless SM, Das Gupta TK: Surgery for metastatic melanoma. Semin Surg Oncol 14:311–318, 1998.
9. Vrouenraets BC, Nieweg OE, Kroon BBR: 35 years of isolated limb perfusion for melanoma: Indications and results. Br J Surg 83:1319–1328, 1996.

65. PAROTID TUMORS

William R. Nelson, M.D.

1. What is the differential diagnosis of a mass in front of the ear in a patient of any age?

A parotid tumor is first choice if the mass is painless, discrete, nontender, and located beneath or anterior to the ear lobe. Slight variations in location are occasionally seen. Diffuse unilateral enlargement of the parotid gland usually indicates parotid duct obstruction, persistent or intermittent, due to calculus in the main duct. On the other hand, bilateral diffuse enlargement may be caused by a long list of conditions beginning with mumps, starch-eaters disease, and fatty infiltration.

2. What if the mass or nodule is located high in the gland in front of the tragus of the ear?

An enlarged parotid lymph node is the most likely diagnosis, although parotid tumors occasionally are found in this location. In a patient with solar-irradiated facial skin and numerous skin keratoses and/or a history of skin cancer around the upper face, metastatic skin cancer in the node must be ruled out.

3. If a parotid tumor is the obvious diagnosis, is salivary cancer likely?

Mixed tumor is by far the most likely diagnosis (80%). The term *benign mixed tumor* has been discarded because this lesion, although histologically benign, may recur locally and act in a locally malignant manner. Approximately 60% of tumors of the parotid are benign. The remaining 40% are made up of a variety of parotid cancers of varying degrees of malignant change.

4. What are the types of benign parotid tumors and their frequency?

- Mixed tumor is the most common (81%), although it has some local malignant potential. The truly malignant form is termed *malignant mixed tumor*.
- Warthin's tumor: 14%
- Benign lymphoepithelial lesion: 1%
- Oxyphil adenoma, oncocytoma, and other rare lesions: < 1% each

5. What are other salivary gland locations? What is the frequency of malignant tumors in these glands?

Submandibular glands: 50% malignant

Minor glands (oral cavity): 70–80% malignant

6. Do mixed tumors ever spread systemically?

Forty-three cases have been recorded. Lung and other organs were the sites of metastatic disease, all with classical microscopic findings of mixed tumor. One may surmise that hidden malignant changes have occurred, but no such findings have been noted. These cases are very rare. Other so-called benign tumors of various organs have been known to spread systemically.

7. What are the types of malignant tumors and their frequency?

- Mucoepidermoid carcinoma: 44% (The low-grade variety of this tumor is "almost benign.")
- Malignant mixed tumor: 17%
- Acinic cell carcinoma: 17%
- Adenocarcinoma: 10%
- Adenoid cystic carcinoma: 9%
- Epidermoid carcinoma: 7%

8. Describe the characteristic behavior of an adenoid cystic carcinoma.

1. Perineural invasion, sometimes producing nerve discoloration, is usually microscopic and must be considered ominous.

2. Frequent and often delayed recurrences, local or systemic. Reappearance 10 years after a tumor-free interval is not unusual.

9. Is it proper to biopsy an apparent parotid tumor?

In the past preoperative biopsy was believed to be rarely indicated. Many surgeons did needle aspiration of tumors that seemed malignant (rapid growth, nerve paralysis, extremely hard masses). In general, moveable, benign-appearing tumors are not biopsied preoperatively. A parotid lobectomy is normally carried out with dissection and preservation of facial nerve, followed by frozen section of the tumor. If a tumor is found to be malignant preoperatively by needle aspiration biopsy, a complete lobectomy can be performed with the knowledge that cancer may involve one or more nerve branches. The decision about nerve branch resection depends on evidence of actual neural invasion. Needle diagnosis obviates the necessity for any type of biopsy during surgery, when tumor spillage may occur. Most authorities advise removal of adjacent upper neck nodes as well. With evidence of lymphatic involvement, of course, a modified neck dissection is indicated. Heller and others have recently advised fine-needle aspiration biopsy in all parotid tumors. In their series, 35% of patients underwent a change in clinical approach after the biopsy report. Not all authors advise this approach.

10. How should you handle a deep lobe parotid tumor?

Deep lobe tumors are uncommon because the deep lobe portion of the parotid is only about ⅕ of the total substance and lies beneath the nerve. Superficial parotid lobectomy is first performed with dissection and preservation of the nerve, followed by removal of the tumor in the deep lobe area along with any remaining deep lobe tissue.

11. Is partial or complete facial nerve (cranial nerve VII) paralysis in the presence of an untreated parotid tumor a sign of cancer?

If the paralysis has developed gradually, cancer is a 98–100% bet. Sudden onset of a unilateral CN VII weakness indicates Bell's palsy, a supposed inflammatory process often reversible. Mixed tumors rarely cause this phenomenon, but it has been reported. CN VII palsy with parotid cancer has an ominous prognosis. Radical surgery plus radiotherapy may control this cancer in rare cases.

12. Is magnetic resonance imaging (MRI) helpful in diagnosing parotid lesions, especially those of the deep lobe?

MRI easily diagnoses deep parotid lesions, some of which protrude into the oral pharynx or oral cavity. It is possible to show infiltration or lack of sharpness in the margins of malignant parotid tumors with MRI; otherwise it is not possible to differentiate between benign and malignant lesions with this technique. Routine MRI is not necessary in the moveable, apparently superficial parotid tumor.

13. Do children develop parotid tumors?

Parotid tumors are uncommon in children but quite similar to those in adults.

14. Can radiation cause parotid tumors?

Major and minor gland neoplasms have developed in patients previously treated for benign conditions of the face and neck. There is no proof that inflammatory disease of the parotid or stones in the parotid duct have produced tumors. One recent report indicates that smoking may play a part in the production of Warthin's tumors.

15. Should all apparently benign parotid tumors be removed?

The only exceptions to removal are longstanding parotid lesions of apparently benign type in aged or infirm patients. Aspiration biopsies are helpful in confirming the diagnosis of mixed tumors or other benign lesions in situations where surgery would be life-threatening. Observation is the treatment of choice.

16. What is the significance of a recent parotid enlargement or mass in a patient who is HIV-positive?

In HIV-positive patients, the most likely diagnosis is a benign lymphoepithelial lesion. If needle biopsy confirms this diagnosis, surgery is not indicated because of the benign nature of the process in the face of eventual AIDS development. If a cyst is present, fluid aspiration decreases or temporarily eliminates the swelling.

17. If cancer is found on frozen section of the removed superficial lobe and tumor, should further surgery be carried out?

Removal of the remaining salivary tissue, including the deep lobe, is usually advocated. Low-grade mucoepidermoid carcinoma does not require radical removal. Careful histologic study, of course, is absolutely essential in determining the type of malignant neoplasm. If cancer is confirmed, a limited upper neck dissection is advised. A classical neck dissection is not performed in parotid cancer unless there is evidence of nodal disease.

18. Is further surgery indicated if a mixed tumor is peeled off the nerve without spillage (with microscopic penetration of the capsule)?

Studies have shown few if any cases of recurrence if the dissection is grossly clean.

19. Is nerve grafting ever indicated at the time of removal of a parotid cancer?

If a branch of the nerve is involved, resection must be performed after negative frozen sections from the nerve ends. A nerve graft from the greater auricular nerve of the opposite side of the neck is usually preferred. The graft is normally sutured in place with magnification.

20. Can a parotid tumor be removed without dissection of the facial nerve?

Nerve dissection should be carried out in nearly all cases. For a Warthin's tumor, which usually develops in the lower part of the parotid, careful local excision has been advocated by some authors because local recurrence is uncommon. Mixed tumors arising in rare anterior locations are commonly excised locally without nerve dissection. Local recurrence and peripheral nerve injury are possible; nerve branch localization and preservation should be attempted.

21. Which facial nerve branch is most commonly injured in parotidectomy?

The most commonly injured nerve is the ramus marginalis mandibularis, the lowest branch of the nerve that innervates the depressor muscles of the lower lip. This nerve must be carefully preserved in the operation. If it is not injured, weakness of the lower lip (a common complication even of careful surgery) resolves within 4–6 weeks.

22. How can a surgeon prevent weakness of facial nerve II (CN VII) due to parotidectomy (when the nerve is preserved)?

If great care is taken with nerve dissection, postoperative palsy should be minimal. Coagulation of bleeding vessels near the nerve, careless suctioning around the nerve itself, and unnecessary pulling and stretching of the nerve may result in several weeks of distressing palsy. Despite the greatest care, some patients develop temporary paralysis.

23. Is there any way to prevent the common problem of anesthesia of the ear lobe after parotid surgery?

The posterior branch of the greater auricular nerve can be preserved in parotidectomy if it is uninvolved with tumor and not adherent to the tumor itself.

24. When should postoperative radiation therapy be advised after parotidectomy for cancer?

In all except very low-grade cancers, many authors advise radiation therapy after total parotidectomy and removal of adjacent upper neck nodes. A radical neck dissection is not done without evidence of nodal involvement. At the M.D. Anderson Hospital and Memorial Sloan-Kettering, aggressive surgery in the treatment of parotid cancer, including upper neck node removal followed by radiotherapy, provides gratifying cure rates.

25. What are the cure rates with surgery for parotid cancer?

In low-grade cancers, cure rates may approach 90%. In one large series of all types of cancers, survival rates at 5, 10, and 15 years were approximately 62%, 54%, and 47%, respectively.

26. Is stage of the tumor or histologic grade more important in the prognosis of adenoid cystic carcinoma?

Sprio and Huvos showed that stage of the tumor is more important than grade. Early stage tumors, even in the face of high-grade histology, were found to have a relatively good prognosis.

27. Does salivary fistula ever develop after superficial parotid lobectomy?

If all except a few fragments of the superficial lobe are removed cleanly, fistulas should not occur. The deep lobe itself is rarely, if ever, the source of salivary leak after removal of the superficial lobe.

28. What is Frey's syndrome?

Frey's syndrome (pronounced as if it were spelled "Fries") is also called gustatory sweating. In some 20% of patients undergoing parotid lobectomy, unpleasant sweating may develop in front of the ear during eating. Some patients merely feel a cool sensation in this region. The cause is regeneration of parasympathetic fibers within the auriculotemporal nerve, which results in stimulation of the sweat glands in the absence of the parotid.

29. When is chemotherapy used after parotidectomy and radiation for locally extensive cancers?

Chemotherapy does not affect the cure rate. Studies from the M.D. Anderson Hospital have shown some definite chemotherapeutic effect, but generally it is of short duration.

30. Can a mixed tumor turn into a true cancer?

Most authors believe that truly malignant mixed tumors can develop from the benign type after many years, but this phenomenon is certainly not common.

31. Is it possible for facial nerve (CN VII) function to return after complete removal when nerve grafting has not been carried out?

Although rare, spontaneous return of facial function has been well recorded in isolated cases.

32. Which tumor suppressor gene is often found in patients with parotid cancer?

The suppressor gene known as p53 has been found in some parotid cancers. These lesions are usually advanced and larger than those without p53.

BIBLIOGRAPHY

1. Blevins NH, Jackler RK, Kaplan MJ, Boles R: Racial paralysis due to benign parotid tumors. Arch Otol Head Neck Surg 118:427–430, 1992.
2. Christensen NR, Jacobsen SD: Parotidectomy: Preserving the posterior branch of the great auricular nerve. J Laryngol Otol 111:556–559, 1997.
3. McGurk M, Renehan A, Gleave EN, Hancock BD: Clinical significance of the tumor capsule in the treatment of parotid pleomorphic adenomas. Br J Surg 83:1747–1749, 1996.
4. Harrison LB, Armstrong JG, Spiro RH, et al: Postoperative radiation therapy for malignant salivary gland malignancies. J Surg Oncol 45:52–55, 1990.
5. Heller KS, Dubner S, Chess Q, Attie JN: Value of fine needle aspiration biopsy of salivary gland masses in clinical decision-making. Am J Surg 164:667–670, 1992.

6. Hoorweg JJ, Hilgers FJM, et al: Metastasizing pleomorphic adenoma: Report of three cases. Eur J Surg Oncol 24:452–455, 1998.
7. Kelley DJ, Spiro RH: Management of the neck in parotid carcinoma. Am J Surg 172:695–697, 1996.
8. Malata CM, Camilleri IG, et al: Malignant tumors of the parotid gland: A 12-year review. Br J Plast Surg 50:600–608, 1997.
9. Spiro RH, Huvos AG: Stage means more than grade in adenoid cystic carcinoma. Am J Surg 164:623–638, 1992.
10. Yugueros P, Loellner JR, Petty PM: Treating recurrence of benign parotid pleomorphic adenomas. Ann Plast Surg 40:573–576, 1998.

66. HODGKIN'S DISEASE AND MALIGNANT LYMPHOMAS

Christina A. Finlayson, M.D.

1. What is the differential diagnosis of lymphadenopathy?

Cervical, axillary, or inguinal lymphadenopathy is a common finding during physical examination. The significance of this finding depends on the character of the lymph nodes and associated symptoms. Infection, autoimmune disease, and malignancy should be considered in the differential diagnosis.

2. What historical information helps to direct the diagnostic investigation of lymphadenopathy?

It is unusual for a patient over the age of 40 to have nonspecific lymphadenopathy; over 70% of enlarged cervical lymph nodes in this age group are malignant. Patients under 40 are more likely to have a nonspecific or infectious etiology, although the mean age of onset of Hodgkin's lymphoma is 32 years.

Duration of symptoms may indicate the cause of the adenopathy. Recent awareness of an enlarged lymph node is more suggestive of infection, although an enlarging lymph node can undergo internal hemorrhage with a rapid increase in size. Travel and occupation history, exposure to pets, geographic area of residence, and sexual history provide clues to infectious agents. A history of smoking is associated with lung, upper gastrointestinal, and head and neck malignancy.

Systemic symptoms, including fever, weight loss, night sweats, and pruritus, are present in 30% of patients with Hodgkin's and 10% of patients with non-Hodgkin's lymphoma.

3. A 25-year-old man presents for evaluation of a 1-cm, soft inguinal lymph node that has been present for 1 month. How should the diagnostic evaluation proceed?

The physical examination must focus on all draining lymph node basins: cervical, submandibular, auricular, occipital, supraclavicular, axillary, epitrochlear, inguinal, and popliteal. Supraclavicular adenopathy is virtually always associated with malignant or granulomatous disease. Peripheral adenopathy in the groin and axilla often is a response to trauma, frequently occult. The limb should be examined thoroughly.

The size and consistency of an enlarged lymph node help to discriminate malignant or granulomatous lymphadenopathy from other causes. A lymph node less than 1 cm in size is usually nonspecific and nonsignificant. Nodes larger than 2 cm are often malignant or granulomatous. Soft lymph nodes do not indicate a particular diagnosis; however, hard nodes are typical of metastatic malignancy.

A period of observation can help. Reexamine the patient in 1 months. If regression has not occurred, biopsy is indicated.

4. A 48-year-old woman presents with a 3-cm, firm lymph node in the left supraclavicular area. How may her evaluation differ from that of the previous patient?

The age of the patient, the size and consistency of the lymph node, and its location virtually exclude the possibility that it can be safely ignored. Malignancy must be excluded. Hodgkin's and non-Hodgkin's lymphomas as well as metastatic disease from a primary intraabdominal, genital, lung, or breast tumor may present with supraclavicular adenopathy. Head and neck tumors rarely metastasize to this location but tend to spread first to cervical lymph nodes.

A period of observation is not appropriate. An early diagnosis with fine-needle aspiration or open biopsy is indicated.

5. Should antibiotics be used during a "watch-and-wait" period when a specific site of infection has not been identified?

Rarely are lymph nodes the target of invading organisms. When infected nodes are present, other signs of inflammation, including warmth, erythema, and pain, accompany the swelling. If a specific infection is not identified, the empiric use of "shot-in-the-dark" antibiotics is without therapeutic or diagnostic benefit.

6. Can fine-needle aspiration be used if lymphoma is in the differential diagnosis?

Fine-needle aspiration (FNA) is an established diagnostic tool in the evaluation of breast, thyroid, and metastatic disease. When a patient presents with lymphadenopathy, often a diagnosis can be established from a lymph node aspirate that implicates a cancer other than lymphoma.

Establishing a definitive diagnosis of lymphoma by FNA is not reliable. The pathologist often requires intact lymph node architecture to reach a diagnosis and to provide accurate tumor typing. The recent addition of flow-cytometry evaluation of the aspirate sample has increased the diagnostic yield of FNA for lymphoma. However, many aspirates appear normal and cannot be processed by flow cytometry. Most patients require surgical biopsy to obtain adequate tissue for histology as well as immunohistochemical evaluation.

7. How should a surgeon do a lymph node biopsy for suspected lymphoma?

The primary role of the surgeon in lymphoma is to diagnose and stage the disease. The cervical lymph nodes are usually the site of involvement (75%), followed by axillary (15%) and inguinal lymph nodes. It is common for a primary node involved with tumor to be accompanied by smaller reactive lymph nodes. Therefore, it is important to select the largest, most suspicious lymph node for biopsy. Because the architecture of the lymph node is important for the pathologist, it should be removed in one piece. Care should be used during the dissection to avoid crushing, clamping, or cauterizing the tissue. The specimen must go to the laboratory fresh, preferably wrapped in saline-soaked gauze. The cellular architecture must not be distorted by placing the node in water or formalin.

Careful communication between the surgeon and pathologist before and during the procedure can avert most misadventures. A frozen section can determine whether an adequate tissue sample has been obtained.

8. What are the clinical differences between Hodgkin's and non-Hodgkin's lymphoma?

Hodgkin's lymphoma usually presents with either a neck mass or a mediastinal mass. It most commonly arises in lymph nodes and rarely involves extranodal sites initially. It tends to spread contiguously to adjacent nodal stations rather than "skipping" to more distant sites. Most patients present with early stage I or II disease. Epitrochlear, popliteal, or mesenteric nodal involvement is unusual. There is a bimodal age distribution with an early peak in the 20s and a later peak in the 60s.

Non-Hodgkin's lymphomas originate from lymphocytes and also are called lymphocytic lymphomas. The incidence of these tumors has increased significantly over the past 20 years. Some of the increase has been attributed to their association with AIDS, but this association does not account for all of the observed increase.

In contrast to Hodgkin's lymphoma, non-Hodgkin's lymphomas are often extranodal and spread noncontiguously. They rarely present as localized disease; bone marrow and liver involvement is common. It is more common for non-Hodgkin's lymphoma to involve the epitrochlear, popliteal, and mesenteric lymph nodes as well as Waldeyer's ring. It accounts for almost all gastrointestinal lymphomas. Most patients present with advanced-stage disease.

9. What is Waldeyer's ring?

The mucosa of the posterior oropharynx covers a bed of lymphatic tissues, some of which aggregate to form the palatine, lingual, pharyngeal, and tubal tonsils. When viewed from the posterior aspect, they form a ring around the pharyngeal wall; hence the term lymphatic ring. It may be the site of primary or metastatic tumor.

10. Why are tumors staged?

Tumors are staged on the basis of extent of disease at the time of initial clinical presentation. With the TNM method of staging, the size of the tumor, the presence of nodal metastases, and the presence of distant metastasis are used to quantify tumor burden. Classification on the basis of extent of disease helps to determine therapy and to predict prognosis.

11. How is lymphoma staged?

History and physical examination elicit systemic symptoms and identify involved lymph node stations. Laboratory evaluation includes complete blood count, creatinine, liver function tests, erythrocyte sedimentation rate, lactate dehydrogenase, and alkaline phosphatase. If a chest radiograph is abnormal, a CT scan of the chest is required. A CT scan of the abdomen and pelvis and bilateral bone marrow aspiration and biopsy are required in all cases. The use of lymphangiography and staging laparotomy is controversial.

12. What staging system is used for Hodgkin's and low-grade non-Hodgkin's lymphomas?

Because lymphoma is a malignancy of the lymph nodes and the initial site of disease is rarely identifiable, the TNM staging system does not apply. Staging, therefore, is based on the distribution of the disease and systemic symptoms. Hodgkin's and low-grade non-Hodgkin's lymphomas use the Ann Arbor Staging Classification:

Stage I	Involvement of a single lymph node region or localized involvement of a single extralymphatic organ or site
Stage II	Involvement of two or more lymph node regions on the same side of the diaphragm *or* Localized involvement of a single extralymphatic organ or site and its regional lymph nodes
Stage III	Involvement of lymph node regions on both sides of the diaphragm, which may include localized involvement of an associated extralymphatic organ or site, involvement of the spleen, or both
Stage IV	Disseminated involvement of one or more extralymphatic organs (including bone marrow) with or without associated lymph node involvement *or* Isolated extralymphatic organ involvement with distant nodal involvement

The subscript E denotes extralymphatic organ involvement, and the subscript S denotes splenic involvement in stage III or IV disease. E and S may be combined with involvement of both an extralymphatic site and the spleen.

Each stage is subdivided into either A or B, depending on associated systemic symptoms. Patients who present without systemic symptoms are classified as A. Patients who present with unexplained weight loss of more than 10% in the 6 months preceding diagnosis, unexplained fever with temperatures above 38°C, or drenching night sweats are classified as B; the systemic manifestations are called B symptoms. Pruritus often is included in the description of B symptoms but does not qualify for B classification when it is the only presenting systemic symptom.

For example, a 24-year-old man who presents with an asymptomatic mass in the neck, no systemic symptoms, and no other sites of disease on staging work is classified as stage IA. A 70-year-old woman who presents with a localized small bowel lymphoma (low-grade) that involves the mesenteric (regional) lymph nodes and has had a temperature of 38.5°C over the past 6 weeks is classified as stage II$_E$B.

13. What staging system is used for intermediate- and high-grade non-Hodgkin's lymphomas?

Intermediate- and high-grade non-Hodgkin's lymphomas are staged according to the National Cancer Institute Modified Staging System:

Stage I Localized nodal or extranodal disease

Stage II Two or more nodal sites of disease or one localized extranodal site plus draining lymph nodes with no poor prognostic features

Stage III Stage II plus one or more poor prognostic features

Poor prognostic features include (1) Karnofsky performance status < 70, (2) B symptoms, (3) any mass > 10 cm in diameter, (4) serum lactate dehydrogenase > 500, or (5) three or more extranodal sites of disease.

14. What is Karnofsky performance status?

Karnofsky performance status is a scale used to quantify a patient's activity level. Activity level reflects the impact of the disease. If the a patient knows that he or she has a disease but it does not interfere with activities, the performance status is 100%. As disease progresses, activity decreases and performance status falls. A bed-bound patient has a performance status of 10%.

15. What is the difference between clinical and pathologic staging?

Clinical staging is based on history, physical examination, and radiographic evaluation. Abnormal lymph nodes identified by abdominal CT scan or lymphangiography imply clinical subdiaphragmatic disease. Pathologic staging requires the histologic evaluation of all potentially involved tissues. **Pathologic staging** of abnormal lymph nodes identified by abdominal CT scan or lymphangiography requires staging laparotomy with biopsies. To identify the method of staging, a lower case "c" for clinical staging or "p" for pathologic staging precedes the staging nomenclature. For example, cIII indicates a tumor staged clinically with abnormal lymph nodes identified by abdominal CT scan or lymphangiography. If a staging laparotomy is performed and biopsy and pathologic confirmation identify involved lymph nodes, the tumor is stage pIII.

16. What is a staging laparotomy?

A midline incision permits attention to lymph node-bearing areas. Splenectomy is performed first, followed by wedge and core biopsies of each lobe of the liver. Lymph nodes are obtained from the celiac, mesenteric, portal, paraaortic, and paracaval areas. In premenopausal women, an oophoropexy is performed. This procedure secures the ovaries behind the uterus and preserves fertility in approximately one-half of women who require pelvic radiation. When the abdomen is closed, bone marrow biopsies are repeated bilaterally. Currently, surgeons are investigating the use of laparoscopy for staging.

17. What are the indications for staging laparotomy?

A staging laparotomy should be performed only when the results may change the clinical stage *and* when a change in stage will alter the planned treatment. Pathologic staging of surgically removed tissue is more accurate than clinical staging. In the Stanford experience, 43% of patients had a change in stage after laparotomy. Approximately 30% of patients in clinical stages (CS) I and II are "upstaged: to pathologic stage III or IV disease after surgery. Conversely, 20% of patients with clinical stage III or IV disease are "downstaged." In some subgroups of patients, risk of subdiaphragmatic disease is so low (< 10%) that staging laparotomy rarely adds significant information and is not indicated. These subgroups include all CSIA females and CSIA males with a high neck presentation, lymphocyte-predominant histology, or mediastinal-only disease.

Obscuring the role of staging laparotomy in treating Hodgkin's disease is its lack of effect on survival because of the highly effective salvage chemotherapy available for patients who relapse Evidence indicates, however, that patients staged surgically have a lower incidence of recurrence and, therefore, are less likely to require a second course of treatment.

Staging laparotomy is not performed for non-Hodgkin's lymphoma.

18. How is Hodgkin's lymphoma treated?

Stage I and IIA disease may be treated with radiation alone if the tumor burden is not bulky and the prognostic factors are favorable. More advanced disease may be treated with combined chemotherapy. The most popular combinations include three or more of the following: mechlorethamine, vincristine, procarbazine, prednisone (MOPP), doxorubicin, bleomycin, vinblastine, and dacarbazine (ABVD).

19. What is the Working Formulation for non-Hodgkin's lymphoma?

Non-Hodgkin's lymphoma is a broad category encompassing any lymphoma that is not Hodgkin's lymphoma. It includes many diverse histologic patterns, each with its own natural history and prognosis. Early attempts to classify these subtypes resulted in six separate classification schemes. The Working Formulation was created to standardize the nomenclature for non-Hodgkin's lymphomas. It categorizes each cytologic description into three general categories: low-grade, immediate-grade, and high-grade. Each category has a similar natural history, treatment plan, and prognosis.

20. How does the natural history for each category of non-Hodgkin's lymphoma differ?

Lymphomas with a low histologic grade tend to be indolent and slow-growing, often waxing and waning in symptoms over a long period. Aggressive lymphomas progress rapidly and, if left untreated, are fatal in a short period. Ironically, chemotherapy has been most successful in the intermediate and aggressive subtypes. Whereas the rare patient with a localized low-grade lymphoma may be cured with radiotherapy, more extensive disease rarely is eradicated with chemotherapy, although the median survival is still measured in years because of the indolent nature of the disease. Intermediate-grade lymphomas often respond to standard combination chemotherapy. Aggressive lymphoma, when treated promptly and aggressively with combination chemotherapy, has a 75% complete response rate and 50% chance of long-term survival.

21. Is there a role for the surgical treatment of lymphoma?

Yes. Localized non-Hodgkin's lymphoma of the gastrointestinal tract most commonly arises from the stomach. It originates in the lymphoid tissue of the submucosa. Surgery has been the mainstay of treatment, and complete resection of early-stage disease is considered curative. More advanced disease may benefit from adjuvant radiation and chemotherapy.

Lymphoma at other locations within the gastrointestinal tract often presents as a surgical emergency. The diagnosis is often made at the time of the operation, and attention is focused on treating perforation, obstruction, or hemorrhage. Resection of the primary tumor should be performed if the disease is localized.

22. What is the risk of a second cancer in patients successfully treated for Hodgkin's lymphoma?

Patients who are successfully treated for lymphoma have a higher life-time risk of developing a second cancer than the average population. The more common of these second cancers are lung, breast, sarcoma, leukemia, and non-Hodgkin's lymphoma. Patients who received radiation therapy to the cervical area require annual thyroid function testing to detect radiation-induced hypothyroidism. Young women who received thoracic radiation require careful screening for breast cancer. Annual mammography should be started 8–10 years after treatment but no later than age 40.

BIBLIOGRAPHY

1. Fisher RI (ed): Non-Hodgkin's lymphoma: Approaches to current therapy. Oncology Suppl 8, 1998 [entire issue].
2. Fleming I (ed): The surgeon and malignant lymphoma. Surg Oncol Clin North Am April, 1993 [entire issue].
3. Hoppe RT (chair): NCCN practice guidelines for Hodgkin's disease. Oncology 13:18–25, 1999.
4. Nynadoto P, Muhonen T, Joensu H: Second cancer among long-term survivors from Hodgkin's disease. Int J Radiat Oncol Biol Phys 42:373–378, 1998.
5. Pangalis G, Vassilakopoulos T, Boussiotis V, Fessas P: Clinical approach to lymphadenopathy. Semin Oncol 20:570–582, 1993.
6. Taylor M, Kaplan H, Nelsen T: Staging laparotomy with splenectomy for Hodgkin's disease: The Stanford experience. World J Surg 9:449–460, 1985.
7. Walsh RM, Heniford BT: Role of laparoscopy for Hodgkin's and non-Hodgkin's lymphoma. Semin Surg Oncol 16:284–292, 1999.
8. Young NA, Al-Saleem TI, Ehya H, Smith MR: Utilization of fine-needle aspiration cytology and flow cytometry in the diagnosis and subclassification of primary and recurrent lymphoma. Cancer 84:252–261, 1998.

67. NECK MASSES

Nathan W. Pearlman, M.D.

1. What causes lumps in the neck?

Enlarged lymph nodes, benign or malignant tumors, congenital abnormalities, and normal anatomy.

2. Normal anatomy?

In some patients, the neck mass is nothing more than a submaxillary gland or omohyoid muscle that has become prominent with aging and loss of surrounding fat. This finding usually is apparent if the other side of the neck is carefully examined.

3. A 34-year-old man presents with a 2–3-cm mass just below the angle of the mandible. What are the likely causes?

Nonspecific lymphadenopathy	Branchial cleft cyst
Infectious mononucleosis	Submaxillary or parotid gland tumor
Intraoral infection	Lymphoma
Carotid body tumor	Metastatic carcinoma

4. The patient seems awfully young for metastatic cancer.

Yest, but it still occurs in this age group, particularly thyroid, tongue, and nasopharyngeal cancer.

5. This is a long list. Is there any way to narrow it?

- Inflammatory nodes and nodes of mononucleosis are mildly tender, relatively soft, bilateral (one side may be more symptomatic than the other) of recent onset. They generally are less than 3 cm in diameter, usually the patient reports a history of a systemic illness, and skin over the tender nodes is normal.
- Lymphadenopathy due to intraoral infection is also of recent onset but exquisitely painful, indurated, and unilateral; overlying skin is often erythematous.
- Carotid body tumors may be tender and unilateral but are longstanding, more rubbery than infectious nodes, and cannot be separated from the carotid pulse.

- A branchial cleft cyst is unilateral, relatively soft, nontender, and longstanding; it also trans-illuminates.
- Nodes of lymphoma are nontender and have the consistency of the submaxillary gland. They may be unilateral or bilateral and of recent onset or several months' duration. In addition, signs of systemic illness may or may not be present.
- Submaxillary or parotid tumors are rubbery and nontender and occupy the position of the contralateral gland.
- Lymphadenopathy due to metastatic cancer is hard, nontender, and often larger than 3–4 cm.
- Tuberculosis can mimic all of these conditions.

6. Why not just remove the mass or lymph node and see what it is?

Open biopsy can unduly complicate further management when it is the *initial* diagnostic maneuver. If lymphoma or an unusual infection is present but not suspected, the node may be mishandled when sent to pathology or microbiology. If metastatic cancer is the problem, the scar tissue created by the biopsy may be difficult to distinguish from tumor on computed tomography (CT) or magnetic resonance imaging (MRI), leading to inaccurate staging. The scar also may resemble cancer at subsequent surgery, potentially resulting in a larger operation than originally needed. A better choice for histologic diagnosis is fine-needle aspiration (FNA), which is 95% accurate and avoids the problems of open biopsy.

7. A complete head and neck exam shows nothing, but FNA of the node reveals squamous cancer. What next?

Examination of mouth, pharynx, larynx, esophagus, and tracheobronchial tree under anesthesia (triple endoscopy). If nothing is seen, blind biopsy of the nasopharynx, tonsils, base of tongue, and pyriform sinuses should be done at the same sitting.

8. Isn't this a bit much?

No. The squamous cancer came from somewhere, and the most likely site is somewhere in the region (e.g., mouth, pharynx). In approximately 15% of patients primary tumor is detected at triple endoscopy when it cannot be found on office examination, and another 10% of patients are found to have a synchronous second primary tumor elsewhere in the aerodigestive tract.

9. Why not just start with triple endoscopy and skip all the other folderol?

Examination with the patient awake provides information about tongue and laryngeal function that cannot be obtained when the patient is asleep, and treatment planning depends on such knowledge. In addition, examination under anesthesia may be a blind search because of collapse of the tongue and pharynx, unless directed by findings on awake examination.

10. What about CT scan or MRI?

Both modalities may provide information about areas difficult to evaluate by physical examination, such as the base of the skull, and are helpful in staging, if cancer is present, but do not replace the measures already outlined.

11. We do all that and still can't find a primary tumor. What now?

There are two options. Most surgeons would treat the patient with a functional or modified radical neck dissection and postoperative irradiation to the neck and likely site of the primary tumor. Alternatively, one may proceed with irradiation alone to the neck and likely primary site, with neck dissection at a later date if the enlarged node(s) persist after treatment.

12. What if the primary tumor never shows up? Does this influence prognosis?

No. Prognosis is determined by the presence of metastatic neck disease, not by whether a small primary tumor is or is not found.

13. If the mass or enlarged node is in the posterior triangle of the neck, is the work-up still the same?

Yes. Although most oral or pharyngeal tumors spread first to nodes in the anterior triangle, it is not uncommon for naso- or hypopharyngeal tumors, thyroid cancers, and lymphomas to present as enlarged nodes in the posterior triangle.

14. What if FNA of the node reveals only lymphocytes or shows adenocarcinoma?

The presence of lymphocytes most likely represents inflammation or lymphoma; but if the "node" is just below the ear lobe, it may be a Warthin's tumor (cystadenoma-lymphomatosa) of the parotid. Adenocarcinoma on FNA usually means metastases from thyroid cancer or a primary site below the clavicles, but it may mean salivary gland cancer if the "node" lay high in the anterior triangle. If only lymphocytes are present, excision of the node may be reasonable, as long as it was *clearly* not in the parotid or submaxillary gland. In the latter case, one should proceed with a parotidectomy or submaxillary gland excision.

15. Lumps in the neck are common, and relatively few patients have cancer. Isn't this a cost-ineffective approach?

No. Most patients with lumps in the neck have benign, self-limiting conditions, which should be apparent on initial history and physical examination. If there is a question, FNA can be done. Only rarely is removal of the mass indicated for diagnosis and/or treatment.

On the other hand, if neck lumps are routinely excised to facilitate work-up (or to see what they are), the physician will constantly be surprised by what is found (e.g., metastatic cancer, lymphoma, tuberculosis). The work-up outlined above will then have to be undertaken anyway—and in a field dirtied by the biopsy. Such a course is *not* cost-effective but, in fact, a waste of time and resources.

BIBLIOGRAPHY

1. Attie JN, Setzon M, Klein I: Thyroid cancer presenting as an enlarged cervical lymph node. Am J Surg 166:428–430, 1993.
2. Lee NK, Byers RM, Abbruzzese JL, Wolfe P: Metastatic adenocarcinoma to the neck from an unknown primary source. Am J Surg 162:306–309, 1991.
3. Rice DH, Spiro RH: Metastatic carcinoma of the neck, primary unknown. Current Concepts in head and Neck Cancer. American Cancer Society, 1989, pp 126–133.
4. Tarantino DR, McHenry CR, Strickland T, Khiyami A: The role of the fine-needle aspiration biopsy and flow cytometry in the evaluation of persistent neck adenopathy. Am J Surg 176:413–417, 1998.

VII. Vascular Surgery

68. PATHOGENESIS OF ATHEROSCLEROSIS
Craig H. Selzman, M.D.

1. What is atherosclerosis?
Literally, atherosclerosis is derived from the Greek words *athere*, meaning porridge or gruel, and *sclerosis*, meaning induration or hardening. It is difficult to define atherosclerosis as a single disease entity because of the wide spectrum of pathologic lesions with diverse patterns of distribution and clinical sequelae.

2. Do you have to be old to have atherosclerosis?
No. The initial or type I lesion, consisting of lipid deposits in the intima, has been well characterized in infants and children.

3. What is a fatty streak?
Fatty streaks or type II lesions are visible as yellow-colored streaks, patches, or spots on the intimal surface of arteries. Microscopically they are characterized by the intracellular accumulation of lipid.

4. What is a foam cell?
A foam cell is any cell that has ingested lipids, thus giving the histologic appearance of a vacuole. In general, a foam cell refers to a lipid-laden macrophage; however, other cells that uptake lipids, particularly vascular smooth muscle cells, also may be considered foam cells.

5. Describe the progression of atherosclerosis.
Although the sequence of events is not always consistent, fatty streaks progress to type III or intermediate lesions. This growth is characterized by extracellular pools of lipid, which generally are clinically occult. However, when the pools coalesce to create a core of extracellular lipid (type IV lesion or atheroma), the blood vessel architecture has been altered sufficiently to become clinically overt. With smooth muscle cell proliferation and collagen deposition, the atheroma becomes a fibroatheroma (type V). The fibroatheroma is susceptible to thrombogenic surface defects with subsequent hemorrhage or thrombus (type V lesion), thus resulting in vessel occlusion, which, in the case of a coronary artery, results in myocardial infarction.

6. Of the one hundred medical students in your class, how many have significant atherosclerosis?
In 1953, Enos reported autopsy findings from 300 American male battle casualties in Korea (average age: 22 years). He noted that 77% of the hearts had some gross evidence of coronary atherosclerosis. About 39% of the men had luminal narrowing, estimated at 10–90%, and 3% had plaques causing complete occlusion of one or more coronary vessels. However, a subsequent study evaluating 105 combat casualties in Vietnam demonstrated that only 45% had evidence of atherosclerosis, and less than 5% were considered severe. Finally, a recent study looking at 105 trauma victims corroborated the Korean War study by demonstrating a 78% incidence of atherosclerosis, with left main or significant two- and three-vessel involvement in 20%. The message: you should have broccoli instead of a chimichanga for dinner on call.

7. What are the classic risk factors for atherosclerotic cardiovascular disease?

Traditional cardiovascular risk factors include tobacco, hyperlipidemia, hypertension, diabetes mellitus, and family history of cardiovascular disease.

8. How do such diverse risk factors produce similar disease?

That is the million-dollar question. Do parallel pathways lead to a final atherosclerotic lesion, or do the apparently dissimilar risk factors activate signals that converge to a few dominant events, promoting the development of atherosclerosis? Certainly, this question has broad therapeutic implications. It would be a lot easier to inhibit a single proximal point in this process rather than to treat multiple divergent, more distal cellular pathologic events.

9. What is the response to injury?

The premise that atherogenesis represents an exaggerated inflammatory, fibroproliferative response to injury has evolved into an attractive unifying hypothesis of vascular disease and repair. Mechanical, metabolic, and toxic insults may injure the vessel wall. The common denominator is endothelial injury. Disruption of the endothelium not only results in endothelial cell dysfunction but also allows adhesion and transmigration of circulating monocytes, platelets, and T-lymphocytes. Within the developing lesion, the activated cells release potent growth-regulatory molecules that may act in both a paracrine and autocrine manner. Under the influence of cytokines and growth factors, vascular smooth muscle cells (VSMCs) adapt to a synthetic phenotype and begin proliferation and migration across the internal elastic lamina into the intimal layer. Stimulated VSMCs allow the deposition of extracellular matrix, thus converting the initial lesion to a fibrous plaque.

10. Does vascular injury mean only direct physical injury, as with an angioplasty catheter?

No. Injury is a catch-all phrase that includes physical injury such as angioplasty, hypertension, and shear forces (atherosclerotic lesions typically occur at bifurcations) as well as other diverse insults, including viruses, bacteria, nicotine, homocysteine, and oxidized low-density lipoproteins.

11. Are lipids important?

The lipid hypothesis of atherosclerosis suggests that the cellular changes in atherosclerosis are reactive events in response to lipid infiltration. Indeed, antilipid therapy is one of the few strategies that has induced regression of atherosclerosis in randomized, prospective clinical trials. Strong evidence is also seen in patients with genetic hyperlipidemias; homozygotes rarely live beyond the age of 26.

12. What is syndrome X?

Syndrome X describes the metabolic phenomenon in healthy, nonobese, nondiabetic people who have hyperinsulinemia associated with elevated blood sugar, high blood pressure, and increased triglycerides with decreased high-density lipoprotein (HDL) cholesterol levels. Clinically such patients develop premature cardiovascular disease. Insulin resistance with elevated insulin levels, with or without overt diabetes, fuels important aspects of atherogenesis, including dyslipidemias, endothelial dysfunction, hypertension, and smooth muscle proliferation.

13. Why would vitamin E be theoretically protective for cardiovascular disease?

Antioxidant therapy with vitamins C and E as well as beta-carotene is intuitively sound. In vitro these agents afford resistance of low-density lipoprotein (LDL) to oxidation as well as reduce elaboration of reactive oxygen species. Reactive oxygen metabolites (as much as 5% of oxygen), such as superoxide and hydrogen peroxide, directly injure vascular cells, impair endothelial vasomotor function, promote platelet aggregation and leukocyte adhesion, and stimulate vascular smooth muscle proliferation. Although descriptive, case-control, and prospective cohort studies have found inverse associations between the frequency of coronary artery disease and dietary intake of antioxidant vitamins, randomized therapeutic trials thus far have exhibited no benefit to wearing sandals and shopping exclusively at health food stores.

14. What is homocysteine?

Homocysteine is an amino acid intermediate in the metabolism of methionine, an essential amino acid in both animal and plant proteins. Excessive homocysteine in the vessel wall reacts with LDPs to create damaging reactive oxygen species. Epidemiologic evidence correlates elevated levels of homocysteine and decreased levels of folate with cardiovascular disease.

15. How does homocysteine rank as a risk factor for atherosclerosis?

It is estimated that 10% of the risk of coronary artery disease in the general population is attributable to homocysteine. An increase in 5 μmol/L in plasma homocysteine concentration (normal: 5–15 μmol/L) raises the risk of coronary disease by as much as an increase of 20 mg/dl in the cholesterol concentration.

16. Should we all take folate?

Folic acid, vitamins B_{12} and B_6, and pyridoxine are important cofactors for the enzymatic processing of homocysteine. Indeed, the reduction in mortality from cardiovascular causes since 1960 has been correlated with the increase in vitamin B_6 supplementation in the food supply. Furthermore, the Food and Drug Administration recently mandated folic acid fortification in flours and cereal products as a method of preventing atherosclerotic-related death. Although these supplements may decrease homocysteine levels, the expected decrease in cardiovascular events has not yet been documented in prospective, randomized clinical trials.

17. What microorganisms have been implicated in atherosclerosis?

Bacteria include *Chlamydia pneumoniae*, *Helicobacter pylori*, streptococci, and *B. typhosus*. Viruses include influenza, herpes virus, adenovirus, and cytomegalovirus.

18. If you have visited a venereal disease clinic, are you at a greater risk for cardiovascular disease?

The initial epidemiologic description linking *Chlamydia* species to atherosclerosis was reported by venerologists in South America in the 1940s. *Chlamydia pneumoniae*, a ubiquitous respiratory organism, is the predominant species subsequently identified in cardiovascular lesions. More than 50% of the population has antichlamydial antibodies (ACA) by the age of 50; yet this 50% of the population does not have sexually transmitted diseases. You are probably safe. You can argue that you acquired ACA by inhaling at the clinic.

19. Is there an *Helicobacter pylori*-peptic ulcer equivalent in atherosclerosis? Should we all take a macrolide a day?

The jury is still out. It is unlikely that eradication of *Chlamydia* sp. will have the same profound effect on disease as eradication of *H. pylori*. However, *C. pneumoniae* may be another piece of the pie, exacerbating the response to injury. Of interest, evidence suggests that antibiotic therapy decreases the number of cardiovascular events in patients with elevated antichlamydial antibody titers.

20. What is the role of the endothelium?

A healthy blood vessel wall is lined by a monolayer of phenomenally metabolically active endothelial cells. The surface area of the endothelium is approximately 5000 m² but comprises only 1% of the total body weight. While acting as a physical barrier to protect the underlying vessel and allowing formed blood elements to flow freely, thus preventing thrombosis, this seemingly bucolic layer is a central control center of vascular physiology. The endothelium is a key docking point for monocytes, neutrophils, and lymphocytes by virtue of its ability to express sticky, cell-specific adhesion molecules. The endothelium is a source for cytokines and peptide growth factors that act in both autocrine and paracrine fashion to promote atherogenesis.

21. What are some of the products of endothelial cells that govern vasomotor tone?

Factors favoring vascular relaxation include nitric oxide and prostacyclin. Conversely, factors favoring vascular constriction include thromboxane, leukotrienes, free radicals, endothelins, and cytokines (e.g., tumor necrosis factor and interleukin-1).

22. What is the importance of vascular thrombosis?

Thrombosis is central to the pathogenesis of acute arterial insufficiency and acute coronary or cerebrovascular syndromes, including unstable angina, non–Q-wave myocardial infarction, acute (ST-elevation) myocardial infarction, and vessel occlusion after vascular intervention (angioplasty).

23. Describe the three main phases of platelet activation involved with thrombus formation.

The three main phases of platelet activation include adhesion, aggregation, and secretion. With exposure of the subendothelial space after vascular injury, platelets adhere to basement membrane proteins, especially collagen. This adhesion depends on binding of endothelial or circulating von Willebrand factor (vWF) to the platelet membrane glycoprotein 1b receptor. Platelet aggregation is an energy-dependent process requiring adenosine triphosphate (ATP). The predominant mechanism of aggregation involves binding of fibrinogen to the platelet glycoprotein IIb–IIIa receptor. Platelet secretion usually follows aggregation. Released products include the contents of dense bodies (serotonin, calcium, ATP) and alpha granules (vWF, fibrinogen, growth factors, platelet factor 4, and coagulation factors).

24. So atherosclerosis is an inflammatory disease?

Yes.

25. Then why don't we just take an aspirin a day?

Good idea. Strategies aimed at limiting the inflammatory cascade offer promise as antiatherosclerosis therapy. Examples in daily use include aspirin, fibrinolytics, HMG-reductase inhibitors, and estrogens. Others in the preclinical arena include gene therapy, anticytokine therapy, and anti-growth factor therapy. Certainly primary prevention is important in limiting the initial injury stimulus. However, the smoldering inflammation involved with atherosclerosis may best be attacked by modifying the vascular cells' response to these insults. Or, if you prefer, a steady diet of broccoli won't make you live any longer—but it will make it seem longer.

BIBLIOGRAPHY

1. Boushey CJ, Beresford SA, Omenn GS, et al: A quantitative assessment of plasma homocysteine as a risk factor for vascular disease: Probable benefits of increasing folic acid intakes. JAMA 274:1049–1057, 1995.
2. Cain BS, Meldrum DR, Selzman CH, et al: Surgical implications of vascular endothelial physiology. Surgery 122:516–526, 1997.
3. Diaz MN, Frei B, Vita JA, et al: Antioxidants and atherosclerotic heart disease. N Engl J Med 337:408–416, 1997.
4. Enos WF, Holmes RH, Beyer J: Coronary disease among United States soldiers killed in action in Korea. JAMA 152:1090–1093, 1953.
5. Gupta S, Leatham EW, Carrington D, et al: Elevated *Chlamydia pneumoniae* antibodies, cardiovascular events, and azithromycin in male survivors of myocardial infarction. Circulation 97:633–636, 1997.
6. Ross R: Atherosclerosis—an inflammatory disease. N Engl J Med 340:115–126, 1999.
7. Stary HC, Chandler AB, Dinsmore RE, et al: A definition of advanced types of atherosclerotic lesions and a histological classification of atherosclerosis. Circulation 92:1355–1374, 1995.

69. ARTERIAL INSUFFICIENCY

Mark R. Nehler, M.D., and William C. Krupski, M.D.

1. Describe claudication and its physiology.

Intermittent claudication consists of reproducible lower extremity muscular pain induced by exercise and relieved by short periods of rest. It is caused by arterial obstruction to affected muscular beds, which restricts the normal exercise-induced increase in blood flow and thus produces transient muscle ischemia. More than one-half of patients with intermittent claudication have never complained of this symptom to their physicians, assuming that difficulty with walking is a normal consequence of aging.

2. List the different nonoperative therapies for intermittent claudication.

Nonoperative treatment for claudication includes risk factor modification, exercise, and pharmacologic therapies. Smoking cessation reliably doubles walking distances. In addition, the need for eventual amputation in patients with lower extremity arterial occlusive disease decreases after smoking cessation. Exercise (defined as walking until onset of leg pain, resting, and then resuming walking) for 30–60 minutes, 3 days per week, also has been demonstrated in multiple randomized trials to increase treadmill walking distance by 120–180% in 6–12 months. Currently, the only drugs approved by the Food and Drug Administration for the treatment of claudication are pentoxifylline (minimally effective) and cilostazol (appears to improve walking distances more reliably).

3. Define critical limb ischemia.

Critical limb ischemia is lower extremity arterial occlusive disease of a magnitude that potentially threatens viability of the limb. Symptoms include rest pain. Foot pain at rest typically occurs at night when the patient is supine and the gravity contribution to foot arterial pressure is no longer present. Pain is relieved with foot dependency or short periods of ambulation.

4. Define the ankle-brachial index. What are its implications?

The ankle-brachial index (ABI) is the highest ankle pressure (anterior tibial or posterior tibial artery) divided by the higher of the two brachial pressures. The normal ABI is slightly greater than 1. An ABI of 0.9–0.5 is typically seen in patients with claudication. Patients with rest pain have an ABI < 0.5, and patients with tissue necrosis often have an ABI of 0.2 or below.

5. Describe the natural history of claudication.

Multiple studies of natural history have documented the benign nature of claudication. Many patients have stable or improved walking distances over time. The cumulative 10-year amputation rate is 10%. Conversely, 40% of patients experience symptom deterioration, and one-half of these require some sort of bypass surgery. Continued smoking and diabetes are major risk factors for progression.

6. Describe the natural history of critical limb ischemia.

In the past it was commonly believed that chronic ischemic rest pain or necrosis inevitably led to either surgical reconstruction or major amputation. This belief is both simplistic and inaccurate. Clearly, continuous ischemic rest pain or progressive gangrenous changes are unstable conditions that require therapy. However, the control groups from several pharmacologic trials for critical limb ischemia noted improvement over time in 40% of patients.

7. What are segmental limb pressures? How are they used?

Just as the ABI is recorded at the ankle, cuffs at the high-thigh, above-knee, and below-knee level can record pressures. Noting the location of arterial pressure drops can determine the anatomic level of obstruction.

8. Describe the natural history of graft occlusions.

Although bypass grafts can dramatically improve lower extremity circulation, they have a limited life expectancy. When the grafts fail, the involved limb is frequently in worse circulatory trouble than before the surgical bypass because of division of major arterial collateral pathways during the operation and thrombus propagation and/or embolization to occlude distal arteries at the time of graft occlusion.

9. What is the prognosis of young patients with vascular disease?

Significant atherosclerosis in young patients (< 40 years) is infrequent. Such patients are almost exclusively heavy smokers with a high incidence of hypercoaguable states (defective fibrinolysis, anticardiolipin antibodies, homocysteinemia, or deficiencies in natural anticoagulants). Those with limb-threatening conditions frequently progress to limb loss despite attempts at revascularization. Reconstructive procedures have limited longevity and require frequent revision. Despite the aggressive nature of their peripheral vascular disease, studies indicate survival, although less than in controls, is not markedly abbreviated.

10. Describe the anatomic distribution of vascular disease in diabetes.

Diabetic patients have several pathologic features of atherosclerosis that make them unique. They have a predilection for calcification of the arterial wall, rendering diagnostic studies (ankle pressure, ABI) unreliable because of false elevation. The digital arteries are usually spared, and the great toe pressure can be used to approximate the ankle pressure. In addition, the distribution of lower extremity atherosclerosis is unique. The inflow arteries (aorta, iliacs, common femorals) are usually spared. Significant occlusive disease most commonly affects the profunda femoris, posterior and anterior tibials, and pedal arteries, with relative sparing of the peroneal artery.

11. What are the implications of renal failure for prognosis of outcome?

Patients with end-stage renal failure who have critical limb ischemia are at the end of life with three-year survival rates of < 30% (similar to patients with metastatic cancer). In addition, the healing potential for partial foot amputations after successful revascularization is limited. Reconstructions are technically difficult because of calcified very distal targets. The combination of these problems has caused many vascular surgeons to shy away from vascular reconstruction in patients with renal failure.

12. Discuss the concept of inflow vs. outflow.

The limb is conceived as a separate circulation network when revascularization procedures are planned. Adequate leg circulation requires blood to enter the leg from the heart (inflow) and reach the foot from the thigh (outflow). In the normal limb, the inflow to the leg is via the aorta, iliacs, and common and deep femoral arteries. The normal outflow to the foot is via the popliteal and three tibial arteries (anterior, posterior, and peroneal). For arterial bypasses to work, they need adequate inflow (blood coming into them) and outflow (a vascular bed to supply).

13. What are the choices for autogenous conduits?

The success of infrainguinal bypass is highly dependent on the conduit (what the graft is made of). The best choices for conduit, in order of preference, are a single-segment greater saphenous vein, spliced pieces of saphenous vein, spliced lesser saphenous veins, arm veins, spliced arm veins, and prosthetic graft with a distal vein cuff. Cryopreserved cadaver veins are expensive and have limited durability. Prosthetic grafts are best used for above-knee popliteal targets because the bend at the knee joint and the size mismatch at more distal arteries markedly decrease their longevity.

14. What are the indications for arteriography?

Arteriography is performed only to plan future operations or interventions. Diagnostic arteriography without intervention is rarely used in lower extremity occlusive disease. Arteriography is expensive and carries a finite risk of bleeding, arterial injury with thrombosis, and renal failure from contrast toxicity to the kidneys (combined incidence: < 2%).

15. Discuss the patency rates of inflow procedures.

The durability of vascular reconstructions is measured by patency. The three types of patency are measured by a life-table method, which accounts for the moderate number of deaths (primarily of cardiac origin) in vascular patients over time. Patency can be primary (the graft has remained functioning without any intervention), assisted primary (the graft has not thrombosed but has required some intervention to keep it functioning), or secondary patency (the graft has thrombosed, but an intervention has reopened it and it is again functioning). The four most common procedures to improve inflow include iliac angioplasty, aortofemoral bypass, femoro-femoral bypass, and axillofemoral bypass. The most durable is the aortofemoral bypass, with a 10-year primary patency of 80%. Five-year primary patency rates for iliac angioplasty, ax-illofemoral, and femorofemoral bypass are 70%, 80%, and 75%, respectively.

16. Discuss the patency rates of infrainguinal bypass procedures.

Infrainguinal bypasses include grafts to the above-knee popliteal, below-knee popliteal, tibial, and pedal arteries. Five-year primary patency for above-knee popliteal grafts with saphe-nous vein and prosthetic grafts are 70% and 60%, respectively. Five-year primary patency rates for below-knee saphenous vein popliteal grafts are 70%; for tibial bypasses, 60%; and for pedal bypass, 50%.

17. What is the primary cause of perioperative mortality?

The majority (> 90%) of all patients with peripheral vascular disease have underlying coro-nary artery disease. Because of the ambulatory limitations of the peripheral vascular disease, a number of patients have no overt coronary symptoms. The most common cause of perioperative mortality in vascular surgery is myocardial infarction.

18. What are the causes of graft failure?

Vascular bypass graft failure is due to different mechanisms, depending on the time course. Early failure (within 30 days) is due to technical problems with the operation (graft kinking or twisting, narrowing of the anastomosis, bleeding, infection, intimal flaps, or embolization). Graft failure at 2–18 months is most often due to fibrointimal hyperplasia at distal anastomoses or venous valve sites within the graft. Late graft failure (> 18 months after implantation) is caused most frequently by recurrent atherosclerosis. Hypercoaguable states are an unusual but important cause of graft failure.

19. What are the therapeutic options for graft failure?

If a vein graft fails immediately after surgery, the correct approach is to explore the distal anastomosis and try to fix the presumed technical problem. If a graft fails weeks to months after implantation, the correct course is somewhat controversial. Exploring the graft to remove throm-bus mechanically and to repair any stenoses has a poor success rate and is not recommended. Using thrombolytic therapy to open the graft and then repair underlying stenoses seems attrac-tive, but the longevity of grafts treated in this manner has been poor; < 50% remain patent at 1 year. Replacing the vein graft with a new bypass provides the most durable alternative if it is technically possible and the patient is an operative candidate. Inflow grafts that occlude are usu-ally managed with operative thrombectomy and revision of the usually encountered distal anasto-motic stenosis.

20. What method of graft surveillance should be used?

Because of the limited options for occluded vein bypass grafts, ultrasound studies are used to detect stenoses within the graft before occlusion. Various criteria have been championed to detect accurately > 50% narrowing within the graft and/or native inflow and outflow arteries.

Natural history data indicate that grafts with > 50% stenoses, left untreated, have high intermediate-term failure rates. Recurrent symptoms and/or changes in the ABI are too insensitive to detect these lesions.

21. What are the therapeutic options for graft stenoses?

Most vein graft stenoses are due to fibrointimal hyperplasia of sclerotic portions of the graft or valve sites. These lesions have a firm rubber consistency and are not amenable to long-term success with percutaneous angioplasty. They are best addressed with open techniques, including resection and interposition grafting or vein patch angioplasty using small segments of saphenous or arm veins.

22. What is the role of iliac angioplasty and stenting?

Iliac artery atherosclerotic lesions that respond best to balloon angioplasty are short (< 3 cm) and confined to the common iliac artery. Nondiabetic patients fare better than diabetic patients. Current reports of initial success exceed 90%. The success rate has improved with the use of stents to treat iatrogenic arterial dissections (splitting the arterial wall at the intima or media layers), but their effect on long-term success is unknown.

23. How is visibility determined in cases of acute ischemia?

The five Ps of acute ischemia include pain, pallor, pulselessness, paresthesia, and paralysis. Early findings with acute ischemia include absent pulse, pain, and pallor. Paresthesia and paralysis are later findings. Classical teaching predicts irreversible muscle ischemia after 6 hours. Perhaps the most sensitive finding that indicates limb nonviability is muscle rigor in the calf. Many acutely ischemic limbs can be managed with initial heparin therapy followed by angiography and/or surgery with thrombolysis on the next day(s).

24. How is thrombus distinguished from embolus in acute ischemia?

The diagnosis of acute thrombotic vs. embolic lower extremity arterial occlusion can be complicated. Findings suggestive of embolus include no prior history of vascular disease, normal contralateral leg circulation, history of cardiac arrhythmia or recent myocardial infarction, or known cardiac thrombus. Patients with embolus frequently have rather profound leg ischemia due to the proximal nature of the occlusion (aortic or femoral bifurcation) and the absence of developed collaterals. Occasionally arteriography is required to differentiate the two.

25. What are the indications for thrombolysis?

Thrombolytic therapy requires a patient without contraindications (bleeding risks) and a thrombus that can be crossed with a wire. The lytic medication (urokinase, streptokinase, or tissue plasminogen activator) needs to be laced directly within the thrombus. An arterial embolus in an extremity that is not severely ischemic and can tolerate the time course of successful thrombolysis is an appropriate indication. Frequently the multiple hours of intraarterial infusion and repeat trips to the angiography suite for angiograms help to determine optimal catheter repositioning for complete thrombus lysis. The use of thrombolytic therapy for graft occlusions is more controversial because of the relatively poor long-term durability of the grafts once flow is restored.

26. What is compartment syndrome?

Reperfusion after acute ischemia may lead to profound tissue swelling in the involved extremity. Edema of the involved muscle can increase the pressure within the four fascia-bound muscle compartments of the lower extremity (anterior, lateral, deep posterior, and superficial posterior) to a level that exceeds capillary perfusion pressure (> 30 mmHg). Muscle death is then inevitable unless pressure is relieved by opening the compartments surgically, a procedure known as fasciotomy. Patients with compartment syndrome complain of intense pain and swelling with associated paresthesia. Pedal pulses usually remain palpable.

BIBLIOGRAPHY

1. Carter SA: The challenge and importance of defining critical limb ischemia. Vasc Med 2:126–131, 1997.
2. Gahtan V: The noninvasive vascular laboratory [review]. Surg Clin North Am 78:507–518, 1998.
3. Nehler MR, Hiatt WR: Exercise therapy for claudication. Ann Vasc Surg 13:109–114, 1999.
4. Nehler MR, Taylor LM Jr, Moneta GL, Porter JM: Natural history, nonoperative treatment, and functional assessment in chronic lower extremity ischemia. In Moore W (ed): Vascular Surgery: A Comprehensive Review. Philadelphia, W.B. Saunders, 1998, pp 251–265.
5. Ouriel K, Veith F: Acute lower limb ischemia: Determinants of outcome. Surgery 124:336–342, 1998.
6. Pomposelli FB Jr, Arora S, Gibbons GW, et al: Lower extremity arterial reconstruction in the very elderly: Successful outcome preserves not only the limb but also residential status and ambulatory function. J Vasc Surgery 28:215–225, 1998.

70. CAROTID DISEASE

Stephen D. Malley, M.D., and B. Timothy Baxter, M.D.

1. What diseases affect the carotid arteries?

Atherosclerosis is by far the most common (accounting for 90% of lesions in the Western world). The carotid also can be affected by fibromuscular dysplasia, inflammatory arteriopathies (e.g., Takayasu's arteritis), extrinsic compression (e.g., neoplasm), and trauma.

2. What are the most common symptoms of carotid artery disease?

- Transient ischemic attack
- Reversible ischemic neurologic deficit
- Cerebrovascular accident
- Amaurosis fugax

3. Define transient ischemic attack, reversible ischemic neurologic deficit, and cerebrovascular accident.

These clinical terms describe a spectrum of cerebral ischemic syndromes. **Transient ischemic attack** (TIA) is a neurologic deficit that lasts less than 24 hours. Most TIAs last only 15–30 seconds. **Reversible ischemic neurologic deficit** (RIND) is a neurologic event that lasts longer than 24 hours and completely resolves within 1 week (usually within 3 days). **Cerebrovascular accident** (CVA), or acute stroke, is a stable neurologic deficit that may show gradual improvement over a long period.

4. Define amaurosis fugax.

Amaurosis fugax is an episode of transient (minutes to hours) monocular blindness, often likened to a window shade pulled across the eye. It is due to decreased blood flow through or embolization into the ophthalmic artery.

5. What are Hollenhorst plaques?

Hollenhorst plaques are bright yellow plaques of cholesterol, usually at a branch point in the retinal vessels, that have embolized from the carotid bifurcation. Clinically, this finding indicates that the atheromatous plaque in the carotid is quite friable. Further embolization may occur with manipulation at the time of surgery.

6. What mechanisms produce neurologic deficits?

1. Embolization from atherosclerotic arteries or the heart
2. Reduced blood flow
3. Occlusive disease with thrombosis
4. Intracranial hemorrhage

7. What is the natural history of a TIA?

The natural history of a TIA is defined by the pathology of the ipsilateral carotid artery. In patients with severe stenosis (> 70%), the risk of ipsilateral stroke within 24 months is 26%. For those with moderate disease (50–69%), the risk is 22% at 5 years. With minimal stenosis (< 30%), the risk is 1% at 3 years.

8. What is the effect of aspirin on TIAs?

Acetylsalicylic acid is a cyclooxygenase inhibitor that affects platelets and decreases the incidence of both TIAs and stroke.

9. What does a carotid bruit signify?

The finding of a carotid bruit is a generalized marker for atherosclerosis; it is more predictive of a cardiac event than a neurologic event. Although a carotid bruit indicates increased risk of neurologic events, it is as likely to occur on the contralateral side as on the side of the bruit.

10. Does the sound of a bruit correlate with the degree of stenosis?

No. As a stenosis progresses, the bruit may actually diminish and disappear as flow decreases.

11. What test should be ordered to evaluate a cervical bruit?

Duplex scanning.

12. When is surgery indicated for symptomatic carotid artery disease?

Surgery is strongly indicated for symptomatic carotid artery disease associated with > 70% stenosis. The absolute risk reduction of stroke is 17% at 2 years. Recent data also suggest a benefit in select patients with symptomatic stenoses of 50–69% (6.5% risk reduction at 5 years). Patients with stenosis of < 50% do not benefit from surgery.

13. Should a patient with asymptomatic stenosis undergo surgery?

The absolute reduction in risk of stroke is 6% over a 5-year period in asymptomatic patients with > 60% stenosis who undergo carotid endarterectomy (CEA) with aspirin vs. those who are treated with aspirin alone (5.1% vs. 11%). Thus, CEA should be performed for asymptomatic carotid disease when the following criteria are met: (1) the patient is expected to live at least 3 years, and (2) the CEA can be performed with a combined stroke and mortality rate of < 3%.

14. What are the complications of carotid endarterectomy?

Intraoperative complications include neurologic deficits and cerebral ischemia. New deficits or exacerbations of old deficits may occur by embolization of debris during vessel manipulation or by poor flushing technique after arteriotomy closure. Cerebral ischemia may result from hypotension or poor protection during cross-clamping. Symptoms may be manifest as TIA or acute stroke. The overall incidence of neurologic deficits during CEA is about 2%. Other complications include hematoma, false aneurysm formation, hypertension, hypotension, and cranial nerve injury.

15. Which cranial nerves (CNS) may be injured during CEA? What are the clinical signs of injury?

Facial nerve (CN VII): injury to the marginal mandibular branch may cause droop of the ipsilateral corner of the mouth.

Glossopharyngeal nerve (CN IX): difficulty in swallowing both solids and liquids.

Vagus nerve (CN X): hoarseness, loss of effective cough.

Superior laryngeal nerve (branch of the vagus): voice fatigue, loss of high-pitch phonation.

Hypoglossal nerve (CN XII): deviation of the tongue to the ipsilateral side, difficulty with speech and mastication.

16. What is the danger of wound hematoma after surgery?

The main danger is airway compromise, which may necessitate emergent decompression by opening of the wound. Whether vacuum drains prevent this complication is under debate.

17. What are the possible causes of postoperative hypertension?
- Denervation of the carotid sinus
- Cerebral renin and/or norepinephrine production
- Preexisting hypertension
- Central neurologic deficit

18. When do neurologic events occur during CEA?
1. Dissection: dislodgement of material from the arterial wall with embolization
2. Clamping: ischemic infarct
3. Postoperatively: intimal flap, reperfusion, external carotid artery clot

19. What is a shunt? When is it used?

A shunt is a conduit, usually made of plastic, that diverts blood flow around the surgically opened carotid artery while endarterectomy is performed. A shunt is used to ensure adequate cerebral protection and to avoid intraoperative cerebral ischemia. Many surgeons routinely use shunts, whereas others use them selectively if at all. The decision to use a shunt is based on intraoperative assessment, including temporary clamping under local anesthesia, measurement of stump pressure, intraoperative electroencephalography, or transcranial Doppler. None of these methods is 100% accurate.

20. What is stump pressure?

Stump pressure is the back pressure of the internal carotid artery after clamping. It is used to assess the adequacy of cerebral perfusion. The "safe" pressure varies from author to author with the mean in the range of 40 mmHg.

21. Does stenosis recur after carotid endarterectomy?

Yes. The reported incidence has been quite variable and ranges from < 2% to as much as 36%. During the first 24 months after operation, restenosis is thought to be secondary to myointimal hyperplasia. Beyond this time, it is due to progression of disease (atherosclerosis). The incidence has been found to be lower when the arteriotomy is closed with a patch angioplasty.

22. What is the most common morbidity associated with recurrent endarterectomy?

The most common morbidity is cranial nerve injury (reported incidence = 2.4–18.9%). Most injuries are transient, however.

23. In which layer of the artery is the carotid endarterectomy performed?

It is performed in the outer layers of the tunica media.

24. What anatomic landmark is useful in identifying the level of the carotid artery bifurcation?

The facial vein.

25. How many branches of the internal carotid artery are located in the neck?

None.

26. When the internal carotid artery is occluded, which branches of the external carotid artery form collaterals and reestablish circulation in the circle of Willis?

Periorbital branches of the external carotid artery form communications with the ophthalmic artery, a branch of the internal carotid.

27. What are the functions of the carotid sinus and the carotid body?

Both are located at the carotid bifurcation and are innervated by the glossopharyngeal and vagus nerves, respectively. The function of the carotid sinus is regulation of blood pressure. Hypertension stimulates efferent impulses to the vasomotor center in the medulla, inhibiting sympathetic tone and increasing vagal tone. The carotid body regulates respiratory drive and acid/base status via chemoreceptors. It also induces bradycardia when manipulated.

28. When was the first successful surgical procedure of the extracranial carotid artery performed? Who is credited?

In 1954 by Eastcott.

CONTROVERSIES

29. What is the role of carotid angioplasty?

Although CEA remains the standard of care for carotid artery disease, percutaneous angioplasty with stenting has been investigated as an alternative. The underlying rationale was to decrease morbidity, hospital costs, and anesthetic risks and to improve long-term patency. Reported rates of success, morbidity, and mortality run the gamut from stroke and death rates comparable to CEA (2.4%) to significantly higher neurologic risk (stroke rate of 8.8%) and higher cost. Currently one randomized trial is under way in Great Britain, and applications for two other studies are being considered in the United States. Carotid angioplasty has no apparent benefit compared with CEA.

BIBLIOGRAPHY

1. Barnett HJM, Taylor DW, Eliasziw M, et al, for the North American Symptomatic Carotid Endarterectomy Trial Collaborators: Benefit of carotid endarterectomy in patients with symptomatic moderate or severe stenosis. N Engl J Med 339:1415–1425, 1998.
2. Beebe HG: Scientific evidence demonstrating the safety of carotid angioplasty and stenting: Do we have enough to draw conclusions yet? J Vasc Surg 27:788–790, 1998.
3. Executive-Committee for the Asymptomatic Carotid Atherosclerosis Study: Endarterectomy for asymptomatic carotid artery stenosis. JAMA 273:1421–1429, 1995.
4. Jordan WD, Voellinger DC, Fisher WS, et al: A comparison of carotid angioplasty with stenting versus endarterectomy with regional anesthesia. J Vasc Surg 28:397–402, 1998.
5. Mansour MA, Kang SS, Baker WH, et al: Carotid endarterectomy for recurrent stenosis. J Vasc Surg 25:877–883, 1997.
6. Moore WS, Kempszinski RF, Nelson JJ, Toole JF, for the ACAS Investigators: Recurrent carotid stenosis: Results of the asymptomatic carotid atherosclerosis study. Stroke 29:2018–2025, 1998.
7. North American Symptomatic Carotid Endarterectomy Trial Collaborators: Beneficial effect of carotid endarterectomy in symptomatic patients with high-grade stenosis. N Engl J Med 325:445–453, 1991.
8. Yadav JS, Roubin GS, Iyer S, et al: Elective stenting of the extracranial carotid arteries. Circulation 95:283–381, 1997.

71. ABDOMINAL AORTIC ANEURYSM

Mark R. Nehler, M.D., and William C. Krupski, M.D.

1. What is the definition of an abdominal aortic aneurysm (AAA)?

An increase in normal aortic diameter of 50% or more. Normal infrarenal aortic diameter is 2.0 cm for men. A definition of AAA as an aorta ≥ 3.0 cm in diameter is appropriate.

2. What is the incidence of AAA?

3.2% in unselected adult patients screened with ultrasound, 5% in patients with known coronary artery disease, and 10% in patients with known peripheral vascular disease.

3. Do AAAs have a genetic component?

Multiple reports describe a familial subgroup of AAAs. Therefore, screening of the patient's first-degree relatives over 50 years of age is recommended. Two prospective studies demonstrated that approximately 30% of first-degree relatives of patients with AAAs also harbor an AAA. The proposed genetic defect has been linked to abnormal type III collagen.

4. Are patients with AAA prone to aneurysms in other vascular beds?

Yes. Forty percent of patients with a popliteal artery aneurysm harbor an AAA, and 75% of patients with a femoral artery aneurysm also have an AAA. Patients with thoracic aneurysms have a 20% chance of having a simultaneous AAA. Five percent of patients develop aortic aneurysms proximal to their graft at ≥ 5 years after infrarenal AAA repair.

5. Can AAAs reliably be detected on physical examination?

No. The aortic bifurcation is at the level of the umbilicus. Therefore, the pulsatile mass of an AAA is located in the epigastrium. Only relatively large AAAs can be detected in thin patients.

6. Can AAAs be detected by radiography?

Plain abdominal or lumbar spine radiographs detect about 20% of occult AAAs. A thin rim of calcification identifies the aneurysmal aortic wall. Most AAAs contain insufficient calcium to be visualized by radiographs.

7. Which imaging method is the best for screening patients for AAA?

Abdominal ultrasound (US) permits accurate measurement within 0.3 cm and provides data in both cross-sectional and longitudinal dimensions.

8. What is the best single imaging modality to plan AAA repair?

The contrast-enhanced computed tomography (CT) scan. Diameter measurements are accurate within 0.2 cm. Venous anomalies (retroaortic or circumaortic left renal vein, inferior vena cava duplication, and left-sided inferior vena cava) that dramatically alter the operative approach are well visualized on CT. Although CT is excellent at detecting aneurysmal rupture or leak (92% accuracy and 100% specificity), it is less useful for predicting suprarenal aneurysm involvement (83% sensitive and 90% specific with a positive predictive value of 48%).

9. What is the manifestation of a symptomatic AAA?

Less than one-third of ruptured aneurysms are diagnosed in advance. The sudden onset of abdominal pain is the most common presenting symptom (82%). A hypotensive elderly man with acute onset of low back pain has a leaking AAA until proved otherwise.

10. What is the appropriate management of a patient with a suspected ruptured AAA?

Hemodynamically unstable patients with a pulsatile abdominal mass should have an electrocardiogram to rule out myocardial infarction immediately before emergent surgical exploration. Do not dawdle.

11. Should all patients presenting with AAA rupture undergo repair?

Patients in profound shock and/or cardiac arrest at the time of presentation have little chance of survival. Extreme age, dementia, metastatic cancer, and other severe end-stage medical problems should force you to reassess this allocation of medical resources.

12. Do all patients with ruptured AAA make it to surgery?

Approximately one-half of patients with a ruptured AAA die before reaching the hospital. One-fourth of those who make it to the hospital die before they get to the operating room.

13. How is a ruptured AAA treated operatively?

The patient should not be anesthetized until he or she is completely prepared and draped and ready for immediate incision because the blood pressure may fall dramatically upon induction of anesthesia. Rapid proximal aortic control is the key to successful outcome of operations for ruptured AAA. Control can be achieved at the diaphragm (in unstable patients with free intraperitoneal bleeding or a retroperitoneal hematoma that extends proximal to the left renal vein) or at the infrarenal aorta (in stable patients with a lower retroperitoneal hematoma). Intraluminal balloon occlusion of the aorta is useful with free intraperitoneal rupture. Once control is obtained, the patient is resuscitated, and clamps are moved to the more standard infrarenal location. Distal control also can be obtained with balloons or packs to prevent iliac venous injury.

14. How should patients with symptomatic nonruptured AAAs be managed?

Symptomatic AAAs expand rapidly and are at high risk for rupture. Therefore, most vascular surgeons agree that symptomatic but intact AAAs should be repaired as early as is conveniently possible.

15. Are there any alternatives to open surgical repair for ruptured AAA?

Endovascular prosthetic grafts have been successfully placed in high-risk patients with symptomatic AAAs or contained ruptures in both the aortic and aortoiliac positions.

16. What are the rupture rates of AAAs?

An AAA with a 5-cm diameter has an annual rupture risk of 4%. The risk of AAA rupture increases exponentially with size (a 7-cm AAA has an annual rupture risk of 20%).

17. How fast do AAAs enlarge?

The average expansion rate of all AAAs is 0.4 cm/year. However, 20% of all AAAs demonstrate no change in size over time. Conversely, 20% expand at a rate greater than 0.5 cm/year. Rapid expansion (0.5 cm/6 months) is predictive of rupture and an indication for repair.

18. Should patients with AAA undergo extensive cardiac testing?

This issue is controversial. The incidence of coexistent coronary disease in such patients is > 50%, and the primary cause of perioperative and long-term mortality is myocardial infarction.

19. When are angiograms helpful in the diagnostic work-up for AAA?

Traditionally, angiography has been indicated when there is concern about the extent of the proximal neck, concomitant visceral occlusive disease, renal artery anomalies, a prior colectomy with need to visualize the visceral circulation, or lower extremity occlusive or aneurysmal disease.

20. What other imaging studies are available?

Spiral CT provides three-dimensional reconstructions with dramatic anatomic images of aneurysmal geometry and visceral arterial anatomy. The major disadvantage is cost. The major advantage is the potential benefit in planning and performing endovascular aortic grafting procedures. Magnetic resonance angiography also has been used to visualize the visceral vessels and aortoiliac system, but the need for patient breathholding to eliminate respiratory artifacts is a problem.

21. Extraperitoneal vs. transabdominal approach—what is the difference?

Elective aortic graft placement can be carried out equally well via a transperitoneal or extraperitoneal approach. The transperitoneal approach provides better pelvic vessel exposure, whereas the extraperitoneal approach provides superior exposure of the suprarenal aorta and may facilitate postoperative pulmonary management.

22. What are endografts? Are they durable?

Endovascular grafts are large graft-covered stents placed via the femoral artery by interventional radiology to exclude the aneurysm without the need for an abdominal incision and cross-clamping of the aorta. Results of endovascular AAA repair have been mixed. The Endovascular

Tube Graft Trial reported an 85% success rate for implantation and no operative deaths. However, perigraft leaks were noted in 44% of cases; one-half of these thrombosed spontaneously in the follow-up period.

23. At what size should asymptomatic AAAs be repaired electively?

When the AAA reaches 5 cm in diameter. The only benefit for repair of an asymptomatic AAA is to prevent subsequent rupture and death. Therefore, all candidates for elective repair must expect to live at least 5 years.

24. Describe the technical aspects of AAA surgery.

The two important decisions are (1) the location of the arterial clamps and (2) the type of graft to place. The vast majority of cases can be managed by placing the arterial clamp below the renal arteries. This placement avoids prolonged ischemia to the kidneys. The aneurysm is opened after clamping proximally and distally. Lumbar artery orifices are oversewn to prevent bleeding from collaterals. The inferior mesenteric artery is often occluded but may require reimplantation when it is patent and not vigorously backbleeding.

25. What are the major noncardiac complications of AAA repair?

Renal failure (elevation in creatinine) and intestinal ischemia (bloody diarrhea).

BIBLIOGRAPHY

1. Armon MP, Whitaker SC, Gregson RH, et al: Spiral CT angiography versus aortography in the assessment of aortoiliac length in patients undergoing endovascular abdominal aortic aneurysm repair. J Endovasc Surg 5:222–227, 1998.
2. Barry MC, Burke PE, Sheehan S, et al: An "all comers" policy for ruptured aortic aneurysms: How can results be improved? Eur J Surg 164:263–270, 1998.
3. Boyle JR, Thompson MM, Nasim A, et al: Endovascular abdominal aortic aneurysm repair in the "hostile abdomen." J R Coll Surg Edinburgh 43:283–285, 1998.
4. Holzenbein TJ, Kretschmer G, Dorffner R, et al: Endovascular management of "endoleaks" after transluminal infrarenal abdominal aneurysm repair. Eur J Vasc Endovasc Surg 16:208–217, 1998.
5. Killen DA, Reed WA, Gorton ME, et al: 25-year trends in resection of abdominal aortic aneurysms. Ann Vasc Surg 12:436–444, 1998.
6. Lawrence PF, Wallis C, Dobrin PB, et al: Peripheral aneurysms and arteriomegaly: Is there a familial pattern? J Vasc Surg 28:599–605, 1998.
7. Porcellini M, Bernardo B, Del Viscovo L, et al: Intraabdominal acute diseases simulating rupture of abdominal aortic aneurysms. J Cardiovasc Surg 38:653–659, 1997.
8. Scott RA, Tisi PV, Ashton HA, Allen DR: Abdominal aortic aneurysm rupture rates: A 7-year follow-up of the entire abdominal aortic aneurysm population detected by screening. J Vasc Surg 28:124–128, 1998.

72. VENOUS DISEASE

Thomas A. Whitehill, M.D., and Mark R. Nehler, M.D.

1. Where does deep venous thrombosis (DVT) originate?

Over 95% of DVTs develop in the deep veins of the lower extremities; the majority originate in the valve sinuses of the calf veins.

2. What is the usual source of a pulmonary embolus?

Calf vein thrombosis may propagate proximally into the deep venous system to involve the popliteal, femoral, and/or iliac veins. These proximal DVTs are the source of over 90% of pulmonary emboli.

3. What is Virchow's triad?

Virchow's triad is defined by (1) hypercoagulability, (2) disruption of an intact venous intimal lining, and (3) stasis of venous blood flow. In most patients with DVT, at least two of these three components are operative.

4. What are the major hypercoagulable syndromes (thrombophilia)?

Factor V Leiden mutation, antithrombin III deficiency, protein C deficiency, protein S deficiency, dysfibrinogenemia, lupus anticoagulant, antiphospholipid syndrome, and abnormalities of fibrinolysis are the major examples. The most common is the factor V Leiden mutation (activated protein C resistance).

5. What causes venous intimal injury?

Venous intimal changes may be secondary to vein wall trauma, infection, inflammation, indwelling catheters, or surgery. Venodilation during anesthesia and surgery may produce microscopic intimal tears as well as stasis. The injured venous intima initiates the release of thromboplastic substances that can activate the coagulation cascade.

6. What causes stasis of venous blood flow?

Venostasis is common in surgical patients; it occurs during anesthesia, after certain types of trauma, and with perioperative immobility.

7. What are the usual clinical risk factors for DVT?

Risk factors include malignancy (especially pancreatic, genitourinary, stomach, lung, colon, and breast cancer), age greater than 40, female sex, obesity, history of previous venous thrombosis or pulmonary embolism, major surgical procedures, pregnancy, limited mobility, and trauma.

8. What signs and symptoms suggest DVT? How can DVT be accurately diagnosed?

DVT can cause calf or thigh pain, tenderness, increased skin temperature, swelling, or superficial venous dilation. None of these signs is highly specific for DVT. Even the well-known Homan's sign (calf pain with dorsiflexion of the foot) is quite unreliable; its accuracy is only 50%. The index of suspicion must remain high. Two noninvasive vascular tests—Doppler ultrasound examination (duplex scanning) and impedance plethysmography (IPG)—detect DVT proximal to the calf veins with over 90% accuracy when used together; unfortunately, they are not as sensitive in detecting calf vein DVT. Venography is still the gold standard.

9. What methods of perioperative DVT prophylaxis should be used? In which surgical patients?

Perioperative DVT prophylaxis is strongly recommended in all high-risk patients who are over 40 years of age and undergoing major general or orthopedic procedures. In general surgical patients, well-applied prophylactic measures decrease the relative risk of DVT by 67% or more. The best prophylaxis for DVT includes preoperative activity and early postoperative ambulation. In addition, intermittent pneumatic compression stockings and heparin are recommended as the patient's risk profile increases.

10. How does heparin work?

Heparin binds to antithrombin III (ATIII), rendering it more active. Low-dose heparin (5000 U administered subcutaneously every 8–12 hours until the patient is fully ambulatory) activates ATIII, inhibits platelet aggregation, and decreases availability of thrombin.

11. What is low-molecular-weight heparin (LMWH)?

LMWH is a fragment of heparin produced by chemical breakdown. It exerts its anticoagulation effect by binding with ATIII and inhibiting several coagulation enzymes, principally factor Xa. It has a longer half-life than regular heparin and can be administered once daily. LMWH gives a more predictable anticoagulant response at high doses and thus can be administered without monitoring.

12. Should the placement of an inferior vena cava (IVC) filter ever be considered?

In patients with a documented, recurrent pulmonary embolism while taking adequate antico-agulation therapy or an absolute contraindication to anticoagulation, an IVC filter can be placed to prevent embolization or propagation of clot to the lungs.

13. What are the characteristics of chronic venous insufficiency and postphlebitic syndrome?

The primary long-term consequence of DVT is venous valvular incompetence with distal ambulatory venous hypertension. After DVT, involved venous segments eventually recanalize to some degree. However, their delicate valves remain scarred or trapped by residual organized thrombus. In addition, the loss of valvular function disables the venomotor pump. The vein walls become thicker and less compliant, causing impedance to proximal blood flow. These factors result in distal venous hypertension whenever the patient is not recumbent. Protein-rich fluids, fibrin, and red blood cells are extravasated and deposited through large pores in the distended microcirculation during periods of venous hypertension. This process leads to inflammation, scarring, fibrosis of the subcutaneous tissues, and discoloration by hemosiderin deposition. The resultant inflammatory reaction, scarring, and interstitial edema create a further barrier to capillary flow and diffusion of oxygen; adequate nutrition to the skin is inhibited. These changes may lead to tissue atrophy and ulceration (venous stasis ulcer).

14. Do all patients with DVT develop postphlebitic syndrome?

No. Recent epidemiologic studies suggest that the incidence of venous ulceration is about 5%. As many as one in five patients have no symptoms and maintain normal noninvasive vascular test data. The median time for the appearance of a first stasis ulcer is $2\frac{1}{2}$ years. Of interest, 50% of patients with venous ulcers have no history of DVT (probably because of previous asymptomatic calf vein DVT).

15. How is postphlebitic syndrome treated?

With proper patient education and compliance, postphlebitic stasis sequelae may be controlled by nonoperative means in well over 90% of patients, particularly if no residual venous outflow obstruction complicates valvular incompetence. Nonoperative treatment consists of graded elastic compression stockings or Unna boots to retard swelling *and* periodic leg elevation during the day. Patients must be clearly taught to elevate their legs above the heart ("toes above your nose") at regular intervals (e.g., 10–15 minutes every 2 hours). Compliance is critical.

16. Distinguish between phlegmasia alba dolens and phlegmasia cerulea dolens.

Iliofemoral venous thrombosis is characterized by unilateral pain and edema of an entire lower extremity, discoloration, and groin tenderness. Three-fourths of the cases of iliofemoral venous thrombosis occur on the left side, presumably because of compression of the *left* common iliac vein by the overlying *right* common iliac artery (May-Thurner syndrome). In **phlegmasia alba dolens** (literally, painful white swelling), the leg becomes pale and white. Arterial pulses remain normal. Progressive thrombosis may occur with propagation proximally or distally and into neighboring tributaries, which function as collaterals. In this setting, the entire leg becomes both strikingly edematous and mottled/cyanotic. This stage is called **phlegmasia cerulea dolens** (literally, painful purple swelling). Hence, when venous outflow is seriously impeded, arterial inflow may be reduced secondarily by as much as 30%. Limb loss is a serious concern; aggressive management (venous thrombectomy and/or catheter-directed lytic therapy) is necessary.

17. What is venous claudication?

When venous recanalization fails to occur after iliofemoral venous thrombosis, venous collaterals develop to bypass the obstruction to venous outflow. These collaterals usually suffice while the patient is at rest. However, leg exercise induces increased arterial inflow, which may exceed the capacity of the venous collateral bed and result in progressive venous hypertension. The pressure build-up in the venous system results in calf pain commonly described as tight, heavy, and/or bursting (venous claudication). Relief is obtained with rest and elevation but is not as prompt as with arterial claudication.

18. How can one distinguish primary varicose veins from secondary varicose veins?

Primary varicose veins result from uncomplicated saphenofemoral venous valvular incompetence and have a greater saphenous distribution, positive tourniquet test, no stasis sequelae (dermatitis or ulceration), and no morning ankle edema (lymphedema).

Secondary varicose veins are most commonly a consequence of deep and perforator venous incompetence secondary to postphlebitic syndrome.

19. Why do people develop primary varicose veins?

The most common cause is congenital absence of venous valves proximal to the saphenofemoral junction. There are normally no valves in the vena cava or common iliac veins and only an occasional valve in the external iliac veins. Thus, the sentinel valve in the common femoral vein just above the saphenofemoral junction is of critical importance. However, anatomic studies reveal that this valve is absent on one or the other side in 30% of patients.

20. How, when, and in whom should varicose veins be treated?

Varicose veins that cause discomfort or serious cosmetic embarrassment require treatment. Better results are obtained with early treatment before continuous retrograde pressure and flow down the superficial system and into communicating perforating veins (whenever the patient is standing) cause secondary, irreversible perforator incompetence. High saphenous vein ligation at an early stage can arrest progression of this gravitational process. The distal varicosities can be managed by selective surgical stripping and/or sclerotherapy.

BIBLIOGRAPHY

1. Clagett GP, Anderson FA, Geerts W, et al: Prevention of venous thromboembolism. Chest 114:531s–560s, 1998.
2. Franks PJ, Sharp EJ, Moffatt CJ: Risk factors for leg ulcer recurrence: A randomized trial of two types of compression stockings. Age Ageing 24:490–494, 1995.
3. Ginsberg JS: Management of venous thromboembolism. N Engl J Med 335:1816–1828, 1996.
4. Milne AA, Ruckley CV: The clinical course of patients following extensive deep venous thrombosis. Eur J Vasc Surg 8:56–59, 1994.
5. Samson RH, Showater DP: Stockings and the prevention of recurrent venous ulcers. Dermatol Surg 22:373–376, 1996.

73. NONINVASIVE VASCULAR DIAGNOSTIC LABORATORY

Darrell N. Jones, Ph.D.

1. What is the role of the vascular diagnostic laboratory (VDL) in the assessment and treatment of patients with suspected vascular disease?

Although traditional evaluation by an experienced clinician remains the foundation of vascular diagnosis, clinical assessment has its limitations. For example, only one-third of cervical bruits are associated with significant carotid artery disease; conversely, as many as two-thirds of patients with severe carotid disease present without a cervical bruit. One-half of patients with extensive deep venous thrombosis (DVT) of the lower extremity lack signs and symptoms referable to the lower extremities, and more than one-half of patients presenting with clinical signs of DVT are venographically normal. As many as 40% of diabetic patients with abnormal clinical diagnosis have no large-vessel peripheral arterial occlusive disease. The VDL provides objective and quantitative data to identify and assess the severity of extracranial cerebrovascular disease, peripheral arterial occlusive disease, and acute and chronic venous disease. The VDL provides quantitative assessment of disease status and functional status of the patient both in disease progression and in response to medical and surgical therapy.

2. What differentiates the VDL from diagnostic radiology and ultrasound?

In addition to its obviously specialized focus, the VDL provides functional information rather than or in addition to the morphologic data provided by radiology tests and general ultrasound images. This information is particularly important for peripheral arterial occlusive disease, in which anatomic information about the site of stenosis or occlusion is of limited value without knowledge of the functional significance.

CEREBROVASCULAR DISEASE

3. Which noninvasive tests should be used to diagnose extracranial carotid artery disease?

Duplex ultrasound has a sensitivity of approximately 97% in detecting carotid artery disease and an accuracy of 95% in correctly classifying carotid stenoses with greater than 50% reduction in diameter. No other noninvasive test has comparable accuracy.

4. What is duplex ultrasound?

Duplex ultrasound uses both image and velocity data (hence the name duplex) in a nearly simultaneous presentation of ultrasound echo images (B-mode ultrasound) and blood velocity waveforms obtained by Doppler ultrasound. The Doppler signals in a duplex ultrasound presentation are obtained from a single small region of the blood vessel using pulsed Doppler. With the sacrifice of precision, velocities can be estimated for many such regions over a large area of the blood vessel at the same time. By assigning colors to the average velocity in each such small region and displaying the colors as part of the echo image, blood flow can be represented. Such a presentation, called colorflow duplex ultrasound, aids the duplex examination but cannot replace the information obtained from the Doppler velocity waveform.

5. Why is blood velocity important in assessing the degree of carotid artery stenosis?

It is often difficult to measure accurately the residual arterial lumen on a B-mode ultrasound image, because the acoustic properties (and hence the image) of noncalcified plaque, thrombus, and flowing blood may be similar. However, the hemodynamic changes produced by arterial narrowing can be used to characterize the degree of narrowing. Current practice classifies the degree of internal carotid stenosis into categorical ranges based entirely on the Doppler velocity data.

6. What are the velocity criteria and categorical ranges of the degree of carotid artery stenosis?

The criteria developed at the University of Washington are the most widely accepted:

0% stenosis	Peak systolic velocity < 125 cm/sec and no velocity disturbance
1–15%	Peak systolic velocity < 125 cm/sec with turbulence during systolic deceleration
16–49%	Peak systolic velocity < 125 cm/sec with turbulence in the entire cardiac cycle
50–79%	Peak systolic velocity > 125 cm/sec and diastolic velocity < 140 cm/sec
80–99%	Diastolic velocity > 140 cm/sec
100%	Absent flow velocity signal

Note that progressive carotid stenosis *increases* the flow velocity signal as the volume of blood is squeezed through a smaller and smaller orifice. The category greater than 80% has been termed critical stenosis because of the high rate of disease progression and high incidence of neurologic symptoms for patients in this category.

VENOUS DISEASE

7. What noninvasive test is used to diagnose acute DVT?

Duplex ultrasound has replaced venous occlusion plethysmography as the accepted standard. Colorflow duplex is useful because it helps to identify small veins from the muscle and fascial layers. The ultrasound assessment involves the following steps:

1. Examine the vein for echogenic thrombus.
2. Compress the vein, using pressure on the ultrasound probe, looking for complete collapse. Inability to compress the vein suggests thrombosis. Partial compression suggests partial thrombosis.
3. Obtain a Doppler signal from the vein. A signal that is phasic with respiration suggests no proximal occlusive thrombus. A signal that is spontaneously present but nonphasic suggests flow around an occlusion via small collateral veins. Absence of a Doppler signal in the vein suggests absence of flow, but smaller veins often have no spontaneous flow and distal compression is required to force the venous blood cephalad.

8. Can duplex ultrasound be used for ongoing surveillance in patients at high risk for DVT?

Diagnosis of DVT in asymptomatic patients presents a dilemma. The sensitivity of duplex ultrasound is reduced from the reported 95% to less than 80% for above-knee detection of DVT in asymptomatic patients. Calf DVT detection is much worse, with sensitivities as low as 10–20% in many reported series. However, few clinicians consider serial ascending contrast venography as a realistic surveillance regimen.

9. Does venous occlusion plethysmography still have a role in the assessment of DVT?

Yes. Venous occlusion plethysmography or impedance plethysmography (IPG) has high sensitivity and specificity for detection of occlusive thrombi above the knee, particularly for iliofemoral occlusive thrombi (95%). Because IPG provides functional information about deep venous outflow from the legs, it provides diagnosis of nonvisualized caval or iliac thrombosis, diagnosis of recurrent acute proximal thrombosis superimposed on chronic thrombosis, and functional evaluation of residual or chronic outflow obstruction.

10. What is IPG?

IPG is the most widely used modality of venous occlusion plethysmography. Changes in calf volume are measured first during tourniquet occlusion of the deep thigh veins and then with release of the tourniquet (a pneumatic cuff). The volume change is estimated from electrical impedance changes secondary to vein filling. Reduced filling or volume increase and delayed outflow are diagnostic of proximal venous obstruction.

11. What noninvasive tests are useful for evaluation of venous incompetence?

Doppler ultrasound is used to detect venous reflux in the deep veins of the legs and also in the greater and lesser saphenous veins. With experience, the test can be done using a simple Doppler (continuous wave vs. pulsed Doppler), but duplex ultrasound is often used to facilitate identification of the vein segments and valves and to position a pulsed Doppler sample reliably. Some laboratories measure the duration of reflux during controlled proximal compression as an indicator of severity of valve incompetence, but unless a valvuloplasty or valve transposition is planned for the identified incompetent valve, such specific measures appear to have little clinical utility.

PERIPHERAL ARTERIAL OCCLUSIVE DISEASE

12. What is the primary test for diagnosis of lower extremity ischemia?

The primary test is the measurement of systolic ankle artery pressures and systolic brachial artery pressure. The ankle/brachial pressure ratio (ABI) should be greater than or equal to 1.0.

Typically, Doppler ultrasound is used as the flow sensor distal to the pressure cuff, but plethysmographic instruments also may be used. Doppler signals are usually monitored at the posterior tibial artery or dorsalis pedis artery.

13. What is gained by measuring pressures at limb levels other than the ankle?

Segmental limb pressure measurements (SLP), performed at the upper thigh, lower thigh, calf, and ankle, localize the arterial segment(s) involved in peripheral arterial occlusive disease.

14. What tests are used for assessing peripheral artery disease in diabetic patients who may have incompressible arteries due to medial calcification?

Pulse volume recording (PVR) is a pneumoplethysmographic technique that tracks the limb volume changes over the cardiac cycle. It measures the pressure changes in segmental pneumatic cuffs as a function of the limb volume changes. The relative PVR amplitudes identify the presence of peripheral artery disease and localize the arterial segment involved. The PVR is unaffected by medial calcification. Great-toe pressure also may be used to diagnose and assess disease severity in diabetic patients, because medial calcification rarely affects the digital arteries.

15. How should the patient with suspected intermittent claudication be evaluated?

The patient first should be evaluated by obtaining ankle pressure indices or segmental limb pressures at rest. The patient with ischemia at rest does not normally need further evaluation. The patient with mild arterial insufficiency at rest or even normal resting pressures should perform an exercise stress test (treadmill walking using either fixed or variable load protocols) followed by ankle pressure indices. The distance that the patient is able to walk allows assessment of functional disability, and the postexercise reduction in ankle pressure, or lack thereof, allows assessment of whether the disability is due to arterial insufficiency rather than musculoskeletal or neurologic pain.

CONTROVERSIES

16. Can carotid endarterectomy be performed on the basis of duplex study alone?

The argument for elimination of arteriography in selected cases is persuasive because the carotid arteriogram alone has a morbidity rate greater than 1%. This rate may represent one-fourth of the usual total morbidity associated with carotid endarterectomy. However, to realize the benefit of surgery based on duplex ultrasound, the duplex study must have a high positive predictive value (PPV). Fortunately, the PPV is high for severe lesions that meet suitably strict criteria (e.g., peak systolic velocities > 290 cm/sec and end-diastolic velocities > 80 cm/sec).

17. Does duplex ultrasound have a role in the diagnosis of peripheral artery disease?

Its role is limited. Peripheral artery disease must be assessed functionally, not anatomically. Duplex ultrasound can be used to localize disease that has already been assessed for its functional significance.

18. Does transcranial Doppler have a role in the noninvasive diagnosis of cerebrovascular disease?

No. Although the technique is widely touted, recent large studies show that the results of Doppler evaluation of the intracranial arteries did not change the clinical management of any patient.

BIBLIOGRAPHY

1. Baker WF: Diagnosis of deep venous thrombosis and pulmonary embolism. Med Clin North Am 82:459–476, 1998.
2. Gerlock AJ, Giyanani VL, Krebs C: Applications of Noninvasive Vascular Techniques. Philadelphia, W.B. Saunders, 1988.
3. Moneta GL, Edwards JM, Papanicolaou G, et al: Screening for asymptomatic internal carotid artery stenosis: Duplex criteria for discriminating 60% to 99% stenosis. J Vasc Surg 21:989–997, 1995.
4. Zierler RE: Arterial duplex scanning. In Rutherford RB (ed): Vascular Surgery, 4th ed. Philadelphia, W.B. Saunders, 1995, pp 120–130.
5. Zierler RE, Sumner DS: Physiologic assessment of peripheral arterial occlusive disease. In Rutherford RB (ed): Vascular Surgery, 4th ed. Philadelphia, W.B. Saunders, 1995, pp 65–117.

VIII. Cardiothoracic Surgery

74. CORONARY ARTERY DISEASE

Joseph C. Cleveland, Jr., M.D.

1. What is angina? What causes angina?

Angina pectoris reflects myocardial ischemia. Patients often describe the sensation as pressure, choking, or tightness. Angina typically is produced by an imbalance between myocardial oxygen supply and myocardial oxygen demand. The classic presentation is a man (male-to-female ratio = 4:1) out shoveling snow on a cold night after a big meal and a fight with his wife.

2. How is angina treated?

The treatment options for angina include medical therapy or myocardial revascularization. Medical treatment is directed toward decreasing myocardial oxygen demand. Strategies include **nitrates** (nitroglycerin, isosorbide), which dilate coronary arteries minimally but also decrease blood pressure (afterload) and therefore myocardial oxygen demand; **beta receptor antagonists**, which decrease heart rate, contractility, and afterload; and **calcium channel antagonists**, which decrease afterload and may prevent coronary vasoconstriction. **Aspirin** (antiplatelet therapy) is also important.

If medical therapy is unsuccessful in alleviating angina, myocardial revascularization with either percutaneous transluminal coronary angioplasty (PTCA), with or without placement of a stent, or coronary artery bypass grafting (CABG) may be appropriate.

3. What are the indications for CABG?

1. **Left main coronary artery stenosis.** Stenosis greater than 50% involving the left main coronary artery is a robust predictor of poor long-term outcome in medically treated patients. A substantial portion of the myocardium is supplied by this artery; thus PTCA is too hazardous. Even if the patient is asymptomatic, survival is markedly improved with CABG.

2. **Three-vessel coronary artery disease (70% stenosis) with depressed left ventricular function or two-vessel coronary artery disease (CAD) with proximal left anterior descending (LAD) involvement.** In randomized trials, patients with three-vessel disease and depressed left ventricular function showed a survival benefit with CABG compared with medical therapy. CABG also confers survival benefit in patients with two-vessel CAD and 95% or greater LAD stenosis. An important caveat, however, in managing patients with depressed left ventricular function is that operative mortality increases when the ejection fraction falls below 30%.

3. **Angina despite aggressive medical therapy.** Patients who have lifestyle limitations because of coronary artery disease are appropriate candidates for CABG. Data from the Coronary Artery Surgery Study (CASS) suggest that patients treated with surgery have less angina, fewer activity limitations, and an objective increase in exercise tolerance compared with medically treated patients.

4. What is done during a CABG procedure?

CABG is an arterial bypass procedure that can be done both on bypass and off bypass. The left internal mammary artery (LIMA) is harvested as a pedicled graft. Cardiopulmonary bypass (CPB) is established by cannulating the ascending aorta and the right atrium, and the heart is arrested with cold blood cardioplegia. Segments of the greater saphenous vein are then reversed

251

and sewn with the proximal (inflow) portion of the bypass graft originating from the ascending aorta and the distal (outflow) portion of the bypass graft anastomosed to the coronary artery distal to the obstructing lesion. The LIMA is typically sewn to the left anterior descending coronary artery. When the anastomoses are finished, the patient is weaned from CPB and the chest is closed. Typically, 1–6 bypass grafts are constructed (hence the terms triple or quadruple bypass).

5. Does CABG improve myocardial function?

Yes. Hibernating myocardium is improved by CABG. Myocardial hibernation refers to the reversible myocardial contractile function associated with a decrease in coronary flow in the setting of preserved myocardial viability. Some patients with global systolic dysfunction exhibit dramatic improvement in myocardial contractility after CABG.

6. Is CABG helpful in patients with congestive heart failure?

Possibly. CABG improves congestive heart failure symptoms that are related to ischemic myocardial dysfunction. Conversely, if heart failure is secondary to longstanding irreversibly infarcted muscle (scar); CABG does not prove beneficial. The critical preoperative evaluation must assess the viability of nonfunctional myocardium. A rest-redistribution thallium scan is useful to determine the segments of myocardium that are still viable.

7. Is CABG valuable in preventing ventricular arrhythmias?

No. Most ventricular arrhythmias in patients with CAD originate from the border of irritable myocardium that surrounds infarcted muscle. Implantation of an automated implantable cardiac defibrillator (AICD) is indicated for patients with life-threatening ventricular tachyarrhythmias.

8. What is the difference between PTCA and CABG?

Six randomized controlled clinical trials have compared PTCA with CABG. Although collectively they analyzed data from over 4700 patients, 75% of patients who originally met inclusion criteria were excluded from participation because they had multivessel CAD, which was not deemed suitable for PTCA.

Several important features emerged from these trials. Overall mortality and myocardial infarction rates were no different for CABG and PTCA in 5 of the 6 studies. Only the German Angioplasty Bypass Surgery Investigational Study showed a higher short-term combined incidence of death and myocardial infarction in the CABG group.

The major difference between the two treatment strategies was freedom from angina and reintervention. Overall 40% of PTCA-treated patients required repeat PTCA or CABG, whereas roughly 5% of CABG-treated patients required reintervention. The CABG-treated patients also experienced fewer episodes of angina compared with PTCA-treated patients.

The unavoidable conclusion is that the recommendation of PTCA or CABG should be individualized for each patient. The two therapies should not be viewed as exclusionary or competitive; some patients may benefit from a combination of PTCA and CABG. CABG results in a more durable revascularization, although with the inherent risk of perioperative complications.

9. What is the rule of thumb for vessel patency?

- Internal mammary graft   90% patency at 10 years
- Saphenous vein graft   50% patency at 10 years
- PTCA of stenotic vessel   60% patency at 6 months
- PTCA + stent of stenotic vessel   80% patency at 6 months

10. What operative and technical problems are associated with CABG?

The operative complications broadly include technical problems with the bypass graft anastomosis, sternal complications, and incisional complications associated with the saphenous vein harvest incision. Technical problems with the coronary artery anastomosis usually lead to myocardial infarction. Sternal complications predictably result in sepsis and multiple organ failure.

Incisions for saphenous vein harvest also may result in problems with edema, infection, and pain postoperatively.

11. What are the risks of CABG? Which comorbid factors increase the operative risk for CABG?

Estimating operative risk is a critical component of counseling patients prior to surgical revascularization. The Society of Thoracic Surgeons (STS) and the Veterans' Administration have developed and promoted two large databases. Factors that increase the risk of CABG include depressed left ventricular ejection fraction, previous cardiac surgery, priority of operation (emergency vs. elective), New York Heart Association Classification, age, peripheral vascular disease, chronic obstructive pulmonary disease, and decompensated heart failure at the time of surgery. These comorbidities figure prominently in outcome. Quite simply, raw mortality data for CABG can be misleading. Surgeon A and surgeon B can perform identical operations but have different raw mortality rates if surgeon A operates on young triathletes with CAD, whereas surgeon B operates on old couch potatoes who smoke 2 packs-per-day of cigarettes. Through assessment of these comorbid factors, a fairer representation of predicted to observed outcome can be determined.

12. What steps are taken if a patient cannot be weaned from CPB?

The surgeon is in fact treating shock. As in hypovolemic shock (a bullet transecting the aorta), the basic principles include the following:

1. Volume resuscitation until left- and right-sided filling pressures are optimized.
2. When filling pressures are adequate, initiate inotropic support.
3. Push inotropic support to toxicity (usually ventricular tachyarrhythmias) and insert an intraaortic balloon pump (IABP). The ultimate extension of CPB includes the placement of a left and/or right ventricular assist device. These devices can support the circulation while allowing for myocardial recovery.

CONTROVERSIES

13. Is there an advantage to surgical revascularization with all arterial conduits?

The logical extension of the observation that an internal mammary artery has superior patency to a saphenous vein has sparked an interest in total arterial revascularization. Instead of using saphenous veins as bypass conduits, some surgeons also use the right internal mammary artery, the gastroepiploic artery, and the radial artery as bypass conduits instead of vein. Convincing data suggest a survival benefit as well as freedom from angina when the left internal mammary artery is used as a conduit. The data supporting total arterial revascularization are much less clear.

14. Do you have to "split the patient in two" to perform CABG? Are less invasive surgical options available?

Paralleling the advent of minimally invasive surgical techniques in general surgery (e.g., laparoscopic cholecystectomy), there is an interest in performing coronary artery surgery with less surgical trauma. It is now possible to perform CABG without the use of CPB through a partial sternotomy. This technique is termed MIDCAB (minimally invasive direct coronary artery bypass). A platform is used to stabilize the epicardial surface of the coronary artery that is to be bypassed. The heart continues to beat beneath this platform; thus the procedure avoids the use of CPB.

A second system called the Heartport system actually uses a percutaneously placed aortic cannula and a venous drainage system. It uses small incisions through which trocars are placed. The heart is placed on CPB, and anastomoses are created with the aid of a camera that is introduced through the small thoracoscopic ports.

The remaining issue with both strategies involves the unknown long-term durability of the bypasses. Early reports demonstrated a much higher rate of graft occlusion, suggesting that both methods may compromise the quality of the total surgical revascularization.

15. What are the options for a patient with continued angina who is deemed not suitable for CABG?

For patients on optimized medical treatment who are not surgical candidates (because of prohibitive comorbidities or poor quality coronary artery targets for bypass), the alternative is a procedure called transmyocardial myocardial revascularization (TMR). TMR uses a laser to burn small holes from the endocardium to the epicardium. Although it was originally believed that the laser brought blood from the endocardial capillary network to the myocardium, it has been repeatedly observed that laser-created channels are filled with thrombus within 24 hours and subsequently occluded. Therefore, it is postulated that the laser energy invokes an inflammatory response with a resultant increase in angiogenic factors (vascular endothelial growth factor, tumor growth factor beta, fibroblast growth factor). Although promising experimental data support TMR, large clinical trials are currently in progress.

BIBLIOGRAPHY

1. Bypass Angioplasty Revascularization Investigation (BARI) Investigators: Comparison of coronary artery bypass surgery with angioplasty in patients with multivessel disease. N Engl J Med 335:217–225, 1996.
2. CABRI Trial Participants: First year results of CABRI (Coronary Angioplasty versus Bypass Revascularization Investigation). Lancet 346:1179–1184, 1995.
3. Gundry SR, Romano MA, Shattuck OH, et al: Seven-year follow-up of coronary artery bypasses performed with and without cardiopulmonary bypass. J Thorac Cardiovasc Surg 115:1273–1277, 1998.
4. Hamm CW, Reimers J, Ischinger T, et al (for the German Angioplasty Bypass Surgery Investigation): A randomized study of coronary angioplasty compared with bypass surgery in patients with symptomatic multivessel coronary disease. N Engl J Med 331:1037–1043, 1994.
5. Henderson JA, Pocock SJ, Sharp SJ, et al: Long-term results of RITA-1 Trial: Clinical and cost comparisons of coronary angioplasty and coronary artery bypass grafting. Randomised intervention treatment of angina. Lancet 352:1419–1425, 1998.
6. King SB III, Lembo NJ, Weintraub WS, et al (for the Emory Angioplasty versus Surgery Trial [EAST]): A randomized trial comparing coronary angioplasty with coronary bypass surgery. N Engl J Med 331:1044–1050, 1994.
7. Rodriguez A, Mele E, Peyregne E, et al: Three-year follow-up of the Argentine Randomized Trial of Percutaneous Transluminal Coronary Angioplasty versus Coronary Artery Bypass Surgery in Multivessel Disease (ERACI). J Am Coll Cardiol 27:1178–1184, 1996.

75. MITRAL STENOSIS

David A. Fullerton, M.D., and Glenn J.R. Whitman, M.D.

1. What is the principal cause of mitral stenosis?

Rheumatic fever is almost always the cause. Symptoms of mitral stenosis usually do not occur for at least 10 years after acute rheumatic fever. Most patients are in their 30s or 40s when they become symptomatic.

2. What are rare causes of mitral stenosis?

Rare causes include systemic lupus erythematosus, malignant carcinoid, and rheumatoid arthritis. Congenital mitral stenosis is a rare lesion that is symptomatic in infancy and early childhood and almost never an isolated cardiac anomaly.

3. What cardiac tumor is often in the differential diagnosis of mitral stenosis because it produces similar symptoms?

Left atrial myxoma.

4. Which gender most commonly gets mitral stenosis?
Women (male-to-female ratio: 2:3).

5. What is Lutembacher syndrome?
Mitral stenosis associated with an atrial septal defect.

6. What is the Gorlin formula?
A formula that relates the gradient across a valve to the flow rate across the valve. It permits a calculation of the cross-sectional area of a valve. In simplified terms, the Gorlin formula states:

$$\text{Valve area} = \text{cardiac output} \div \sqrt{\text{mean pressure gradient}}$$

7. What is the normal size of the mitral valve?
The normal cross-sectional area is 4–6 cm^2. Mild mitral stenosis is < 2 cm^2, and severe mitral stenosis < 1 cm^2.

8. During which phase of the cardiac cycle does blood normally flow through the mitral valve?
Diastole.

9. What is the pathophysiology of mitral stenosis?
As the mitral valve becomes more narrowed, a higher pressure gradient is required to move the blood through the mitral valve from the left atrium into the left ventricle; left atrial pressure progressively increases as the mitral valve becomes stenotic. Increased left atrial pressure is transmitted retrograde into the pulmonary veins and pulmonary capillaries and ultimately into the pulmonary arteries. A left atrial pressure of approximately 25 mmHg increases pulmonary capillary pressure enough to produce pulmonary edema.

For example, to maintain adequate left ventricular filling across a 1–2 cm^2 valve, a pressure gradient of 20 mmHg is required. A normal left ventricular end-diastolic pressure of 5 mmHg results in a left atrial pressure of 25 mmHg. Left atrial pressure rises further if flow rate across the valve increases (increased cardiac output). Hence, with increased cardiac output in the presence of mitral stenosis, left atrial pressure rises further and promotes pulmonary edema. It gives the patient a sensation of dyspnea.

10. What hemodynamic conditions precipitate symptoms in patients with mitral stenosis?
1. **Tachycardia.** Because blood flows through the mitral valve during diastole, anything that shortens the duration of diastole (tachycardia) means less time for blood to move through a stenotic mitral valve.
2. **Loss of atrial kick.** A pressure gradient is required to move the blood through the stenotic valve, and presystolic atrial contraction contributes about 30% of the necessary gradient. Loss of the atrial kick means less left atrial pressure to move the blood into the left ventricle. In either situation, blood backs up in the left atrium, raising left atrial pressure higher.

11. What is the first symptom of mitral stenosis?
Dyspnea, which initially occurs under two conditions:
1. **Exertion.** Left atrial pressure rises secondary to more blood flowing across a stenotic valve in less time (higher cardiac output and shorter diastole with tachycardia).
2. **Atrial fibrillation.** With time, the increased left atrial pressure distends the left atrium, and the patient goes into atrial fibrillation. With loss of the atrial kick and a tachycardiac ventricular response to the fibrillating atrium, left atrial pressure rises.

12. What complications may result from mitral stenosis?
Hemoptysis may occur from severe pulmonary venous congestion. Thromboembolism may occur in patients in atrial fibrillation. Endocarditis may result if deformed valve becomes

infected. Pulmonary hypertension frequently develops because of (1) retrograde transmission of increased left atrial pressure, (2) reflex pulmonary vasoconstriction initiated by left atrial distension, and (3) hypertrophy of the pulmonary arteries leading to remodeling of the pulmonary vasculature.

13. Which patients with mitral stenosis should be anticoagulated?

Patients in atrial fibrillation. Clot tends to form in the fibrillating atrium, particularly in the left atrial appendage. Without anticoagulation the risk of thromboembolism is at least 20%. The emboli may go anywhere, but 50% go to the brain. A coronary embolism may cause a myocardial infarction.

14. What are the physical findings of mitral stenosis?

By auscultation one may hear an opening snap followed by a low-pitched diastolic rumble best heard at the left ventricular apex.

15. How is the diagnosis confirmed?

By Doppler echocardiography, which can quantify the severity of the mitral stenosis.

16. What is the medical therapy of mitral stenosis?

- **Beta blockers** (metoprolol or atenolol) slow the ventricular rate to about 50–70 beats per minute.
- **Digoxin** slows the ventricular rate in patients with atrial fibrillation. It may be used in addition to beta blockers and does not affect the heart rate in patients not in atrial fibrillation.
- **Diuretics** (furosemide) relieves pulmonary edema.
- **Coumadin** may be used if the patient is in atrial fibrillation.

17. What is the natural history of mitral stenosis?

Data from the period before widespread availability of mitral valve surgery suggest that the mortality rate after diagnosis is approximately 50% over 10 years.

18. What are the indications for procedural intervention in mitral stenosis?

Patients who are symptomatic with moderate-to-severe mitral stenosis, even if medical therapy attenuates the symptoms; the disease may progress rapidly, increasing the risks of intervention.

19. What types of procedures are available for the treatment of mitral stenosis?

Balloon valvuloplasty, surgical mitral commissurotomy, and mitral valve replacement.

20. Which patients may be appropriate candidates for balloon mitral commissurotomy?

Patients without calcification of the mitral anulus or leaflets, no mitral regurgitation, and little or no stenosis or fusion of the mitral chordae tendineae. These features usually can be determined by echocardiography. In appropriately selected patients, balloon mitral commissurotomy is the treatment of choice in most centers.

21. What are the benefits and drawbacks to balloon mitral commissurotomy?

It is an alternative to a surgical procedure and has the potential for less morbidity. The mortality rate is 4%. Complications include stroke (3%), cardiac perforation (4%), severe mitral regurgitation requiring operation (2%), and persistent atrial septal defect (20%). The need for a subsequent valve operation is approximately 10% at 5 years.

22. What are the benefits and drawbacks of an open surgical mitral commissurotomy?

Mitral commissurotomy is an excellent procedure that permits accurate repair of the valve under direct vision. It affords an opportunity to eliminate all areas of stenosis. Left atrial thrombus may be removed, and the left atrial appendage may be oversewn. Thirty percent of patients with mitral stenosis have some element of mitral regurgitation, which may be repaired at the same time with a mitral anuloplasty ring. The mortality rate of mitral commissurotomy is 0–2%, and the recurrence rate is 2% per year.

23. What are the benefits and drawbacks of mitral valve replacement?
Mitral valve replacement is curative in that it completely eliminates mitral stenosis. However, it is associated with a higher operative mortality rate (6%). After mitral valve replacement, the patient is subject to the risks of all prosthetic valves, including endocarditis, thromboembolism, and risks of hemorrhage from anticoagulation. If the surgical procedure requires removal of the entire mitral valve apparatus, left ventricular function may deteriorate over the long term.

BIBLIOGRAPHY
1. Carabello BA, Crawford FA Jr: Valvular heart disease. N Engl J Med 337:32–41, 1997.
2. Essop MR, Kontozis L, Savelis P: Preoperative left ventricular systolic dysfunction correlates with the adverse postoperative consequences of annular-papillary disconnection in the course of mitral valve replacement for stenosis. J Heart Valve Dis 7:431–437, 1998.
3. Loulmet DF, Carpentier A, Cho PW, et al: Less invasive techniques for mitral valve surgery. J Thorac Cardiovasc Surg 115:772–779, 1998.
4. Ben Farhat M, Ayari M, Maatouk F, et al: Percutaneous balloon versus surgical closed and open mitral commissurotomy: Seven-year follow-up results of a randomized trial. Circulation 97:245–250, 1998.
5. Cotrufo M, Renzulli A, Vitale N, et al: Long-term follow-up of open commissurotomy versus bileaflet valve replacement for rheumatic mitral stenosis.
6. Aagaard J, Andersen UL, Lerjerg G, Andersen LI, Thomsen KK: Mitral valve replacement with total preservation of native valve and subvalvular apparatus. J Heart Valve Dis 6:274–278, 1997.
7. Cesnjevar RA, Feyrer R, Walther F, et al: High-risk mitral valve replacement in severe pulmonary hypertension—30 years experience. Eur J Cardiothorac Surg 13:344–351, 1998.

76. MITRAL REGURGITATION

David A. Fullerton, M.D., and Glenn J.R. Whitman, M.D.

1. What causes mitral regurgitation?
Competency of the mitral valve depends on an intact mitral valve apparatus, which is composed of (1) mitral leaflets, (2) chordae tendineae, (3) mitral valve anulus, and (4) papillary muscles. Abnormalities of any component of the mitral valve apparatus may produce mitral regurgitation. The most common causes of mitral regurgitation are rheumatic fever, endocarditis, rupture of the chordae tendineae, senile mitral anular calcification, papillary muscle dysfunction from ischemia, and left ventricular dilation, which stretches the mitral anulus.

2. What is the pathophysiology of mitral regurgitation?
In mitral regurgitation the left ventricle may eject blood via two routes: (1) antegrade, through the aortic valve, or (2) retrograde, through the mitral valve. The amount of each stroke volume that is ejected retrograde into the left atrium is termed the **regurgitant fraction**. The greater the regurgitant fraction, the greater the total volume that the left ventricle must pump to maintain adequate antegrade blood flow through the aortic valve. The ultimate results are volume overload of the left ventricle and progressive left ventricular dilation. Over time, the contractile function of the ventricle declines.

3. What are the symptoms of mitral regurgitation?

Dyspnea on exertion is typically the first symptom, followed by loss of exercise tolerance and progressive symptoms of heart failure. Symptoms derive from (1) left atrial hypertension and (2) contractile dysfunction of the left ventricle. As with mitral stenosis, left atrial hypertension is transmitted retrograde into the pulmonary veins and capillaries. With chronic, severe mitral regurgitation leading to left ventricular dysfunction, symptoms of pulmonary edema and congestive heart failure predominate.

4. What determines left atrial pressure in mitral regurgitation?

Left atrial pressure in mitral regurgitation is determined by the compliance of the left atrium. Chronic mitral regurgitation is associated with progressive dilation of the left atrium and an increase in left atrial compliance; thus left atrial pressure may not rise with chronic mitral regurgitation. Conversely, acute mitral regurgitation into a normally compliant left atrium may create an immediate increase in left atrial pressure.

5. What hemodynamic conditions exacerbate mitral regurgitation?

- **Increased left ventricular afterload.** Increased systemic arterial blood pressure increases the impedance against which the left ventricle must pump to eject blood antegrade. The regurgitant fraction is therefore increased.
- **Tachycardia.** Because mitral regurgitation occurs during systole, tachycardia (more systoles per minute) increases the regurgitant fraction.
- **Volume overload.** Left ventricular distension secondary to volume overload stretches the mitral anulus, impairs coaptation of the mitral valve leaflets, and increases mitral regurgitation.

6. How is mitral regurgitation diagnosed?

On auscultation a holosystolic murmur is best heard at the apex with radiation to the left axilla. The best test is color-Doppler echocardiography, especially transesophageal echocardiography. The regurgitant jet may be accurately visualized and quantitated. Echocardiography also allows determination of which abnormality of the mitral valve apparatus is responsible for the regurgitation.

7. What is the medical therapy for mitral regurgitation?

- Afterload reduction with **angiotensin-converting enzyme inhibitors** is the mainstay of medical therapy. The goal is to optimize antegrade flow from the left ventricle by lowering the impedance of left ventricular ejection through the aortic valve, minimizing retrograde ejection.
- **Diuretics** (furosemide) lower left ventricular preload. Volume loading of the left ventricle dilates the mitral anulus, exacerbating mitral regurgitation.
- **Digoxin** provides ventricular rate control for patients in atrial fibrillation. Rapid ventricular response to atrial fibrillation increases the regurgitant fraction because greater time is spent in systole.
- **Coumadin** is used for patients in atrial fibrillation.

8. What are the indications for surgery in patients with mitral regurgitation?

Surgery is indicated when (1) patients have persistent symptoms despite medical therapy; (2) mitral regurgitation worsens by echocardiography during serial follow-up; or (3) left ventricular systolic function worsens. Because mitral regurgitation lowers the total impedance of left ventricular ejection, the left ventricular ejection fraction should be greater than normal in the presence of mitral regurgitation. An ejection fraction < 55% in the presence of mitral regurgitation suggests left ventricular dysfunction.

9. What surgical procedures are available to correct mitral regurgitation?

1. **Mitral valve repair.** Mitral valve repair is the preferred surgical procedure. Repair of the valve permits preservation of the mitral apparatus, which maintains continuity between the left

ventricular muscle and the mitral anulus via the chordae tendineae. Loss of this continuity by resection of the apparatus places the left ventricle at a mechanical disadvantage that over time leads to left ventricular dilation and dysfunction.

2. **Mitral valve replacement.** Inability to repair the regurgitant valve mandates replacement. If replacement is necessary, efforts should be made to preserve the posterior leaflet of the mitral valve. In most series, mitral valve replacement is required in less than 30% of cases.

10. What are the other advantages of mitral valve repair over replacement?

Repair is associated with (1) lower operative mortality, (2) less risk of thromboembolism, (3) less risk of endocarditis, (4) less need (if any) for chronic anticoagulation, and (5) better long-term left ventricular function.

11. How is the mitral valve repaired?

The redundant portion(s) of the valve leaflet(s) is resected, the leaflet is reapproximated, and the mitral anulus is plicated and reinforced with a prosthetic anuloplasty ring. The anuloplasty ring is sewn around the perimeter of the anulus on the left atrial side of the valve. In so doing, the mitral leaflets are supported by competent chordae tendineae, and the circumference of the mitral anulus is decreased. Competency of the repaired valve is assessed intraoperatively using transesophageal echocardiography.

12. What is the operative mortality of mitral valve repair vs. mitral valve replacement.

Repair, 2%; replacement, 6%.

13. How durable are mitral valve repairs?

The risk of requiring another mitral valve operation because of failure of the repair is approximately 2% per year.

14. What is systolic anterior motion (SAM) of the mitral valve?

SAM is a complication of mitral valve repair. After mitral valve repair, the anterior leaflet of the mitral valve may billow into the left ventricular outflow tract during systole, creating two problems: (1) dynamic left ventricular outflow tract obstruction and (2) mitral regurgitation (anterior displacement of the anterior leaflet causes it to be foreshortened). SAM should be suspected if cardiac output is low after mitral valve repair and may be diagnosed by echocardiography. Because it is exacerbated by an increased contractile state of the myocardium, inotropic agents should be avoided. SAM is treated by volume-loading and beta-blocking agents to provide a negative inotropic influence. If these measures fail, the valve should be replaced.

BIBLIOGRAPHY

1. Bolling SF, Pagani FD, Deeb GM, Bach DS: Intermediate-term outcome of mitral reconstruction in cardiomyopathy. J Thorac Cardiovasc Surg 115:381–388, 1998.
2. Carabello BA, Crawford FA Jr: Valvular heart disease. N Engl J Med 337:32–41, 1997.
3. Cooper HA, Gersh BJ: Treatment of chronic mitral regurgitation. Am Heart J 135:925–935, 1998.
4. Cosgrove DM, Sabik JF, Navia JL: Minimally invasive valve operations. Ann Thorac Surg 65:1535–1538, 1998.
5. Dore A, Suave C, Amyot R, et al: Mitral valve repair: Intermediate to long-term echocardiographic follow-up. Can J Cardiol 14:931–934, 1998.
6. Espada R, Westaby S: New developments in mitral valve repair. Curr Opinion Cardiol 13:80–84, 1998.
7. Spencer FC, Galloway AC, Grossi EA, et al: Recent developments and evolving techniques of mitral valve reconstruction. Ann Thorac Surg 65:307–313, 1998.
8. Tavel ME, Carabello BA: Chronic mitral regurgitation: When and how to operate. Chest 113:1399–1401, 1998.

77. AORTIC VALVULAR DISEASE

Peter A. Seirafi, M.D., and David N. Campbell, M.D.

1. What are the two most common causes of aortic stenosis?
Congenital anomaly and rheumatic fever.

2. What is the most common cause of aortic insufficiency?
Connective tissue disease, such as Marfan's syndrome, and aortic dissection.

3. What is the most common anatomic anomaly in congenital aortic stenosis?
Bicuspid aortic valve.

4. What is the most common presentation in infancy for both aortic stenosis and aortic insufficiency?
Congestive heart failure.

5. What are the most common symptoms in adults with aortic stenosis?
Syncope, dyspnea on exertion, and angina.

6. What physical findings suggest aortic stenosis?
In infants, systolic crescendo-decrescendo (diamond-shaped) murmur, poor peripheral pulses. **In adults,** systolic crescendo-decrescendo murmur, delayed pulse upstroke (pulsus parvus et tardus—this lingo will dazzle the medical chief resident on rounds).

7. What physical findings suggest aortic insufficiency in adults?
Aortic insufficiency water-hammer pulse (wide pulse pressure) and low diastolic blood pressure.

8. What is the most feared complication of aortic stenosis?
Sudden death.

9. How is the diagnosis of aortic insufficiency confirmed?
By cardiac catheterization. **In critically ill infants,** the diagnosis may be made by Doppler echocardiography; then the child can be taken directly to the operating room for valvotomy. **In children,** associated lesions such as patent ductus arteriosus and coarctation of thoracic aorta must be identified. **In adults,** the status of the coronary arteries is important to assess because atherosclerotic heart disease commonly coexists, especially in older patients with angina.

10. How is the diagnosis confirmed?
Aortic insufficiency is often confirmed by echocardiography alone in patients under 40 years of age (when you do not need to worry about coexistent coronary artery disease).

11. When is an operation indicated for aortic stenosis?
Development of symptoms, progression of left ventricular hypertrophy, or measured peak-to-peak systolic gradient of 60 mmHg.

12. When is an operation indicated for aortic insufficiency?
End-systolic left ventricular dimension by echocardiography > 55 mm, percentage fractional shortening < 75%, or end-diastolic diameter > 70 mm.

13. Is aortic valvotomy for congenital aortic stenosis curative?

Usually not. Most children need aortic valve replacement later in life.

14. Can aortic valvotomy be used for calcific aortic stenosis?

No. Aortic valve replacement is the procedure of choice in adults (see question 17).

15. Can valve repair be used to treat aortic insufficiency?

Usually not.

16. What are the technical details of aortic valve replacement?

Aortic valve replacement is done on cardiopulmonary bypass. Because the left ventricle is quite thickened, special care must be taken to avoid ischemic injury to the myocardium. The left ventricle should be vented to decrease wall tension, and the heart should be quieted with cold potassium cardioplegia. Care must be taken during debridement of the calcified valve and anulus to prevent dislodgment of calcium particles into the ventricle, which later may be ejected as calcium emboli. Finally, when suturing the valve, the surgeon must take care to avoid obstruction of the left coronary orifice.

17. What is the Ross procedure?

The patient's own pulmonary valve and proximal pulmonary artery are harvested (autograft) and moved to the aortic valve position to replace the aortic valve. The right ventricular outflow tract is reconstructed with a pulmonary allograft (harvested and frozen from a human cadaver).

18. If a valve prosthesis is necessary in a child, what type of valve should be used?

A mechanical valve should be used in children under 15 years of age because of the high incidence of rapid calcification in porcine valves. Calcification of a porcine valve occurs rapidly in young adults between the ages of 15 and 30; therefore, use of a porcine valve in this group is really a problem.

19. What are the techniques to manage a small aortic anulus?

1. **Konno aortoventriculoplasty.** The ventricular septum is split along the aortic anulus. A patch is then sewn into the split to enlarge the aortic anulus, usually by two valve sizes or more.

2. **Ross-Konno procedure.** The native valve is removed and the septum is split. A segment of right ventricle is taken with the pulmonary autograft to patch the septum. The Ross procedure is then completed.

3. **Patch plasty through the aortic anulus toward the mitral valve.** An incision is carried through the center of the noncoronary anulus toward the anulus of the mitral valve but not onto the valve. A V-shaped patch is then sewn into position to enlarge the anulus about one valve size.

4. **Manouguian patch plasty into the anterior leaflet of the mitral valve.** The incision described above is extended onto the mitral valve. This extension allows the anulus to be enlarged about two valve sizes.

20. What is valve size?

Prosthetic valves are provided in numbers relating to valve diameter. Thus, a no. 21 valve is 21 mm in diameter. Area increases exponentially with valve diameter; an increase of two valve sizes is a big deal.

21. What is the operative mortality rate?

In good-risk patients, less than 3%; in patients with poor ventricular function, 15–20%.

22. What are the complications of aortic valve replacement?

• Low cardiac output (5%): higher for patients with preoperative congestive heart failure
• Bleeding requiring reexploration (5%)
• Heart block (2%)
• Stroke (1%); due to air or calcium left in the heart after closure of the aortotomy

23. What are the long-term results of aortic valve replacement?

Long-term results are excellent, unless the patient has had preoperative congestive heart failure or severe coronary artery disease. The 10-year survival rate is 75%.

24. Can balloon valvotomy be used for adult calcific aortic stenosis?

No. Balloon valvotomy has been used for adult calcific aortic stenosis, but long-term results are poor. Initially, it was hoped that balloon valvotomy could replace surgery and provide long-term palliation in older patients who are at higher surgical risk because of decreased ventricular function. However, it is exactly this group who do poorest after balloon valvotomy; fewer than 50% are alive at 1 year.

25. What are the indications for balloon valvotomy?

Because of the early hemodynamic deterioration, balloon valvotomy is used primarily as a bridge to aortic valve replacement or transplantation in critically ill patients. Temporary improvement in ventricular function suggests that the patient will benefit from aortic valve replacement. It also has been used to relieve symptoms of women in the second trimester of pregnancy who have severe aortic stenosis. The major use of balloon valvotomy remains in infants and young children who have congenital aortic stenosis and a normal-sized anulus. In such circumstances, the intermediate results are similar to surgical valvotomy.

CONTROVERSIES

26. Should valvotomy with inflow occlusion be used in infants under 3 months of age?
For:
1. Low mortality rate (20%).
2. Low incidence of low cardiac output.
Against:
1. Time-limited; procedure must be performed rapidly.
2. 20% incidence of significant aortic regurgitation.

27. Should knife valvotomy with cardiopulmonary bypass be used in infants under 3 months of age?
For: Allows plenty of time to perform operation.
Against: Higher postoperative incidence of low cardiac output.

28. Is balloon valvotomy in the catheterization lab appropriate for infants, children, and young adults?
For: Avoids an operation.
Against: Often not successful in infants with a small aortic anulus.

29. Should a tissue valve be used in young adults between ages 15 and 30?
For: Anticoagulation is not necessary; thus the risk of significant bleeding complications in active patients is avoided. For women in the childbearing years the advantages are real.
Against: Somewhat higher incidence of early valve dysfunction due to valve calcification; thus valve replacement may be necessary before 10 years.

30. Should the Ross procedure be done?
For:
1. Avoids mechanical valves even in small children, thus avoiding anticoagulation.
2. May be a life-time aortic valve.
Against:
1. Destroys a normal pulmonary valve, thus giving the patient two valve diseases over a lifetime.
2. Significant surgical learning curve with high morbidity.

BIBLIOGRAPHY

1. Bernal J, Fernandez-Vals M, Rabasa J, et al: Repair of non severe rheumatic aortic valve disease during other valvular procedures: Is it safe? J Thorac Cardiovasc Surg 115:1130, 1998.
2. Crumbely AJ III, Crawford FA Jr: Long-term results of aortic valve replacement [review article with 161 refs]. Cardiol Clin 9:353, 1991.
3. Davidson CJ, Harrison JK, Pieper KS, et al: Determinants of one-year outcome from balloon aortic valvuloplasty. Ann J Cardiol 68:75, 1991.
4. Elkins RC: Congenital aortic valve disease: Evolving management. Ann Thorac Surg 59:269, 1995.
5. Ettedgui JA, Tallman-Eddy T, Neches WH, et al: Long-term results of survivors of surgical valvotomy for severe aortic stenosis in early infancy. J Thorac Cardiovasc Surg 104:1714, 1992.
6. Jaggers J, Harrison J, Bashore T, et al: The Ross procedure: Shorter hospital stay, decreased morbidity, and cost effective. Ann Thorac Surg 65:1553, 1998.
7. Keane JF, Driscoll EJ, Gersony WM, et al: Second natural history study of congenital heart defects. Results of treatment of patients with aortic valvar stenosis. Circulation 87:116, 1993.
8. Konno S, Imai Y, Lida Y, et al: A new method for prosthetic valve replacement in congenital aortic stenosis associated with hypoplasia of the aortic valve ring. J Thorac Cardiovasc Surg 70:909, 1975.
9. Logeais Y, langanay T, Roussin R, et al: Surgery for aortic stenosis in elderly patients. A study of surgical risk and predictive factors. Circulation 90:2891, 1994.
10. Manouguian S, Abu-Aishah N, Neitzel J: Patch enlargement of the aortic and mitral valve rings with aortic and mitral double valve replacement. J Thorac Cardiovasc Surg 78:394, 1979.
11. Natsuaki M, Itoh T, Tomita S, Naito K: Reversibility of cardiac dysfunction after valve replacement in elderly patients with severe aortic stenosis. Ann Thorac Surg 65:1634, 1998.
12. Pentely G, Morton M, Rahimtoola SH: Effects of successful, uncomplicated valve replacement on ventricular hypertrophy, volume, and performance in aortic stenosis and in aortic incompetence. J Thorac Cardiovasc Surg 75:383, 1978.
13. Rao PS: Balloon aortic valvuloplasty in children [review article with 78 refs]. Clin Cardiol 13:458, 1990.
14. Straumann E, Kiowski W, Langer I, et al: Aortic valve replacement in elderly patients with aortic stenosis. Br Heart J 71:449, 1994.
15. Stelzer P, Weinrauch S, Tranbaugh R: Ten years experience with the modified Ross procedure. J Thorac Cardiovasc Surg 115:1901, 1998.
16. Schafers H, Fries R, Langer F, et al: Valve-preserving replacement of the ascending aorta: Remodeling versus reimplantation. J Thorac Cardiovasc Surg 116:990, 1998.

78. TUBERCULOSIS, PLEURAL EFFUSION, AND EMPYEMA

Marvin Pomerantz, M.D., and James R. Mault, M.D.

TUBERCULOSIS

1. How is tuberculosis treated?

Tuberculosis is primarily a medically treated disease. Conversion of the purified protein derivative (PPD) skin test requires 6 months of isoniazid (INH) therapy. With this therapy active disease is almost always prevented.

Active disease is treated with 6 months of INH and rifampin and 2 months of pyrazinamide. Because of the toxicity of these drugs, patients often try to avoid taking them. Noncompliance may result in the development of drug-resistant organisms. To prevent complication, directly observed therapy is increasingly used. (Like kids, you must watch your patients swallow.)

2. How many people worldwide die yearly from tuberculosis?

Three million people.

3. What is the most common indication for surgical therapy in patients with tuberculosis in the United States?

Multidrug-resistant tuberculosis (MDR-TB) exists when the infecting organism is resistant to both INH and rifampin. Most often these organisms are also resistant to other first-line drugs (streptomycin, ethambutol, pyrazinamide). Patients with MDR-TB and significant cavitary disease or destroyed lung with or without positive sputum require surgical resection.

4. What are other indications for surgery in patients with tuberculosis?

Massive hemoptysis (> 600 ml in 24 hours), bronchostenosis, bronchopleural fistula, trapped lung, and exclusion of cancer.

5. Is there a predilection for one-lung destruction in patients with MDR-TB?

For reasons that are unclear, in 75% of patients with MDR-TB and only one destroyed lung, the left lung is destroyed.

6. Are there other mycobacterial pulmonary infections?

Atypical mycobacterial infections, nontuberculosis mycobacterial infections, and infection with mycobacteria other than tuberculosis (MOTT) are synonyms. The most common of these organisms are the *Mycobacterium avium* complex (MAC). Others include *M. chelonae* and abscesses *M. kansaii*, *M. fortuitum*, and *M. xenopi*. These infections are more indolent than tuberculosis. Indications for surgery are similar to tuberculosis.

7. Does surgery for mycobacterial infections eliminate the need for medical therapy?

No.

PLEURAL EFFUSION

8. What is a pleural effusion?

Normal adults have approximately 1 ml/kg of lubricating fluid in the pleural spaces. Dynamic exchange of this fluid takes place across the pleural space. However, once production of fluid exceeds the clearance capacity of the pleural lymphatics, the fluid accumulates as an effusion. Pleural fluid is generated at a rate of 10 L per 24 hours in the combined hemithoraces.

9. How does a pleural effusion present?

Shortness of breath, chest pain, fever, and occasionally hemoptysis. History should emphasize recent infections, especially pneumonia.

10. What is the initial management of a pleural effusion?

Thoracentesis or a tube thoracostomy to evacuate the effusion completely. The fluid obtained is allocated for cultures (aerobic, anaerobic, acid-fact bacilli [AFB], fungal), cytology, and cell count with analysis of pH, lactate dehydrogenase (LDH), and glucose. Bronchoscopy is indicated in patients with persistent unexpanded fields after drainage of the effusion to exclude endobronchial obstruction.

11. What does an air-fluid level on an initial chest radiograph indicate?

A chest radiograph demonstrating an air-fluid level before any drainage procedure may represent a bronchopleural fistula. These fistulas may resolve with chest tube drainage or require open thoracotomy for definitive repair.

12. What is indicative of an infected pleural effusion?

Pleural effusion becomes infected usually by bacteria derived from adjacent infected lung parenchyma (pneumonia). Indirect indications of bacteria are a glucose less than two-thirds of systemic blood sugar, pH less than 7.2, elevated white blood cell count, and an elevated LDH in the fluid.

EMPYEMA

13. What is an empyema?
When an infected pleural effusion persists, an inflammatory process isolates the infection in the pleural cavity. A walled-off or loculated infected pleural effusion is an empyema. This diagnostic distinction is important because an empyema may not resolve with simple drainage.

14. What do you do if a pleural effusion recurs?
The first recurrence requires repeat drainage by thoracentesis or tube thoracotomy. A second recurrence should undergo exploration with video-assisted thoracoscopic surgery (VATS) and possible pleuradesis. With a suspicion of malignancy, pleural biopsies and cytology should be obtained.

15. How should a loculated effusion be treated?
An infected loculated effusion less than 14 days old should undergo VATS decortication (resection of the thickened, adherent peel). The probability of conversion to open thoracotomy increases with the age of the effusion.

16. What is a decortication?
The cortex is the outside wall or peel of the empyema (like an orange). Thus decortication is the surgical release and removal of the abscess cavity walls. After successful decortication, healthy lungs must expand to fill the entire pleural space; otherwise, the effusion will recur.

17. Under what two conditions should an empyema not be surgically drained?
Pure tuberculous and poststaphylococcal pneumonia empyema in children do not require surgical drainage and should resolve with antibiotics alone.

BIBLIOGRAPHY

1. American Thoracic Society: Diagnosis and treatment of disease caused by nontuberculous mycobacteria [official statement approved by the Board of Directors, march 1997]. Am J Respir Crit Care Med 156(2 Pt 2):S1–S25, 1997.
2. Angelillo Mackinlay TA, Lyons GA, Chimondeguy DJ, et al: VATS debridement versus thoracotomy in the treatment of loculated postpneumonia empyema. Ann Thorac Surg 61:1626–1630, 1996.
3. Bradford WZ, Daley CL: Multiple drug-resistant tuberculosis. Infect Dis Clin North Am 12:157–172, 1998.
4. Cassina PC, Hauser M, Hillejan L, et al: Video-assisted thoracoscopy in the treatment of pleural empyema: Stage-based management and outcome. J Thorac Cardiovasc Surg 117:234–248, 1999.
5. Fallon WF Jr, Wears RL: Prophylactic antibiotics for the prevention of infectious complications including empyema following tube thoracostomy for trauma: Results of meta-analysis. J Trauma 33:110–116; discussion, 6–7, 1992.
6. Hanna JW, Reed JC, Choplin RH: Pleural infections: A clinical-radiologic review. J Thorac Imag 6:68–79, 1991.
7. Heffner JE, Brown LK, Barbieri C, DeLeo JM: Pleural fluid chemical analysis in parapneumonic effusions. A meta-analysis. Am J Respir Crit Care Med 151:1700–1708, 1995 [published erratum appears in Am J Respir Crit Care Med 152:8231, 1995].
8. Hoff SJ, Neblett WW, Edwards KM, et al: Parapneumonic empyema in children: Decortication hastens recovery in patients with severe pleural infections. Pediatr Infect Dis J 10:104–199, 1991.
9. Lawrence DR, Ohri SK, Moxon RE , et al: Thoracoscopic debridement of empyema thoracis. Ann Thorac Surg 64:1448–1450, 1997.
10. Mandal AK, Thadepalli H, Mandal AK, Chettipally U: Outcome of primary empyema thoracis: Therapeutic and microbiologic sepsis. Ann Thorac Surg 66:1782–1786, 1998.
11. Mannheimer SB, et al: Risk factors and outcome of human immunodeficiency virus-infected patients with sporadic multidrug-resistant tuberculosis in New York City. Int J Tuberc Lung Dis 1:19–25, 1997.
12. Mault JR, Pomerantz M: Mycobacterium tuberculosis and other mycobacteria. Chest Surg Clin North Am 9:227–238, 1999.
13. Meyer DM, Jessen ME, Wait MA, Estrera AS: Early evacuation of traumatic retained hemothoraces using thoracoscopy: A prospective, randomized trial. Ann Thorac Surg 64:1396–1400; discussion, 1400–1401, 1997.
14. Pomerantz M, Brown J: Surgery in the treatment of multidrug-resistant tuberculosis. Clin Chest Med 18:123–130, 1997.

15. Pomerantz M, Brown J: Surgery of pulmonary mycobacterial disease. In Kaiser LR, Kron IL, Spray TL (eds): Mastery of Cardiothoracic Surgery. Philadelphia, Lippincott-Raven, 1998, pp 265–271.
16. Puskas JD, Mathisen DJ, Grillo HC, et al: Treatment strategies for bronchopleural fistula. J Thorac Cardiovasc Surg 109:989–995; discussion, 95–96, 1995.
17. Richardson JD, Carillo E: Thoracic infection after trauma. Chest Surg Clin North Am 7:401–427, 1997.
18. Ridley PD, Braimbridge MV: Thoracoscopic debridement and pleural irrigation in the management of empyema thoracis. Ann Thorac Surg 51:461–464, 1991.
19. Smith JA, Mullerworth MH, Westlake GW, Tatoulis J: Empyema thoracis: 14-year experience in a teaching center. Ann Thorac Surg 51:39–42, 1991.
20. Somers J, Faber LP: Historical developments in the management of empyema. Chest Surg Clin North Am 6:403–418, 1996.
21. Wait MA, Sharma S, Hohn J, et al: A randomized trial of empyema therapy [see comments]. Chest 111:1548–1551, 1997.
22. Wallenhaupt SL: Surgical management of thoracic empyema. J Thorac Imag 6:80–88, 1991.
23. Wiedeman HP, Rice TW: Lung abscess and empyema. Semin Thorac Cardiovasc Surg 7:119–128, 1995 [published erratum appears in Semin Thorac Cardiovasc Surg 7:247, 1995].

79. LUNG CANCER

James M. Brown, M.D., and Marvin Pomerantz, M.D.

1. How common is lung cancer?

The indicence of lung cancer is approximately 180,000 new cases annually. Although the male-to-female ratio was 8:1 in 1980, the incidence in women has increased to such a degree that the ratio is now less than 2:1. The mortality rate from lung cancer has not decreased. Overall there is a 10% 5-year survival rate. Because of the link to smoking the increase in smoking among teenagers is worrisome. Moreover, the incidence of lung cancer in nonsmokers also is increasing.

2. What risk factors are thought to be important in the development of lung cancer?

The prominent risk factors are smoking and age; 90% of patients have a smoking history. Previously smoking was thought to be associated only with squamous cell carcinoma of the lung; recently, however, there has been an alarming increase in the incidence of adenocarcinoma, especially in nonsmokers. Other potential inciting agents include chemicals (aromatic hydrocarbons, vinyl chloride), radiation (radon gas and uranium), asbestos and metals (chromium, nickel, lead, and arsenic), and environmental factors (air pollution, coal tar, petroleum products).

3. Do genes and heredity play a role in lung cancer?

Yes. A family history of lung cancer probably increases the risk of getting lung cancer. Furthermore, a large array of biomarkers has been identified in lung cancer cells and lung cancer tissue. An example is the K-*ras* gene. K-*ras* encodes for a protein called p21, which is involved in cellular growth and signal transduction. Mutations in the K-*ras* gene that lead to its activation have been associated with a reduced 5-year survival rate in patients with resectable lung cancer. Other important biomarkers in lung cancer include the p53 tumor suppressor gene, the epidermal growth factor gene *c-erb-2*, the apoptosis inhibitor *bcl-2*, markers of angiogenesis, and markers of cell proliferation. As more lung cancer specimens are examined for these markers, links are made with patient prognosis. No single marker yet has a clear meaning with respect to prognosis or a given patient's outcome.

4. What are the major histologic types of lung cancer and their relative frequency?
Non–small-cell carcinomas   80%
1. Adenocarcinoma   45%
   This ominous type of lung cancer is increasing dramatically in nonsmokers.

2. Squamous cell carcinoma   40%

This type of lung cancer, also referred to as epidermoid, is associated histologically with keratin pearls and is promoted by smoking and other inhaled irritants.

3. Large-cell carcinoma   15%

Bronchoalveolar carcinoma is the lung cancer associated with frothy bronchorrhea on "multiple-guess" examinations. It is a subtype of adenocarcinoma. Intuitively malignant overgrowth of surfactant-secreting cells produces frothy sputum. Although this symptom is rarely encountered clinically, it is common on examinations.

Small-cell carcinoma 20%

The most important distinction is between small-cell and non–small-cell carcinoma because of fundamental differences in tumor biology and clinical behavior. Patients with small-cell lung cancer are classified as having either limited or extensive disease. **Limited** means that all known disease is confined to one hemithorax and regional lymph nodes, including mediastinal, contralateral hilar, and ipsilateral supraclavicular nodes. **Extensive** describes disease beyond these limits, including brain, bone marrow, and intraabdominal metastases.

5. Does lung cancer screening make sense?

Unfortunately, no. Even chest radiographs performed in 40–60-year-old male smokers have not increased the curability rate of patients presenting with lung cancer. Although other methods have been developed to screen for lung cancer, such as the use of biomarkers or positron emission tomography, no method is yet useful for mass screening.

6. How do patients with lung cancer present?

Increasingly, primary lung cancer is discovered on routine chest radiograph. Occasionally patients have a cough, streaky hemoptysis, or recurrent pneumonia. As many as 10% of patients complain of a paraneoplastic syndrome.

7. What is a paraneoplastic syndrome?

Paraneoplastic syndromes of lung cancer may be **metabolic** (hypercalcemia, Cushing's syndrome), **neurologic** (peripheral neuropathy, polymyositis, or Lambert-Eaton syndrome, which is like myasthenia gravis), **skeletal** (clubbing, hypertrophic osteoarthropathy), **hematologic** (anemia, thrombocytosis, disseminated intravascular coagulation), or **cutaneous** (hyperkeratosis, acanthosis nigricans, dermatomyositis). Of interest, the presence of a paraneoplastic syndrome does not influence the ultimate curability of the lung cancer.

8. Does the staging system for lung cancer havoc prognostic and therapeutic importance?

Yes. The classification system is based on clinical and pathologic data for non–small-cell lung cancer. Patients often are staged clinically in conjunction with CT scans.

Stage I:	Intraparenchymal disease with or without extension to the visceral pleura, at least 2 cm from the carina, and no lymph node or metastatic spread.
Stage II:	Primary tumor is similar to that of stage I with extension to interbronchial lymph nodes (N1), or tumor invades chest wall without nodal involvement.
Stage IIIa:	Extension of tumor into hilar or mediastinal lymph nodes (N2) or chest wall with N1 nodes.
Stage IIIb:	All elements of IIIa plus extension to mediastinal structures (heart or great vessels) and/or contralateral hilar, paratracheal, or supraclavicular lymph nodes (N3).
Stage IV:	Malignant pleural effusion or metastatic disease (M1)

9. Describe the work-up of a patient with a mass on chest radiograph.

Surgical resection remains the most effective way to cure lung cancer. Therefore, early evaluation stresses the patient's candidacy for a thoracotomy and subsequently focuses on the diagnosis and staging of the pulmonary neoplasm. The diagnosis can be made only 60% of the time by sputum cytology; less than 85% of the time by bronchoscopy with biopsy; and only 80–90% of the time with CT scan-guided needle biopsy. Thus, the mainstay of diagnosis is wedge resection of the pulmonary lung mass. CT scanning of the chest (looking for mediastinal lymph nodes) and abdomen (looking for adrenal metastases) is standard. Other procedures, such as bone or brain scanning, are omitted unless the patient complains of specific symptoms. The patient's ability to withstand a thoracotomy requires cardiac evaluation (history of myocardial infarction, congestive heart failure, and angina) and pulmonary reserve (bedside spirometry determines FEV_1).

10. What are the lower limits of pulmonary function reserve that allow resection of lung cancer?

1. The forced expiratory volume in one second (FEV_1) should be more than 1 liter/second; the room air arterial blood gas indicates that the partial pressure of oxygen (PO_2) and partial pressure of carbon dioxide (PCO_2) are on the proper side of 50 (PO_2 above 50 and PCO_2 below 50).
2. The patient should be able to walk up one flight of stairs.
3. In borderline cases, ventilation-perfusion scanning can be used to predict how much functioning lung will remain after operation.

11. How is lung cancer treated?

The most effective treatment for lung cancer is surgical resection. Unfortunately, 50% of patients initially present with clearly advanced disease, and only 25% of all patients are candidates for resection. Fortunately, preoperative chemotherapy with a cisplatinum-containing regimen has increased the number of stage III patients who are candidates for resection. This recently innovative therapy may translate into improved survival rates. For stage III lung cancer several clinical trials have shown an advantage to preoperative chemotherapy and radiation treatment called neoadjuvant therapy. Even lower-stage disease or tumors at high risk of recurrencemay benefit from newer chemotherapeutic regimens.

12. Does radiation therapy have a place in the therapy of lung cancer?

Radiation therapy is effective palliative but not curative therapy for lung cancer. Specifically, patients who present with a superior vena cava syndrome or a blocked bronchus with distal pneumonia frequently can be "opened up" with radiation therapy. Radiation is also excellent for the palliation of pathologic bone pain. Some—but not all—clinical trials have shown some benefit from preoperative chemoradiation treatment in advanded-stage lung cancer.

13. What is the survival rate of patients treated for lung cancer?

For stage I, non–small-cell carcinoma, the 5-year survival rate is 60–80% after complete resection. The 5-year survival rates for stage II, stage IIIa, and stage IIIb are 50%, 15%, and 5%, respectively. The 5-year survival rate for small-cell carcinoma remains dismal: 7% of patients with limited disease and only 1% of patients with extensive disease survive 5 years.

14. What is mediastinoscopy?

Mediastinoscopy is a staging procedure in which the paratracheal, subcarinal, and proximal peribronchial lymph nodes are sampled from a small incision made in the suprasternal notch.

15. What are the indications for mediastinoscopy?

Mediastinal staging is indicated in patients with either apparent or documented lung cancer who have:

1. Known lung cancer with mediastinal lymph node accessible by cervical mediastinal exploration and > 1 cm, as assessed by CT scan.
2. Adenocarcinoma of the lung and multiple mediastinal lymph nodes < 1 cm.
3. Central or large (> 5 cm) lung cancers with mediastinal lymph nodes < 1 cm.

4. Lung cancer in patients who are high risks for thoracotomy and lung resection.

If the mediastinoscopy is negative, the surgeon should proceed with thoracotomy, biopsy, and curative lung resection. Mediastinoscopy benefits only a patient who is proved to have unresectable lung cancer. A positive mediastinoscopy spares the patient a thoracotomy.

16. Is malignant pleural effusion and/or recurrent nerve involvement with tumor an absolute contraindication to surgical resection for lung cancer?

A malignant pleural effusion is an absolute contraindication to surgical resective therapy. Conversely, both King George V and Arthur Godfrey had successful surgical resections in the face of recurrent nerve involvement with tumor.

BIBLIOGRAPHY

1. Dristin L: The price of prevention. Sci Am 124–127, 1995.
2. Johnston MR: Selecting patients with lung cancer for surgical resection. Semin Oncol 15:246–254, 1988.
3. Martini N, Flelinger BJ: The role of surgery in N2 lung cancer. Surg Clin North Am 667:1037, 1987.
4. McGee JM: Screening for lung cancer. Semin Surg Oncol 5:179, 1989.
5. Minna JD, Pass H, Glatstrein E, Ihde DC: Cancer of the lung. In Devita VT, Hellman S, Rosenberg SA (eds): Cancer: Principles and Practice of Oncology, 2nd ed. Philadelphia, J.B. Lippincott, 1989.
6. Moosa AR, Schimpff SC, Robson MD (eds): Comprehensive Textbook of Oncology. Baltimore, Williams & Wilkins, 1991, pp 732–785.
7. Mountain EF: Revision in the international system for staging lunc cancer. Chest 111:1710, 1997.
8. Parker SH, et al: Cancer statistics. 47:5, 1997.
9. Pass HI: Adjunctive and alternate treatment of bronchogenic lung cancer. Chest Surg Clin North Am 1:1, 1991.
10. Shields TW: General Thoracic Surgery, 4th ed. Baltimore, Williams & Wilkins, 1994, pp 1095–1277.
11. Strauss GM: Prognostic markers in resectable non–small-cell lung cancer. Hematol Oncol Clin North Am 1:409, 1997.
12. Sonett JR, et al: Safe pulmonary resection after chemotherapy and high-dose thoracic radiation. 68:316, 1999.

80. SOLITARY PULMONARY NODULE

James M. Brown, M.D., and Marvin Pomerantz, M.D.

1. What is a solitary pulmonary nodule?

A solitary pulmonary nodule or "coin lesion" is < 3 cm and discrete on chest radiograph. It is usually surrounded by lung parenchyma.

2. What causes a solitary pulmonary nodule?

The most common causes of a pulmonary nodule are either neoplastic (carcinoma) or infectious (granuloma). Pulmonary nodules also may represent lung abscess, pulmonary infarction, arteriovenous malformations, resolving pneumonia, pulmonary sequestration, hamartoma, and others. As a general rule of thumb, likelihood of malignancy is comparable to the patient's age. Thus, lung cancer is rare (although it does occur) in 30-year-olds, whereas in 50-year-old smokers the chances of malignancy may be as high as 50–60%.

3. How does a solitary pulmonary nodule present?

Typically, a solitary nodule is picked up incidentally on routine chest radiograph. In several large series, more than 75% of lesions were surprise findings on routine chest radiograph. Less than 25% of patients had symptoms referable to the lung. Solitary nodules are now seen on other sensitive imaging tests such as computed tomography (CT).

4. How frequently does a solitary pulmonary nodule represent metastatic disease?

Less than 10% of solitary nodules represent metastatic disease. Accordingly, an extensive work-up for a primary site of cancer other than the lung is not indicated.

5. Can a tissue sample be obtained by fluoroscopic or CT-guided needle biopsy?

Yes, but the results do not change the treatment. If the needle biopsy tissue indicates cancer, the nodule must be removed. If the needle biopsy is negative, the nodule still must be removed.

6. Are radiographic findings important?

Only relatively. The resolution of modern CT scanners allows the best identification of characteristics that suggest cancer:

1. Indistinct or irregular spiculated borders of the nodule.
2. The larger the nodule, the more likely it is to be malignant.
3. Calcification in the nodule generally is associated with benign disease. Specifically, central, diffuse, or laminated calcifications are typical of a granuloma, whereas calcifications with more dense and irregular popcorn patterns are associated with hamartomas. Unfortunately, eccentric foci of calcium or small flecks of calcium may be found in malignant lesions.
4. Nodules can be studied using a CT scanner by measuring their change in relative radiodensity after injection of contrast. This information improves the accuracy of predicting the presence of malignancy.

7. What social or clinical findings suggest that a nodule is malignant rather than benign?

Unfortunately, none of the findings are sufficiently sensitive or specific to influence the work-up. Both increasing age and a long smoking history predispose to lung cancer. Winston Churchill should have had lung cancer—but he did not. Thus, the fact that the patient is the president of the spelunking club (histoplasmosis), has a sister who raises pigeons (cryptococcosis), grew up in the Ohio River Valley (histoplasmosis), works as sexton for a dog cemetery (blastomycosis), or just took a hiking trip through the San Joaquin Valley (coccidioidomycosis) is interesting associated history but does not affect the work-up of a solitary pulmonary nodule.

8. What is the most valuable bit of historic data?

An old chest radiograph. If the nodule is new, it is more likely to be malignant, whereas if the nodule has not changed in the past 2 years, it is less likely to be malignant. Unfortunately, even this observation is not absolute.

9. If a patient presents with a treated prior malignancy and a new solitary pulmonary nodule, is it safe to assume that the new nodule represents metastatic disease?

No. Even in patients with known prior malignancies, less then 50% of new pulmonary nodules are metastatic. Thus, the work-up should proceed exactly as for any other patient with a new solitary pulmonary nodule.

10. How should a solitary pulmonary nodule be evaluated?

A complete travel and occupational history is interesting but does not affect the evaluation. Because of the peripheral location of most nodules, bronchoscopy has a diagnostic yield of less than 50%. Even in the best hands, sputum cytology has a low yield. CT scanning is recommended because it can identify other potentially metastatic nodules and delineate the status of mediastinal lymph nodes. As indicated above, percutaneous needle biopsy has a diagnostic yield of approximately 80% but rarely alters the subsequent management.

The critical step in the evaluation is to determine whether the patient is capable of withstanding curative surgical therapy. Cardiac, lung, hepatic, renal, and neurologic function must be deemed stable. If the patient is not likely to survive for several years, there is simply no point in surgical excision of an asymptomatic pulmonary nodule.

The mainstay of management in patients who can tolerate surgery is resection of the nodule for diagnosis by either a minimally invasive thoracoscopy approach or a limited thoracotomy.

11. If the lesion proves to be cancer, what is the appropriate surgical therapy?

Although several series have suggested that wedge excision of the nodule is sufficient, an anatomic lobectomy remains the procedure of choice. A solitary nodule that turns out to be cancer should be early-stage disease and has a 65% 5-year survival rate if there are no notable metastases. Unfortunately, the recurrence rate even for stage I tumors or a small nodule is 30% over 5 years. Recurrences are splilt between local and distant.

BIBLIOGRAPHY

1. Cummings SR, Lillington GA, Richard RJ: Managing solitary pulmonary nodules: The choice of strategy is a "close call." Am Rev Respir Dis 134:453–460, 1986.
2. Ginsberg RJ, et al: Randomized trial of lobectomy versus limited resection T.N. non-small cell lung cancer. Ann Thorac Surg 60:615, 1995.
3. Higgins GA, Shield TW, Keehn RJ: The solitary pulmonary nodule: Ten-year follow-up of Veterans Administration–Armed Forces Cooperative Study. Arch Surg 10:570–575, 1975.
4. Khouri NF, Meziane MA, Zerhouni EA, et al: The solitary pulmonary nodule: Assessment, diagnosis and management. Chest 91:128–133, 1987.
5. McKenna RJ, Libshitz HI, Mountain CE, McMurtrey MJ: Roentgenographic evaluation of mediastinal nodes for preoperative assessment in lung cancer. Chest 88:206–210, 1985.
6. Mountain CF: Value of the new TNM staging system for lung cancer. Chest 96:47s–49s, 1989.
7. Neff TA: When the x-ray shows a "spot" on the lung. Med Times 106:65–69, 1978.
8. Neff TA: The science and humanity of the solitary pulmonary nodule. Am Rev Respir Dis 134:433–434, 1986.
9. Nesbitt J, et al: Survival in early stage non-small cell lung cancer. Ann Thorac Surg 60:466, 1995.
10. Ray JF, Lawton BR, Magnin GE, et al: The coin lesion story: Update 1976. Chest 70:332–336, 1976.

81. DISSECTING AORTIC ANEURYSM

David N. Campbell, M.D.

1. Why is the term *dissecting aortic aneurysm* really incorrect?

The correct term should be **dissecting aortic hematoma** because the lesion is not an aneurysm. Blood dissects between the middle and outer layers of the media of the aorta.

2. How is the diagnosis made?

Suspicion is the most important factor because no one feature is common to patients presenting with aortic dissections. In any patient who presents with severe knifelike, ripping chest and back pain, the diagnosis of aortic dissection should be considered.

3. Once the diagnosis is entertained, how should the patient be managed?

The other diagnosis to be strongly considered is acute myocardial infarction. Two-thirds of patients are hypertensive, and blood pressure must be controlled. An electrocardiogram often rules out an infarction, but some aortic dissections tear off a coronary artery and thus involve both acute infarction and aortic dissection.

4. What is the most significant diagnostic clue?

A new aortic valvular diastolic murmur, indicating aortic valvular regurgitation. Blood flow from the dissecting hematoma encircles the lumen of the blood vessel and constricts it or actually cleaves the takeoff of the subclavian or femoral vessels (with a loss of pulse). Neurologic findings, including paraplegia and hemiplegia, also may be present. Hypertension is common, as are differential blood pressures in the four extremities.

5. What chest radiograph findings are helpful in diagnosis?

Widened mediastinum and loss of aortic knob silhouette—a hematoma surrounding the aorta makes the aortic outline blurry.

6. How is the diagnosis confirmed? What is the role of transesophageal echocardiography?

The literature reports the high accuracy of transesophageal echocardiography (TEE) in the diagnosis of aortic dissections. In some institutions patients undergo operation with this diagnostic tool only. However, the aortogram is still the gold standard. If time allows and the patient is stable, an aortogram should be obtained to confirm the diagnosis, type of dissection (ascending vs. descending), status of the aortic valve, and status of the coronary arteries. In fact, both modalities may be complementary: the TEE confirms the diagnosis, whereas the aortogram defines location, aortic valve status, and coronary arteries.

7. What are the types of dissection?

The following classification has both therapeutic and prognostic valve:

Ascending (type A) involves only the ascending or both the ascending and descending aorta.
Descending (type B) involves only the descending aorta.

8. Who cares whether a dissection involves the ascending (type A) or descending (type B) aorta?

Ascending dissections require early surgical correction to avoid extension into the coronary or carotid arteries and rupture into the pericardium (tamponade).

Descending dissections do not involve the ascending aorta and may be managed medically or surgically (see Controversies).

9. What is the key to medical management?

Blood pressure should be lowered to 100–110 mmHg (systolic) with a combination of sodium nitroprusside and propranolol. Propranolol is particularly important because it decreases the contractility of the myocardium (dp/dt), thereby decreasing the shearing force and preventing propagation of the dissection down the aorta. Conceptually, you should lower the blood pressure as much as you can, but the patient must continue to make urine.

10. Can trimethaphan camsylate (Arfonad) be used instead of propranolol or nitroprusside?

No.

11. What are the principles and advantages of surgical management?

Ascending dissection

1. To close off the hematoma by obliterating *the most proximal* intimal tear.
2. To restore competency of the aortic valve.
3. To restore flow to any branches of the aorta that have been sheared off and receive blood flow from a false lumen.
4. To protect the heart during these maneuvers and to restore coronary blood flow if a coronary artery has been sheared off.
5. To look for tears in the transverse aortic arch.

Technique. Use of deep hypothermia circulatory arrest with or without retrograde cerebral perfusion is in vogue at present. This technique allows the arch to be inspected and the distal anastomosis of the Dacron graft to be sewn accurately to the distal ascending aorta in open fashion. Whether to replace or repair the aortic valve is controversial.

Descending dissection

1. To close off the hematoma by obliterating the most proximal intimal tear.
2. To restore blood flow to branches of the aorta fed by the false channel.

Technique. Surgery is performed using partial cardiopulmonary bypass, or the "clamp and run" technique, in which the aorta is cross-clamped and the graft is sewn in as fast as possible (see Controversies).

12. What are the operative complications?

1. Hemorrhage (20%): very common because of the use of heparin and the poor quality of aortic tissue (like wet Kleenex).

2. Renal failure (20%).

3. Pulmonary insufficiency (30% higher in repair of descending dissections).

4. Paraplegia: often presents before operation; as a surgical complication, it usually occurs only with descending dissections.

5. Acute myocardial infarction or low cardiac output (30%).

6. Bowel infarction (5%).

7. Death (15%): higher for acute than chronic dissections and higher for repair of ascending dissections.

13. What are the long-term results?

Of patients who survive the operation, two-thirds die within 7 years because of comorbid cardiac and cerebrovascular disease.

CONTROVERSIES

14. Which is preferred: surgical or medical management of descending dissections?
Initial surgical management

1. Approximately 25% of patients initially treated medically need an operation eventually.

2. Operative mortality is much less today (20%) than in the past.

3. Medical management has the same in-hospital mortality (20%).

Initial medical management

1. Avoids unnecessary operation and its attendant cost and complication rate.

15. What is the preferred management of aortic insufficiency in ascending dissections?
Replacement of aortic valve

1. Easy (valved conduits now available).

2. Eliminates aortic insufficiency completely.

3. Should be done in patients with Marfan's syndrome.

Repair of aortic valve

1. With native valve reconstruction, when done correctly, the need to replace the valve at a later time is only 10%.

2. Avoids need for anticoagulation, which is necessary when a mechanical valve is used to replace the aortic valve.

16. What is the preferred repair of descending dissections?

1. **Partial left atrial-to-femoral artery bypass**

For:

• Allows unloading of the heart.

• Allows distal perfusion to avoid visceral ischemia.

• Allows as much time as needed to complete anastomosis.

Against: requires heparinization.

2. **Simple aortic cross-clamping**

For: Fast

Against: Placement of the graft has to be done in less than 30 minutes or the complication rate, particularly paraplegia, increases significantly.

BIBLIOGRAPHY

1. Banning AP, Masani ND, Ikram S, et al: Transesophageal echocardiography as the sole diagnostic investigation in patients with suspected thoracic aortic dissection. Br Heart J 72:461–465, 1994.

2. Barron DJ, Livesey SA, Brown IW, et al: Twenty-year follow-up of acute type A dissection: The incidence and extent of distal aortic disease using magnetic resonance imaging. J Card Surg 12:147–159, 1997.

3. Blanchard DG, Kimura BJ, Dittrich HC, DeMaria AN: Transesophageal echocardiography of the aorta. JAMA 272:546–551, 1994.

4. Chirillo F, Cavallini C, Longhini C, et al: Comparative diagnostic valve of transesophageal echocardiography and retrograde aortography in the evaluation of thoracic aortic dissection. Am J Cardiol 74:590–595, 1994.

5. Cigarroa JE, Isselbacher EM, DeSanctis RW, Eagle KA: Diagnostic imaging in the evaluation of suspected aortic dissection. Old standards and new directions. N Engl J Med 328:35–43, 1993.

6. Costelli JS, Buket S, Djukanovic B: Aortic arch operation: Current treatment and results. Ann Thorac Surg 59:19–27, 1995.

7. Glower DD, Fann JI, Speier RH, et al: Comparison of medical and surgical therapy for uncomplicated descending aortic dissection. Circulation 82(Suppl IV):39–46, 1990.

8. LeMaire SA, Coselli JS: Aortic root surgery in Marfan syndrome: Current practice and evolving technique. J Card Surg 12(Suppl):137–141, 1997.

9. Nienaber CA, von Kodolitsch Y, Nicolas V, et al: The diagnosis of thoracic aortic dissection by noninvasive imaging procedures. N Engl J Med 328:1–9, 1993.

10. Okita Y, Takamoto S, Ando M, et al: Mortality and cerebral outcome in patients who underwent aortic arch operations using deep hypothermic circulatory arrest with retrograde cerebral perfusion: No relation of early death, stroke, and delirium to the duration of circulatory arrest. J Thorac Cardiovasc Surg 115:129–138, 1998.

11. Pansini S, Gagliardotto PV, Pompei E, et al: Early and late risk factors fin surgical treatment of acute type A aortic dissection. Ann Thorac Surg 66:779–784, 1998.

12. Safi HJ, Milelr CC, Reardon MJ, et al: Operation for acute and chronic aortic dissection: Recent outcome with regard to neurologic deficit and early death. Ann Thorac Surg 66:402–411, 1998.

13. Wheat MW Jr, Palmer RF, Bartley TB, Seelman RC: Treatment of dissecting aneurysms of the aorta without surgery. J Thorac Cardiovasc Surg 50:364–373, 1995.

IX. Pediatric Surgery

82. HYPERTROPHIC PYLORIC STENOSIS

Denis D. Bensard, M.D.

1. What is the incidence of pyloric stenosis?

Hypertrophic pyloric stenosis (HPS) is the most common pathologic cause of nonbilious vomiting in infants. A familial pattern is well documented. Offspring of an affected parent have an increased incidence of HPS (10%); the highest rate occurs in males born to an affected mother (20%).

2. Describe the typical presentation of HPS.

A healthy infant who initially fed normally presents at 2–6 weeks of age with a history of "projectile" vomiting. The emesis is nonbilious, although blood or "coffee grounds" may be observed if esophagitis or gastritis is present. After vomiting the infant appears hungry and will refeed immediately. With time dehydration and malnutrition worsen, leading the parents to seek medical evaluation. The parents frequently report multiple formula changes with no apparent improvement in symptoms.

3. What are the physical findings?

Affected infants are dehydrated. The abdomen is nondistended. A palpable pyloric tumor, known as the "olive," confirms the diagnosis. The pyloric tumor is palpable in 50% of patients, but ultrasound has now supplanted palpation to confirm the diagnosis. Associated findings are rare, but mild jaundice occurs in 5% of infants as a result of reduced glucuronyl transferase activity.

4. How is the diagnosis confirmed?

Ultrasonographic criteria include pyloric diameter > 1.4 cm, wall width > 4 mm, and pyloric channel length > 1.6 cm. Alternatively, a barium upper gastrointestinal (UGI) examination may be used to confirm the diagnosis. Diagnostic criteria include gastric outlet obstruction, a "string" sign demonstrating pyloric channel narrowing, and "shoulder" sign or pyloric "tit" in high-grade obstruction. If a UGI study is used, a nasogastric tube should be placed and the stomach irrigated with saline to remove the barium and thus reduce the risk of aspiration during the induction of anesthesia. Recent analyses demonstrate that UGI is the most cost-effective initial radiologic diagnostic test.

5. Describe the likely electrolyte abnormalities.

Electrolytes often are normal, but persistent vomiting produces a hypokalemic, hypochloremic metabolic alkalosis due to the loss of gastric acid (hydrochloric acid). Earlier consideration of the diagnosis has led to a significant reduction in this classic electrolyte abnormality at presentation. Repeated vomiting of gastric acid results in significant loss of chloride and hydrogen ion. The kidneys compensate by preserving hydrogen ions at the expense of potassium. If the condition remains uncorrected, paradoxical aciduria ensues, resulting in the triad of hypokalemia, hypochloremia, and metabolic alkalosis. Adequate fluid resuscitation begins with intravenous administration of 0.45% saline solution. Once urinary flow has been established,

20–40 mEq/L of potassium chloride is added to the intravenous solution to correct the potassium deficit, augment chloride replacement, and correct dehydration.

6. What procedure is recommended for the correction of HPS?

The Fredet-Ramstedt pyloromyotomy is generally accepted as the surgical procedure of choice. Medical management, although reportedly effective in some patients, is associated with a higher failure rate and longer hospitalization compared with surgical management. Endoscopic balloon dilation and laparoscopic pyloromyotomy have not yet approached the success of open pyloromyotomy. The standard pyloromyotomy is performed through a supraumbilical transverse incision over the right rectus muscle. The pylorus is delivered through the muscle-splitting incision, and a superficial incision is made longitudinally over the pyloric muscle in an avascular area. The incision extends onto the antrum for a short distance. The muscle fibers are spread to expose the underlying mucosa. At the conclusion of the pyloromyotomy, the gastric mucosa should bulge upward into the cleft, and the pyloric muscle walls should move independently of one another. Air should be injected into the stomach via the nasogastric tube to identify inadvertent mucosal perforation.

7. What should be done if a perforation is identified?

The mucosa should be closed with several fine sutures and covered with an omental patch. If the mucosal injury is too extensive, the myotomy should be closed with sutures, and a second, parallel myotomy should be made at 45–180° from the original myotomy.

8. When can postoperative feeding begin? What are the limitations?

If is necessary to begin with frequent, small-volume feedings (15–30 ml every 2–3 hours) and advance gradually. Small amounts of vomiting are common (20%) and should not cause alarm unless persistent. Incomplete pyloromyotomy is generally not considered unless symptoms of gastric outlet obstruction continue for 7–10 days postoperatively.

9. Describe several hypotheses about the pathogenesis of HPS.

Recent studies of the abnormal pyloric complex demonstrate improper innervation of pyloric smooth muscle, excessive contraction of circular pyloric smooth muscle (decreased nitric oxide synthase), increased extracellular matrix proteins (collagen), and increased expression or local synthesis of growth hormones (insulinlike growth factor-1, transforming growth factor beta-1, platelet derived growth factor).

BIBLIOGRAPHY

1. Chen EA, Luks FI, Gilchrist BF, et al: Pyloric stenosis in the age of ultrasonography: Fading skills, better patients? J Pediatr Surg 31:829, 1996.
2. Georgeson KE, Corbin TJ, Griffen JW, et al: An analysis of feeding regimens after pyloromyotomy for hypertrophic pyloric stenosis. J Pediatr Surg 28:1478, 1993.
3. Hulka F, Campbell TJ, Campbell JR, et al: Evolution in the recognition of infantile hypertrophic pyloric stenosis. Pediatrics 100:E9, 1997.
4. Hulka F, Campbell JR, Harrison MW, et al: Cost-effectiveness in diagnosing infantile hypertrophic pyloric stenosis. J Pediatr Surg 32:1604, 1997.
5. Hulka F, Harrison MW, Campbell TJ, et al: Complications of pyloromyotomy for infantile hypertrophic pyloric stenosis. Am J Surg 173:450, 1997.
6. Ohshiro K, Puri P: Pathogenesis of infantile hypertrophic pyloric stenosis: Recent progress. Pediatr Surg Int 13:237, 1998.
7. Poon TS, Zhang AL, Cartmill T, et al: Changing patterns of diagnosis and treatment of infantile hypertrophic pyloric stenosis: A clinical audit of 303 patients. J Pediatr Surg 31:1611, 1996.

83. INTESTINAL OBSTRUCTION OF NEONATES AND INFANTS

Denis D. Bensard, M.D., and Jeffery Pence, M.D.

1. What signs or symptoms suggest intestinal obstruction in the neonate?

Signs and symptoms vary according to the level of obstruction. Proximal intestinal obstruction leads to the early onset of vomiting (bilious vomiting is always ominous), generally with minimal abdominal distention. In contrast, neonates with distal intestinal obstruction present after the first day of life with vomiting and pronounced abdominal distention. The failure to pass meconium suggests intestinal obstruction.

2. What is the differential diagnosis of intestinal obstruction in neonates?

Look for an anal opening, which eliminates the diagnosis of imperforate anus. Next obtain an abdominal radiograph. The extent of gaseous distention of the bowel implicates a proximal or distal bowel obstruction. No attempts should be made to distinguish small- and large-bowel obstruction.

Proximal	Duodenal atresia, stenosis
(minimal bowel gas)	Malrotation with midgut volvulus
	Jejunal atresia
Distal	Ileal atresia
(significant bowel gas)	Meconium ileus/plug
	Hirschsprung's disease

3. When are contrast studies of the gastrointestinal (GI) tract indicated?

If peritonitis or pneumoperitoneum is present, proceed to exploratory laparotomy without delay. In malrotation, the upper GI demonstrates distention of the proximal duodenum, corkscrewing of the distal duodenum, and lack of fixation. In duodenal atresia the upper GI demonstrates filling of a blind ending and a distended duodenum. Contrast enema is extremely helpful in the delineation of distal bowel obstruction and, in the case of meconium ileus, may even be therapeutic.

Disorder	Barium Enema
Ileal atresia	Microcolon; no reflux into terminal ileum
Meconium ileus	Microcolon; reflux into terminal ileum with filling defects
Meconium plug	Normal colon; large filling defect of left colon
Hirschsprung's disease	Narrowed rectosigmoid; dilated proximal colon

4. Describe intestinal atresia. How do duodenal atresia and intestinal atresia differ?

Atresia can occur anywhere in the GI tract: duodenal (50%), jejunoileal (45%), or colonic (5%). Duodenal atresia arises from a failure of recanalization during the 8–10th week of gestation; jejunoileal and colonic are caused by an in utero mesenteric vascular accident.

Duodenal atresia is associated with onset of bilious vomiting (85% of atresia distal to the ampulla of Vater) with absence of significant abdominal distention within the first day of life. Approximately 25% of infants have trisomy 21. Diagnosis is based on the classic abdominal radiograph suggesting duodenal obstruction: "double bubble" (distended stomach and first/second portions of duodenum). If air is seen distally, malrotation with midgut volvulus or duodenal stenosis may be present, but an upper GI must be obtained to rule out malrotation with midgut volvulus. Surgical correction of the anomaly is performed by duodenoduodenostomy.

Jejunoileal atresia is associated with onset of bilious vomiting at 2–3 days of life with moderate-to-severe abdominal distention. Abdominal radiograph exhibits dilated loops of bowel with air-fluid levels. Barium enema reveals microcolon and no reflux of contrast into dilated bowel. Associated anomalies are uncommon. Surgical correction involves end-to-end anastomosis with or without limited intestinal resection.

Colonic atresia is associated with onset of bilious vomiting at > 2 days of life, no passage of meconium, and moderate-to-severe abdominal distention. Abdominal radiograph reveals dilated loops of bowel with air-fluid levels suggesting distal intestinal obstruction. Barium enema demonstrates a microcolon with cutoff in colonic segment. Approximately 20% of patients have an associated anomaly of the heart, musculoskeletal system, abdominal wall, or GI tract. Surgical management includes limited colonic resection with primary anastomosis.

5. Describe malrotation with midgut volvulus. Is it a surgical emergency?

During the 6–12th week of gestation the intestine undergoes evisceration, growth, return to the abdominal cavity, and counterclockwise rotation with fixation. Malrotation is an error in both rotation and fixation that results in abnormal fixation and a narrow based mesentery prone to twisting (volvulus). Twisting of the midgut on its blood supply (superior mesenteric artery) produces vascular occlusion (strangulation) and obstruction (malrotation with midgut volvulus). The risk of strangulation implies a surgical emergency, for delay places the infant at risk of losing the entire midgut and death. Typically, a previously well neonate or child without a history of previous surgery presents with bilious vomiting, abdominal distention, and variable degrees of shock. Abdominal radiograph may demonstrate a "double bubble" and distal intestinal air. If the infant is acutely ill, no further studies are needed and surgical exploration is indicated. If the diagnosis is in question and the infant is stable, an upper GI, not a barium enema, is performed. Barium enema may demonstrate malrotation, but midgut volvulus cannot be excluded. Surgical treatment is correction of the rotational anomaly with or without intestinal resection, depending on the degree of ischemic injury to the bowel.

6. What is meconium ileus? How does it differ from meconium plug?

Meconium ileus (MI) is the obstruction of the terminal ileum by highly viscid, tenacious meconium. MI is nearly always associated with cystic fibrosis (CF), although it has been reported in premature infants without CF. CF is an autosomal recessive disorder. A three base pair deletion on chromosome 7 results in defective chloride transport in the apical membrane of epithelial cells. The combination of hyperviscous mucus secreted by the abnormal intestinal glands and pancreatic insufficiency leads to abnormal meconium, which obstructs the lumen of the terminal ileum. Fifteen percent of neonates with CF present with MI. Symptoms of feeding intolerance, bilious emesis, and abdominal distention begin in the second to third day of life. On palpation, the abdomen feels soft but doughlike. Abdominal radiographs demonstrate multiple dilated loops of bowel without air-fluid levels (distal obstruction) and may show a ground-glass appearance in the right lower quadrant (Neuhauser's sign). Contrast enema demonstrates a microcolon with multiple, small filling defects of the terminal ileum (inspissated meconium). Unlike most forms of neonatal intestinal obstruction, surgery is reserved for cases refractory to nonoperative treatment or complex MI (atresia, volvulus, perforation). Sixty percent of infants with simple MI can be treated successfully with gastrograffin enema(s) and rectal irrigation. If an operation is indicated, the objective is to remove the obstructing meconium by limited resection or enterostomy with evacuation of the meconium and irrigation of the distal bowel.

Meconium plug syndrome is the obstruction of the colon by thickened meconium; unlike MI, it is rarely associated with CF (< 5%). Meconium plug may be seen in Hirschsprung's disease; therefore all patients should undergo suction rectal biopsy to exclude this diagnosis. Similarly, affected infants should undergo sweat chloride testing or genetic testing to rule out CF.

7. What is Hirschsprung's disease? Hirschsprung's enterocolitis?

The intestine is innervated by cells originating in the neural crest. During the 5–12th week of gestation neural crest cells migrate in a craniocaudal direction and disperse within the wall of the intestine (intermuscular, to Auerbach's plexus; submucosal, to Meissner's plexus). **Hirschsprung's**

disease is a disorder of abnormal enteric innervation arising from the failure of normal craniocaudal migration of the neural crest. This abnormal enervation results in a contracted state of bowel and produces a functional rather than mechanical obstruction. Although it typically is an isolated disorder, 10% of affected patients have trisomy 21. Neonates exhibit progressive abdominal distention, feeding intolerance, and delayed or absent meconium within the first 48 hours of life. Older patients may have a history of chronic constipation, abdominal distention, and failure to thrive. Physical examination is remarkable only for abdominal distention, and abdominal radiograph suggests distal intestinal obstruction. Barium enema facilitates the diagnosis. Because the disease always affects the most distal bowel with a variable involvement of proximal bowel, the characteristic radiographic appearance is a spastic, contracted rectum and sigmoid colon with dilated proximal bowel. Delayed passage of contrast (> 24 hours) supports the diagnosis. Suction rectal biopsy documenting the absence of ganglion cells confirms the diagnosis. Surgical correction is performed by excision of the aganglionic (distal colorectal) segment and coloanal anastomosis.

Hirschsprung's enterocolitis describes an inflammatory condition of the bowel arising through stasis, bacterial overgrowth, and mucosal injury. If left untreated, the disease can be rapidly progressive with onset of sepsis, shock, and even death (10%). This condition most commonly occurs before definitive treatment but also may occur after resection and pull-through.

8. What is intussusception? What are the therapeutic options?

Intussusception is the peristalsis of proximal bowel into distal bowel. The invagination of bowel upon itself results in swelling, vascular compromise, and obstruction. Nearly two-thirds of cases occur in the first 2 years of life. The cause is thought to be the hypertrophy of lymphoid tissue in the terminal ileum (idiopathic) and invagination of the ileum into the cecum (ileocolic). The diagnosis should be suspected in a previously well infant, 6–9 months of age, with vomiting, crampy abdominal pain, and bloody stools. The abdomen is often distended, and a mass may be palpable in the right lower quadrant or midabdomen. Abdominal radiograph demonstrates distal intestinal obstruction and may suggest a paucity of bowel or mass in the right lower quadrant (Dance's sign). Barium or air enema is both diagnostic and therapeutic. Injection of contrast demonstrates colonic obstruction with no reflux into proximal bowel. Controlled hydrostatic reduction with barium (column height: < 30 cm) or air (pressure: < 120 cm H_2O) is successful in reducing the intussusception in 90% of cases. Hydrostatic reduction should not be attempted in any patient with signs of sepsis or peritonitis because of the risk of perforation. If hydrostatic reduction is unsuccessful, operation is indicated with manual reduction. Rarely resection with primary anastomosis is required. The risk of recurrent intussusception is 5%.

9. What examples of neonatal obstruction can escape early detection and present later in life?

Although most conditions are identified within the first week to month of life, lesions other than atresia may be identified in children and even adults.

Duodenal stenosis. Unlike duodenal atresia, stenosis results in narrowing but not complete obstruction of the duodenum. Thus infants fed formula or pureed foods may not become symptomatic until childhood. Children with intermittent abdominal pain and symptoms of gastric outlet obstruction require an upper GI, particularly if they have trisomy 21.

Malrotation. One-third of patients with malrotation are identified after the first month of life. Children present with intermittent abdominal pain, and malrotation is generally identified by an upper GI series. Malrotation with midgut volvulus should be suspected in any ill child with signs of intestinal obstruction and no previous history of abdominal surgery.

Meconium ileus. Patients with CF often suffer constipation. The combination of constipation and right lower quadrant pain suggests distal intestinal obstruction syndrome. Gastrograffin enema may be both diagnostic and therapeutic.

Hirschsprung's disease. One-third of patients are diagnosed after the first year of life. A long history of constipation refractory to therapy mandates rectal biopsy, particularly in patients with trisomy 21.

Intussusception. One-third of cases occur after 2 years of age. A pathologic lead point (polyp, tumor, hematoma, Meckel's diverticulum) is present in one-third of older patients.

BIBLIOGRAPHY

1. Aquino A, Domini M, Rossi C, et al: Correlation between Down's syndrome and malformation of pediatric surgical interest. J Pediatr Surg 33:1380, 1998.
2. Dalla Vecchia LK, Grosfeld JL, West KW, et al: Intestinal atresia and stenosis: A 25 year experience with 277 cases. Arch Surg 133:490, 1998.
3. Fuchs JR, Langer JC: Longterm outcome after neonatal meconium obstruction. Pediatrics 101:E7, 1998.
4. Long FR, Kramer SS, Markowitz RI, et al: Radiographic patterns of intestinal malrotation in children. Radiographics 16:547, 1996.
5. Maxson RT, Franklin PA, Wagner CW: Malrotation in the older child: Surgical management, treatment, and outcome. Am Surg 61:135, 1995.
6. Reding R, de Ville de Goyet J, Gosseye S, et al: Hirschsprung's disease: A 20 year experience. J Pediatr Surg 32:1221, 1997.
7. Hackam DJ, Filler RM, Pearl RH: Enterocolitis after the surgical treatment of Hirschsprung's disease: Risk factors and financial impact. J Pediatr Surg 33:830, 1998.
8. Daneman A, Alton DJ, Ein S, et al: Perforation during attempted intussusception reduction in children—a comparison of perforation with barium and air. Pediatr Radiol 25:81, 1995.

84. IMPERFORATE ANUS

Frederick M. Karrer, M.D., and Denis D. Bensard, M.D.

1. What is imperforate anus?

A congenital defect wherein the opening of the anus is absent or misplaced, usually fistulizing anteriorly to the perineum or genitourinary tract. Anorectal malformations range from slight anterior malpositioning of the anus to complex cloacal deformities. Children with anorectal malformations commonly have other congenital anomalies, such as the VACTERL association.

2. What is the VACTERL association?

V = Vertebral defects
A = Anorectal malformations
C = Cardiac anomalies
T = Tracheoesophageal fistula
E = Esophageal atresia
R = Renal anomalies
L = Limb defects

The incidence of renal anomalies increases with the severity of the imperforate anus—from 10% with low lesions to 75% with high lesions.

3. How do you determine the severity of the defect in males?

The key is whether the male infant has a high or low lesion. Low lesions are characterized by a fistula to the perineum somewhere along the midline raphe between the anus and the penis. After 24 hours most infants with low lesions demonstrate meconium at the fistula. Other signs of a low lesion include white "pearls" along the raphe or a raised loop of skin, the so-called bucket-handle deformity. Males with high lesions typically have a flat bottom without a good buttocks crease and may have meconium at the urethral meatus or on urinalysis.

4. How do you assess the lesion in females?

Most females (> 90%) have a rectovestibular or rectovaginal fistula, which usually can be determined by careful perineal examination. Females with cloacal deformities (one orifice) have a high incidence of genitourinary obstruction such as hydrocolpos or bladder obstruction. In low lesions the anal opening is displaced anteriorly on the perineum. The normal location of the anus is halfway between the vaginal orifice and the coccyx.

5. How do you treat infants with anorectal malformations?

Infants with high lesions should be managed initially with a sigmoid colostomy and later with a pull-through procedure (posterior sagittal anorectoplasty). Infants with low lesions usually can be managed with dilatation and immediate or delayed anoplasty.

6. What is posterior sagittal anorectoplasty?

Posterior sagittal anorectoplasty is a procedure performed through a longitudinal incision in the midline of the perineum, which permits visualization of the pelvic musculature and sphincters and clear exposure of the rectum and fistula. After closure of the fistula, the rectum is repositioned within the sphincteric muscle complex, and a neoanus is created.

7. What are the results after surgical reconstruction?

Continence, defined as voluntary bowel movements with no soiling, depends on the type of lesion. Continence approaches 100% for low lesions but is rare with the highest lesions such as vaginal fistulas in females or bladder-neck fistulas in males. Constipation is present in almost one-half of patients but is more frequent with the simpler defects.

BIBLIOGRAPHY

1. de Vries PA, Pena A: Posterior sagittal anorectoplasty. J Pediatr Surg 17:638–643, 1982.
2. Pena A: Anorectal malformations. Semin Pediatr Surg 4:35–37, 1995.

85. TRACHEOESOPHAGEAL MALFORMATIONS

Denis D. Bensard, M.D., and David A. Partrick, M.D.

1. What are tracheoesophageal fistula and esophageal atresia?

The trachea and esophagus appear as a ventral diverticulum arising from the primitive foregut during the third week of gestation. The trachea and esophagus undergo separation by the ingrowth of ectodermal ridges during the fourth week of gestation. Failure of separation results in anomalous connection of the trachea to the esophagus (tracheoesophageal fistula [TEF]) with or without incomplete formation of the esophagus (esophageal atresia [EA]).

2. Describe the three most common variants and the relative incidence of each type.

• Proximal esophageal atresia with distal tracheoesophageal fistula ("proximal pouch with distal fistula") (85%)
• Isolated esophageal atresia (10%)
• Tracheoesophageal fistula without esophageal atresia ("H fistula") (5%)

3. What other anomalies occur with tracheoesophageal malformations?

TEF/EA results from an insult during the critical phase of embryogenesis (3–8 weeks' gestation). Up to 70% of infants with tracheoesophageal malformation suffer one or more concomitant anomalies. Cardiovascular anomalies are the most prevalent (35%), followed by anomalies of the gastrointestinal (24%), genitourinary (20%), skeletal (13%), and central nervous (10%) systems. Twenty-five percent of infants born with tracheoesophageal malformation have one or more components of the VACTERL association (see question 2 in chapter 84).

4. Does the presence of other anomalies alter management and outcome?

Healthy infants without concomitant anomalies generally undergo early repair with a nearly 100% survival rate, whereas infants who are severely premature or have life-threatening anomalies typically undergo delayed repair. Infants with lethal anomalies, such as trisomy 18, receive palliative care only.

5. Describe the clinical presentation, diagnosis, and preoperative management of EA with distal TEF.

EA/distal TEF, the most common variant of tracheoesophageal malformation, results in a pathologic connection of the distal esophagus to the airway and a blind-ending proximal esophageal pouch. Early in the newborn period the infant demonstrates excessive salivation (inability to swallow secretions), choking, or regurgitation with feeding (inability to swallow feeds). Respiratory distress quickly ensues because of aspiration of secretions or feeds from the esophageal pouch and reflux of gastric acid into the airways and lungs via the distal TEF.

The inability to pass a nasogastric tube into the stomach supports the clinical diagnosis. A plain radiograph with a nasogastric tube demonstrates the tube in the blind-ending proximal esophageal pouch and an air-filled stomach secondary to the anomalous connection of the distal esophagus to the airway. The infant should be maintained in a semiupright position, and sump catheter drainage of the proximal esophageal pouch should be initiated to minimize contamination of the lungs due to aspiration or reflux. Endotracheal intubation is avoided to reduce the risk of worsening gastric distention resulting from ventilation through the TEF.

6. Describe the clinical presentation, diagnosis, and preoperative management of isolated EA.

The second most common variant of tracheoesophageal malformation results in blind-ending proximal and distal esophageal pouches with no communication to the airway. Like EA/TEF, isolated EA is associated with excessive salivation, choking, and regurgitation. Unlike TEF, the abdomen is scaphoid, and no air is detectable within the gastrointestinal (GI) tract by clinical examination or radiograph. Once the diagnosis is suspected, the inability to pass a nasogastric tube into the stomach and a gasless abdomen (by radiograph) confirm the diagnosis. Contrast study is generally helpful to assess the length of the proximal pouch, because most infants have little esophagus within the thorax and considerable distance between the blind ends (long-gap EA). Preoperative management, unlike EA/TEF, is directed to the identification of associated anomalies and determination of gap length. The infant is placed in a semiupright position, and sump catheter drainage of the proximal esophageal pouch is maintained to minimize aspiration. Gastrostomy is generally performed within the first 24 hours of life to permit feeding and assessment of the distal esophageal length. Typically infants with EA undergo delayed repair to permit growth of the esophagus and reduction of gap distance.

7. Describe the clinical presentation, diagnosis, and preoperative management of TEF without EA.

The third most common variant of tracheoesophageal malformation results in normal tracheal and esophageal continuity with a pathologic communication of the airway and GI tract. Infants demonstrate repeated choking or cyanotic spells with feeding due to the reflux of feeds from the esophagus to the lungs via the anomalous connection. Older infants and children may present with recurrent bouts of pneumonia or unexplained reactive airway disease resulting from the intermittent contamination of the lungs via the fistula. Chest radiograph may demonstrate pneumonia (right upper lobe), but this finding is nonspecific. Video esophagography is performed in an attempt to demonstrate the fistulous connection, but up to 50% of cases escape detection.

8. How are tracheoesophageal malformations corrected surgically?

The goals of surgical therapy are restoration of esophageal continuity (the best conduit) and elimination of pathologic connection of the esophagus to the airway. Correction of EA with or without TEF requires thoracotomy, ligation of TEF, and end-to-end esophageal anastomosis. The first successful procedure was performed by Cameron Haight in 1941. At 5–7 days postoperatively an esophagogram is performed; if no leak is visualized, oral feedings are started and the pleural drain is removed.

TEF without EA can be approached via a cervical incision, avoiding thoracotomy. Bronchoscopy permits intubation of the fistulous tract with a catheter that facilitates subsequent identification during neck exploration. Once identified, the fistulous tract is divided and healthy tissue is interposed to prevent fistulous reformation.

9. What are the early and late complications of surgical repair?

Early complications

Anastomotic disruption	5%
Recurrent TEF	5%
Anastomotic leak	15%
Tracheomalacia	15%

Early complications are related to basic surgical principles of wound healing. Anastomotic disruption generally results from poor blood supply and tension.

Late complications

Anastomotic stricture	25%
Gastroesophageal reflux	50%
Esophageal dysmotility	100%

Most strictures (50%) respond to 1–3 dilatations performed in the first 6 months of life. Refractory strictures require identification of associated gastroesophageal reflux (GER), which may worsen stricture formation. Of interest, the incidence of GER also appears related to gap length (i.e., the greater the gap distance, the greater the risk of significant GER).

BIBLIOGRAPHY

1. Brown AK, Tam PK: Measurements of gap length in esophageal atresia: A simple predictor of outcome. J Am Coll Surg 182:41, 1996.
2. Saing H, Mya GH, Cheng W: The involvement of two or more systems and the severity of associated anomalies significantly influence mortality in esophageal atresia. J Pediatr Surg 33:1596, 1998.
3. Somppi E, Tammela O, Ruuska T, et al: Outcome of patients operated on for esophageal atresia: 30 years' experience. J Pediatr Surg 33:1341, 1998.
4. Spitz L: Esophageal atresia: Past, present, and future. J Pediatr Surg 31:19, 1996.
5. Teich S, Barton DP, Ginn-Pease ME, et al: Prognostic classification for esophageal atresia and tracheoesophageal fistula: Waterston versus Montreal. J Pediatr Surg 32:1075, 1997.
6. Torfs CP, Curry CJ, Bateson TF: Population-based study of tracheoesophageal fistula and esophageal atresia. Teratology 52:220, 1995.
7. Tovar JA, Diez Pardo JA, Murcia J, et al: Ambulatory 24-hour manometric and pH metric evidence of permanent impairment of clearance capacity in patients with esophageal atresia. J Pediatr Surg 30:1224, 1995.

86. CONGENITAL DIAPHRAGMATIC HERNIA

Denis D. Bensard, M.D., and Frederick M. Karrer, M.D.

1. What is the most common type of congenital diaphragmatic hernia (CDH)?

Congenital abnormalities of the diaphragm include posterolateral defect (Bochdalek hernia), anteromedial defect (Morgagni hernia), and eventration (central weakening) of the diaphragm. The Bochdalek hernia is the most common variant and generally occurs on the right (80%). The posterior lateral diaphragmatic defect permits herniation of the bowel into the thorax, compression of the developing lung, and resultant lung hypoplasia.

2. What signs and symptoms suggest CDH?

Neonatal respiratory distress is the most common manifestation of CDH. At birth or shortly thereafter, the infant develops severe dyspnea, retractions, and cyanosis. On physical examination, breath sounds are diminished on the ipsilateral side, heart sounds can be heard more easily in the contralateral chest, and the abdomen is scaphoid because of the herniation of abdominal viscera into the chest. As the infant struggles to breathe, air enters the bowel, which becomes distended and further compromises ventilation. If the herniation is allowed to progress, the mediastinum shifts, impairing venous return and cardiac output.

3. How is the diagnosis confirmed?

If CDH is suspected, a plain chest radiograph demonstrates multiple loops of air-filled intestine in the ipsilateral thorax. If, however, films are obtained before entry of significant amounts of air into the bowel, a confusing pattern of mediastinal shift, cardiac displacement, and opacification of the hemithorax may be observed. Insertion of a nasogastric tube, injection of air or contrast, and repeat chest radiograph should confirm the diagnosis.

4. Are other anomalies associated with CDH?

Fifty percent of infants with CDH have associated anomalies. Fewer than 10% of patients with multiple major concurrent anomalies survive. If CDH is diagnosed in utero (before 25 weeks), the anomalies are often life-threatening. Excluding intestinal malrotation and pulmonary hypoplasia, cardiac anomalies (63%) are the most frequent, followed by genitourinary (23%), gastrointestinal (17%), central nervous system (14%), and other pulmonary (5%) anomalies.

5. What therapeutic measures should be initiated before transport or operation?

Perhaps the easiest and most effective palliative intervention is decompression of the stomach with a nasogastric tube, which prevents further distention of the bowel, and thus improves ventilation. Endotracheal intubation permits adequate ventilation and oxygenation and prevents further bowel distention. Because the lungs are hypoplastic and at risk for further injury from barotrauma, ventilatory pressures are kept low (< 30 mmHg) and the infant is ventilated at a rapid rate (40--60 breaths/minute). Venous access is rapidly obtained, fluids administered, and acidosis corrected.

6. What is the "honeymoon period"?

Up to 65% of neonates with CDH are stillborn or die shortly after birth, whereas 25% are diagnosed after the neonatal period. If the patient develops symptoms after the first 24 hours of life, the survival rate is nearly 100%. The degree of respiratory symptoms appears to be related to the degree of lung hypoplasia. Minimally symptomatic or asymptomatic neonates have already demonstrated sufficient lung volume compatible with survival. The honeymoon period describes the interval of time in which a neonate demonstrates adequate oxygenation and ventilation in the absence of maximal medical therapy. Regardless of subsequent deterioration, a honeymoon period suggests that pulmonary function is compatible with survival.

7. Describe the operative approach.

The infant must be stabilized before surgical repair is attempted, but the optimal timing of surgery remains unclear. CDH results in a physiologic derangement of the lungs that is not reversed by surgical reconstruction of the diaphragm. Thus, repair of CDH is not a surgical emergency. In a multicenter report of current surgical management of CDH, Clark et al. reported that the average age at repair was after the first day of life: with extracorporeal membrane oxygenation (ECMO), 170 hr; without ECMO, 73 hr. A transthoracic or transabdominal approach may be used for surgical repair of CDH. The transabdominal approach is the favored initial approach for the following reasons: (1) reduction of the herniated abdominal viscera is simplified; (2) the diaphgramatic defect may be repaired with unobstructed vision and without tension; (3) coincident malrotation with or without obstruction is easily identified and corrected; and (4) if the abdominal cavity does not initially accommodate the reduced viscera, it may be stretched or a ventral hernia may be created with a prosthetic patch. The transthoracic approach is generally reserved for repair of recurrent diaphragmatic hernia or for older children (age > 1 year).

8. What is the most feared complication of diaphragmatic hernia? Is it correctable? If so how?

In CDH one or both lungs are hypoplastic, the pulmonary vascular bed is reduced, and the pulmonary arteries exhibit thickened muscular walls that are hyperreactive. Thus, patients with CDH are particularly prone to the development of pulmonary hypertension. If CDH is uncorrected, the infant rapidly develops persistent fetal circulation (PFC), the most feared complication. PFC arises from a sustained increase in pulmonary artery pressure. Blood is shunted away from the lungs, and the unoxygenated blood is diverted to the systemic circulation (right-to-left shunt) through the patent ductus arteriosus and patent foramen ovale. PFC results in hypoxemia, profound acidosis, and shock. PFC is triggered by acidosis, hypercarbia, and hypoxia, all potent vasoconstrictors of the pulmonary circulation. Various strategies are used to prevent the onset of PFC:

1. Oxygen monitoring or arterial sampling (preductal in the right upper extremity, postductal in the lower extremity) detects the shunting of unoxygenated blood to the systemic circulation.

2. Optimal ventilation to prevent hypercarbia is enhanced by rapid, low-pressure mechanical ventilation, adequate sedation, and, if necessary, pharmacologic paralysis.

3. Hypoxemia is avoided by adequate ventilation and high concentrations of inspired oxygen (generally $FiO_2 = 100\%$).

4. Metabolic acidosis is managed by restoring adequate tissue perfusion with intravenous fluids or blood, inotropes, and sodium bicarbonate.

If these maneuvers fail, supplemental therapies include administration of pulmonary vasodilators via the ventilatory circuit (nitric oxide) or systemic circulation (priscoline, prostaglandin E_2), high-frequency ventilation, and, finally, ECMO. Additional early complications include lung injury and pneumothorax due to barotrauma or bleeding, particularly if the defect is repaired on ECMO.

9. What is the survival rate among patients with CDH?

The overall survival rate is 60%. The major determinants of survival are the degree of pulmonary hypoplasia and associated major congenital anomalies. Among infants surviving the early newborn period without significant lung dysfunction, the survival approaches 100%. Moreover, in centers where salvage therapies, such as ECMO or nitric oxide, are used, survival rates have not improved; in fact, they have decreased because of inclusion of more severely affected patients. At the University of Michigan, examination of data before and after the introduction of ECMO demonstrated a fall in the overall survival rate from 75% to 59%. Furthermore, expansion of inclusion criteria for ECMO resulted in only a 27% increase in survival for patients who were previously considered unsalvageable.

10. Does in utero intervention have a role in treatment of CDH?
To date, fetal surgery for CDH remains experimental. In a prospective trial reported in 1997, the results of intrauterine repair of CDH were compared with conventional postnatal surgery with similar outcome. The investigators concluded that because open fetal surgery does not improve survival or outcome, prenatally diagnosed CDH should be treated postnatally.

BIBLIOGRAPHY

1. Clark RH, Hardin WD, Hirschl RB, et al: Current surgical management of congenital diaphragmatic hernia: A report from the congenital diaphragmatic hernia study group. J Pediatr Surg 33:1004, 1998.
2. Collaborative UK ECMO (extracorporeal membrane oxygenation) trial: Follow-up to 1 year of age. Pediatrics 101:E1, 1998.
3. Fauza DO, Wilson JM: Congenital diaphragmatic hernia and associated anomalies: Their incidence, identification, and impact on prognosis. J Pediatr Surg 29:1113, 1994.
4. Harrison MR, Adzick NS, Bullard KM, et al: Correction of congenital diaphragmatic hernia in utero VII: A prospective trial. J Pediatr Surg 32:1637, 1997.
5. Harrison MR, Mychaliska GB, Albanese CT, et al: Correction of congenital diaphragmatic hernia in utero IX: Fetuses with poor prognosis (liver herniation and low lung-to-head ratio) can be saved by fetoscopic temporary tracheal occlusion. J Pediatr Surg 33:1017, 1998.
6. Nobbuhara KK, Lund DP, Mitchell J, et al: Long-term outlook for survivors of congenital diaphragmatic hernia. Clin Perinatol 23:873, 1996.
7. Steimle CN, Meric F, Hirschl RB, et al: Effect of extracorporeal life support on survival when applied to all patients with congenital diaphragmatic hernia. J Pediatr Surg 29:997, 1994.
8. Weber TR, Kountzman B, Dillon PA, et al: Improved survival in congenital diaphragmatic hernia with evolving therapeutic strategies. Arch Surg 133:498, 1998.

87. ABDOMINAL TUMORS

Frederick M. Karrer, M.D., and Denis D. Bensard, M.D.

1. What are the most common malignant solid abdominal tumors in children?
Neuroblastomas, Wilms' tumors, and hepatoblastomas, in that order. Neuroblastomas are derived from neural crest tissue; in the abdomen they originate from the adrenal glands and paraspinal sympathetic ganglia. Wilms' tumors derive from the kidney, and hepatoblastomas originate in the liver.

2. Is it tough to differentiate Wilms' tumor from neuroblastomas clinically?
Yes. Both tumors present as an asymptomatic abdominal mass. The differences are summarized below:

	WILMS' TUMOR	NEUROBLASTOMA
Age at presentation	3–4 yr	1–2 yr
Extend across midline	Rare	Common
Surface on palpation	Smooth	Knobby
X-ray calcifications	No	Yes

In addition, because neuroblastomas produce hormones, affected children exhibit flushing, hypertension (catecholamine release), watery diarrhea, periorbital ecchymosis, and abnormal ocular movements.

3. How are Wilms' tumors and neuroblastomas treated?

	WILMS' TUMOR	NEUROBLASTOMA
Primary surgical excision	Important (likely)	Important (less likely)
Chemotherapy	Enormous impact	Less responsive

4. What are the major prognostic factors in neuroblastomas and Wilms' tumor?

In **neuroblastomas** age at presentation is the major prognostic factor. Children younger than 1 year have an overall survival rate greater than 70%, whereas the survival rate for children older than 1 year is under 35%. Shimada proposed a histologic classification based on evaluation of histologic parameters (tumor differentiation, mitosis-karyorrhexis index [MKI]) as well as age. Aneuploid tumors, tumors with low MKI, and tumors with fewer than 10 copies of the n-*myc* gene also have better outcomes.

Age is also important in children with **Wilms' tumors**, but the prognosis is better because the tumors are more readily excised and much more sensitive to chemotherapy.

5. What are the differences between hepatoblastomas and hepatocellular carcinomas? How are the tumors treated?

Hepatoblastomas usually occur in infants and young children, whereas hepatocellular carcinoma usually occurs in children over 10 years of age. Hepatocellular carcinoma usually is associated with cirrhosis and hepatitis B and is histologically identical to the adult form. Surgical resection is the primary therapy for both tumors. Hepatoblastomas often have a good response to adjunctive chemotherapy, whereas hepatocellular carcinoma rarely responds to chemotherapy.

CONTROVERSY

6. Should patients with hepatoblastoma receive preoperative chemotherapy to shrink the tumor?

Preoperative chemotherapy does shrink tumors, resulting in easier hepatic resection and lower surgical morbidity. This benefit must be weighed against the considerable toxicity of chemotherapeutic agents.

BIBLIOGRAPHY

1. Reynolds M: Pediatric liver tumors. Semin Surg Oncol 16:159–172, 1999.
2. Shamberger RC, Guthrie KA, Ritchey ML, et al: Surgery related factors and local recurrence of Wilms' tumor in National Wilms' Tumor Study 4. Ann Surg 229:292–297, 1999.
3. Shimada M: Tumors of the neuroblastoma group. Pathology 2:43–59, 1993.

88. CONGENITAL CYSTS AND SINUSES OF THE NECK

Frederick M. Karrer, M.D., and Denis D. Bensard, M.D.

1. What are branchial cleft anomalies?

Cysts, sinuses, and fistulas that result from incomplete obliteration of the first, second, or third branchial clefts, which are present in early fetal development.

2. Which anomaly is the most common?

Second branchial cleft anomalies are by far the most common. When complete, the tract originates internally from the tonsillar fossa and exits along the anterior border of the sternocleidomastoid muscle. First branchial remnants, which are less common, extend from the external auditory canal and exit anterior to the ear or along the angle of the mandible. Third clefts, which are quite rare, run from the pyriform sinus to a point near the suprasternal notch.

3. How do branchial cleft anomalies present?

Complete tracts or sinuses present with intermittent drainage of a mucoid fluid on the neck. Cysts usually present later as either a sterile or infected mass. Complete surgical excision is the treatment of choice.

4. What are the major operative hazards of branchial cleft remnant excision?

The second branchial cleft tracts through the bifurcation of the carotid artery. The facial nerve is in proximity to the first branchial cleft.

5. What is a thyroglossal duct cyst?

A thyroglossal duct cyst is the most common congenital cyst found in the neck. It is caused by failure of normal obliteration of the migration tract of the thyroid gland. Embryologically, the thyroid descends from the base of the tongue to its normal location in the neck.

6. How do thyroglossal duct cysts present?

They present as a paramidline mass in the upper neck; if infected, they may present with fever, tenderness, and erythema.

7. How are thyroglossal duct cysts treated?

The best treatment is complete excision, along with the tract. Because embryologically the thyroid descends before formation of the hyoid cartilage, the tract may pass right through the hyoid. Therefore, complete tract removal requires excision of the central portion of the hyoid and dissection up to the base of the tongue (Sistrunk procedure).

8. What is a cystic hygroma?

A cystic hygroma is a congenital lymphatic malformation with a predilection for the neck. It is a benign lesion that usually presents as a soft mass in the posterolateral neck. Excision is often challenging because the lymph cysts do not respect fascial planes and often intertwine with the neurovascular structures in the neck. Near-total excision is the treatment of choice.

BIBLIOGRAPHY

1. Brown RL, Azizkhan RG: Pediatric head and neck lesions. Pediatr Clin North Am 45:889–905, 1998.
2. Telander RL, Filston HC: Review of head and neck lesions in infancy and childhood. Surg Clin North Am 72:1429–1447, 1992.

X. Transplantation

89. LIVER TRANSPLANTATION

Thomas E. Bak, M.D., Michael E. Wachs, M.D., and Igal Kam, M.D.

1. When and where was the first liver transplant performed? By whom?
On March 1, 1963 at the University of Colorado in Denver by Thomas Starzl.

2. Have graft and patient survival rates improved for liver transplantation?
Yes. The 1-year patient survival rate has improved to 87% with a graft survival rate of 79%.

3. What are the most common indications for liver transplantation in the United States?
Noncholestatic cirrhosis characterizes over one-half of recipients. Underlying diseases include viral hepatitis, alcoholic cirrhosis (Laennec's cirrhosis), and Budd-Chiari syndrome. Cholestatic cirrhosis accounts for an additional 15%, with primary sclerosing cholangitis and primary biliary cirrhosis heading the list of underlying diseases. Other indications include biliary atresia, acute hepatic necrosis, malignant neoplasms, and metabolic disease.

4. How many liver transplants are done yearly in the United States?
Over 4000. However, the waiting list is over 8000 and continues to grow. The median waiting time is over 1 year, and many patients die on the waiting list. Donor shortages continue to be the limiting constraint on the number of transplants performed.

5. What are the major recent advances in liver transplant surgery?
Patients now are routinely transplanted without venovenous bypass and without t-tube biliary drainage. Operative times have been reduced to an average of 5–6 hours. Postoperative intensive care stays are frequently not required, and even the need for blood and blood product transfusions has been eliminated in some cases.

6. How long can a liver be kept "on ice"?
With the improvement of cold preservation solutions, livers can now be safely transplanted up to 24 hours after procurement. Optimal cold ischemia time, however, should be less than 12 hours.

7. What are the common postoperative complications of liver transplantation?
Primary nonfunction (10%), hepatic artery thrombosis (5% in adults, up to 10% in children), and biliary complications (10%).

8. What is the "piggy-back" technique?
The recipient's sick liver is carefully resected off the vena cava, which is left in situ. The upper donor cava is then sewn to a common cuff of native hepatic veins. The donor's lower cava is ligated. With this method, it is possible to do the complete transplant without caval occlusion, thus decreasing intraoperative hemodynamic instability.

9. Is living-donor liver transplantation an option?
Yes. Left lateral lobe resection with transplantation into children has been well established and has greatly reduced waiting lists at many pediatric centers. Experience is building rapidly in

the use of adult-to-adult donation of a full hepatic lobe. Although this is a major operation, it can be done safely. Both donor and recipient lobes of the liver regenerate rapidly.

10. How has TIPS improved liver transplantation?

Transjugular intraheptic portosystemic shunts (TIPS) can be used in potential transplant recipients as a bridge to transplantation. This procedure is highly effective in controlling portal hypertension without the need for a major abdominal operative shunt. A prior portacaval shunt complicates the surgical procedure but is not a contraindication to liver transplantation.

CONTROVERSIES

11. Should liver transplants be performed for alcoholic liver disease?

Transplant centers have strict criteria that alcoholic patients must meet before they are listed. The recidivism rate (transplant patients who start drinking again) remains low. Financially, the cost is comparable to, if not lower than, continued medical management of end-stage liver disease. We currently provide care for other self-inflicted medical problems, such as those due to cigarette smoking. The public must realize that people are not pulled off bar stools and taken to the hospital for transplantation.

12. Should patients with hepatic malignancies be transplanted?

Patients with hepatocellular carcinoma have been transplanted with success, although their survival rate is considerably lower than that of recipients transplanted for other causes. Other hepatic malignancies, including cholangiocarcinoma, generally are considered contraindications to transplantation. Whether scarce donor livers should be allocated to such patients continues to be a complex issue.

BIBLIOGRAPHY

1. Broelsch CE, Burdelski M, Rogiers X, et al: Living donor for liver transplantation. Hepatology 20:495–555, 1994.
2. DiMartini A, Jain A, Irish W, et al: Outcome of liver transplantation in critically ill patients with alcoholic cirrhosis. Transplantation 66:298, 1998.
3. Stegall MD, Wachs ME, et al: Prednisone withdrawal 14 days after liver transplantation with mycophenolate. Transplantation 64:1755, 1997.
4. Teperman L, Gopalan V, et al: Steroid withdrawal is safe and feasible in stable liver transplant recipients. Transplantation 65:S14, 1998.
5. Wachs ME, Bak TE, Karrer FM, et al: Adult living donor liver transplantation using a right hepatic lobe. Transplantation 66:1313, 1998.

90. KIDNEY AND PANCREAS TRANSPLANTATION

Thomas E. Bak, M.D., Michael E. Wachs, M.D., and Igal Kam, M.D.

1. What are the common indications for kidney transplantation?

End-stage renal disease due to hypertension, diabetes, glomerulonephritis, and polycystic kidney disease.

2. What are graft survival rates for kidney transplantation?

For cadaveric kidney transplants, the graft survival rate at 1 year is 87%. The 5-year survival rate is around 62%. For living donor kidney transplants, the graft survival rate at 1 year improves to 93%, with a 5-year survival rate of 77%.

3. How long can a kidney be kept "on ice"?

Kidneys can survive and function after longer cold ischemia time than other solid organs. Function can be maintained up to 72 hours, although optimal function is achieved if cold ischemia time is kept under 24 hours.

4. Where is the transplanted kidney placed?

Most commonly, the kidney is placed in the iliac fossa. The peritoneal cavity is reflected superiorly, and the external iliac vessels are anastomosed to the donor renal artery and vein.

5. Are the native kidneys routinely removed during transplantation?

Not usually. Indications for nephrectomy include chronic infection, symptomatic polycystic kidney disease, intractable hypertension, and heavy proteinuria.

6. What are the advantages of living donation?

The long wait for a cadaveric kidney can be eliminated. Overall, long-term graft survival is better with living related kidneys. In addition, dialysis-related complications can be minimized or avoided altogether.

7. What new technique makes living donation more attractive?

Laparoscopic donor nephrectomy can now be performed safely. This procedure decreases the recuperation time for the donor. A subcostal, muscle-splitting incision is avoided, and the kidney is taken out of the abdomen through a small lower midline incision.

8. What are the indications for kidney-pancreas transplantation?

In general, all type I diabetics who have poorly controlled diabetes despite optimal medical management should be considered as along as they are acceptable surgical risks. A kidney-only transplant should be used if the patient would have difficulty in tolerating the more stressful pancreatic transplant. A pancreas-only transplant can be performed for unstable diabetic patients without end-stage renal disease.

9. Can a patient undergo pancreas transplantation before or after a kidney transplant?

Yes. Patients can receive a simultaneous kidney-pancreas transplant, which is the most common course. The operation is done through a midline abdominal incision with the pancreas and kidney placed on opposite iliac vessels. One also may receive a pancreas-only transplant or pancreas-after-kidney transplant. The survival rate for these grafts is similar. Some centers have even performed living donor pancreas transplants.

10. How is the duodenal cuff drained after pancreas transplant?

The cuff is drained either through the bladder or enterically into the small bowel. Bladder drainage avoids the severe complication of enteric leakage but has a higher incidence of metabolic, infectious, and hydration complications. Bladder drainage sometimes requires conversion to enteric drainage. Many centers, therefore, now do primary enteric drainage.

11. What complications are commonly seen with pancreas transplant?

Leakage from the duodenal cuff, graft venous thrombosis, infection, rejection, and graft pancreatitis are potential complications. The incidence of these complications is decreasing as more experience is gained. Pancreas graft survival now approaches kidney graft survival.

CONTROVERSIES

12. Is HLA matching still important?

Somewhat. Historically, human leukocyte antigen (HLA) matching was an important consideration in matching cadaver kidneys to recipients. With improved immunosuppressive agents, many transplant surgeons believe that HLA matching is much less important. Six-antigen-match kidneys are still shared nationally and have a small improvement in long-term graft survival rates. Donor organ quality remains the primary determinant of how well the transplanted organ functions.

13. Does pancreas transplantation halt the progression of diabetic disease?

This assumption is still unproved. Logically, we expect it to do so. Regression of neuropathy and eye dysfunction has been reported. Recently, long-term recipients have exhibited some regression of microscopic nephropathy. Definite answers require study of long-term outcomes in younger pancreatic recipients.

BIBLIOGRAPHY

1. Donovitch G: Handbook of Kidney Transplantation, 2nd ed. Boston, Little, Brown, 1996.
2. Fioretto P, Steffes MW, Sutherland DER, et al: Reversal of lesions of diabetic nephropathy after pancreas transplantation. N Engl J Med 339:69–75, 1998.
3. Sutherland DER, Bartlett ST, Gaber AO, Stock P: Symposium: Pancreatic transplantation. Contemp Surg 51:253–272, 1997.
4. Tekemoto S, Teresaki P, Cecka JM, et al: Survival of nationally shared HLA-matched kidney transplants from cadaveric donors. N Engl J Med 327:834, 1992.

91. HEART TRANSPLANTATION

Daniel R. Meldrum, M.D.

1. Who performed the first experimental heart-lung transplant?

Alexis Carrel, a French-born American surgeon, developed the vascular techniques required for heart-lung transplantation and performed the first experimental heart-lung transplant in 1907. He transplanted the lungs, heart, aorta, and vena cava of a 1-week-old cat into the neck of a large adult cat. For these and other outstanding accomplishments, Carrel received the Nobel Prize in 1912 (the first Nobel Prize awarded to a scientist working in an American laboratory).

2. Who performed the first successful experimental heart-lung transplant?

V.P. Demikhov performed the first successful heart-lung transplant in a dog in 1962.

3. Who developed the surgical strategy required for human heart transplantation?

Norman Shumway.

4. Who performed the first human heart transplant? When?

C.N. Bernard performed the first human heart transplant in December, 1967, although Dr. Shumway set the stage by developing the technique in animals. Shumway and the Stanford group performed the first heart transplant in the United States and also accomplished the first successful clinical series.

5. Approximately how many heart transplants are performed annually? Is the number increasing or decreasing?

In 1983 approximately 300 heart transplants were performed. By 1988, the number had rapidly increased to approximately 3000 and remains relatively stable between 3500–4000.

6. What anastomoses (surgical connections) must be performed for a combined heart and lungs transplant?

The operation requires only a right atrial-to-cava (inflow) anastomosis and an aortic (outflow) anastomosis with a connection at the trachea. Heart-lung transplant is less complicated (fewer anastomoses) than heart transplant alone, which may explain why heart-lung transplant was attempted first.

7. What anastomoses (surgical connections) must be performed for a heart transplant?
Left atrial, right atrial, aortic, pulmonary.

8. Who is an acceptable cardiac donor?
Acceptable cardiac donors meet the following criteria:
1. Requirements for brain death
2. Consent from next of kin
3. ABO compatibility with recipient
4. Approximately the same size as recipient
5. Absence of history of cardiac disease
6. Normal echocardiogram
7. Normal heart by inspection during organ recovery

9. Who is an acceptable cardiac recipient?
Although selection criteria are evolving as a result of improved techniques and outcomes, the following criteria are standard: age between newborn and 65 years; irremediable New York Heart Association Functional Class IV cardiac disease; normal renal, hepatic, pulmonary, and CNS function; pulmonary vascular resistance less than 6–8 Wood units; and absence of malignancy, infection, recent pulmonary infarction, and severe peripheral vascular or cerebrovascular disease. Diabetes is a relative contraindication; the steroids used in posttransplant immunosuppression make diabetes difficult to manage.

10. What are the most common indications for heart transplant in adults and in children?
In adults, coronary artery disease (ischemic cardiomyopathy) and idiopathic cardiomyopathy are the most common indications for heart transplantation, each accounting for approximately 45% of transplants.

In children, congenital heart disease and cardiomyopathy are the most common indications for heart transplantation; hypoplastic left heart is the most common congenital malformation requiring heart transplantation.

11. What percent of potential recipients die while waiting for a heart transplant?
Twenty percent.

12. At what point does donor heart ischemic time influence mortality?
Donor ischemic time greater than 6 hours definitely increases mortality. Ischemic times between 4 and 6 hours stun the donor heart. Most transplant teams try to keep ischemic times (from donor harvest to perfusion in the recipient) to less than 4 hours.

13. Who pioneered hypothermic myocardial preservation?
Henry Swan at the University of Colorado.

14. How is cardiac allograft rejection prevented?
Pharmacologically induced immunosuppression is performed by using one of two protocols. The first is triple therapy, which combines cyclosporine, azathioprine, and prednisone. The second major protocol incorporates the monoclonal antibody OKT3 into the triple therapy protocol. OKT3 is substituted for cyclosporine for the first 2 weeks after transplant.

15. What is OKT3?
OKT3 is a mouse monoclonal antibody that binds to and blocks the T-cell CD3 receptor. A monoclonal antibody is an antibody generated from the clones of a single cell. For instance, a single B-cell, which recognizes the CD3 receptor as an antigen (foreign), is immortalized in cell

culture and able to secrete the monoclonal antibody in limitless supply. The CD3 receptor, which is common to all T-cells, is important for antigen recognition and T-cell activation; therefore, OKT3 is highly immunosuppressive.

16. What complications are associated with the use of OKT3?

OKT3 may have severe side effects, including pulmonary edema and high fevers, that result from transient cytokine release, which may occur when OKT3 binds to the T-cell activation site. Because OKT3 is an antigen (an antibody from a different species [mouse]), patients develop anti-OKT3 antibodies fairly quickly; the result is desensitization. Therefore, OKT3 is used judiciously.

17. What is cardiac preconditioning?

Cardiac preconditioning, first termed ischemic preconditioning, is a phenomenon by which a brief antecedent ischemic episode renders the heart more tolerant of a subsequent ischemic event. Pharmacologic preconditioning is based on using drugs to access the same endogenous protective mechanisms that occur during ischemic preconditioning. Purinergic (adenosine A_1) agonists have shown promise experimentally and clinically. Evidence indicates that preconditioning also decreases myocardial inflammation after ischemia and reperfusion injury.

18. Does HLA mismatch influence the incidence of rejection after heart transplantation? Is HLA typing routinely done before heart transplantation?

Yes and no. In a multiinstitutional, multivariate analysis of 1719 cardiac transplant recipients by Jarcho et al., HLA mismatch increased the incidence of rejection, but HLA typing is not routinely done before heart transplantation because it takes too long. In addition, with 3 of 6 mismatches there was still only a trend toward increased rejection-related deaths (p = 0.14). If longer organ preservation times can be achieved, donor/recipient HLA matching will become feasible and should improve survival rates. Again, ABO compatibility does influence graft survival.

19. What are the major complications of heart transplantation?

Allograft rejection (days to weeks)
Infection (months)
Transplant coronary artery disease (years)

20. What is the incidence of transplant coronary artery disease? What are the risk factors?

Nearly 50% of patients have angiographic evidence of coronary artery disease by 5 years after transplant. However, only approximately 10% develop > 70% occlusions (severe stenosis). Severe stenosis is highly predictive of the need for retransplanation. Risk factors for transplant coronary artery disease include male donor or recipient, older donor age, and donor hypertension.

21. How is cardiac allograft rejection diagnosed?

Clinical suspicion is raised by new-onset cardiac arrhythmia, fever, or hypotension. Diagnosis depends on endomyocardial biopsy, which is performed at regular intervals to detect histologic evidence of rejection before signs or symptoms occur. Radionuclide ventriculography and echocardiography are useful adjuncts in following the hemodynamic manifestations of rejection. Electrocardiography is not useful in the diagnosis of rejection.

22. Can one heart be successfully transplanted twice?

Yes. Meiser et al. transplanted the same heart a second time on March 19, 1991, 42 hours after the initial transplantation. Second transplant of the same heart has since been reported by others.

23. What is "domino heart transplant"?

The good heart from a heart-lung recipient is transplanted into a patient requiring a heart transplant. Some patients with primary lung dysfunction have secondary irreversible cardiac dysfunction (i.e., Eisenmenger's syndrome); others, however, such as patients with cystic fibrosis, have good cardiac function. Patients with good cardiac function may serve as donors and increase the donor pool.

24. Is the heart capable of making tumor necrosis factor (TNF)? What does TNF have to do with heart transplantation?

TNF, typically described as a macrophage/monocyte-derived inflammatory cytokine, is also produced in large quantities by the heart. TNF released by the heart following ischemia-reperfusion probably contributes to immediate injury (dysfunction) and possibly to later rejection. Anti-TNF strategies may offer a promising therapeutic strategy for the future of heart transplantation.

25. What is the overall 30-day mortality rate after heart transplant? What is the breakdown in mortality between adult and pediatric patients?

The registry of the International Society for Heart and Lung Transplantation, which has data about approximately 45,000 heart transplants, has recorded a 30-day mortality rate of 10%. The 30-day mortality rate for adult recipients is about 8%; for pediatric recipients it is slightly higher.

26. What are the 5- and 10-year actuarial survival rates for heart transplant recipients?

75% and 50%, respectively.

27. What work remains to be done in heart transplantation?

The future of heart transplantation is bright. Knowledge gained in experimental myocardial ischemia-reperfusion injury and protection is accelerating. New, exciting ways to manipulate myocardial immunology (signal transduction, gene therapy, and chimerism) will further extend donor ischemic times and improve postoperative myocardial function and graft tolerance. Ultimately, genetic alteration of donor hearts will increase the donor pool.

BIBLIOGRAPHY

1. Baumgartner H, Porenta G, Lau YK, et al: Assessment of myocardial viability by dobutamine echocardiography, positron emission tomography and thallium-201 SPECT: Correlation with histopathology in explanted hearts. J Am Coll Cardiol 32:1701, 1998.
2. Baumgartner WA: Heterotopic transplantation: Is it a viable alternative? Ann Thorac Surg 54:401, 1992.
3. Baumgartner WA, Traill TA, Cameron DE, et al: Unique aspects of heart and lung transplantation exhibited in the "domino-donor" operation. JAMA 261:3121, 1989.
4. Costanzo MR, Naftel DC, Pritzker MR, et al: Heart transplant coronary artery disease detected by coronary angiography: A multiinstitutional study of preoperative donor and recipient risk factors. Cardiac Transplant Research Database. J Heart Lung Transplant 17:744, 1998.
5. Gay WA: Heart transplantation. In Sabiston D, Spencer F (eds): Surgery of the Chest. Philadelphia, W.B. Saunders, 1995, pp 2103–2116.
6. Hosenpud JD, Bennett LE, Keck BM, et al: The Registry of the International Society for Heart and Lung Transplantation: Fifteenth official report—1998. J Heart Lung Transplant 17:656, 1998.
7. Kobashigawa JA: Advances in immunosuppression for heart transplantation. Adv Card Surg 10:155, 1998.
8. Kupiec-Weglinski JW: Graft rejection in sensitized recipients. Ann Transplant 1:34, 1996.
9. Kuvin JT, Kimmelstiel CD: Infectious causes of atherosclerosis. Am Heart J 137:216, 1999.
10. Leier CV, Binkley PF: Parenteral inotropic support for advanced congestive heart failure. Prog Cardiovasc Dis 41:207, 1998.
11. Meldrum DR: Tumor necrosis factor in the heart [review]. Am J Physiol 274:R577, 1998.
12. Meldrum DR, Dinarello CA, Meng X, et al: Ischemic preconditioning decreases post-ischemic myocardial TNF: Potential ultimate effector mechanism of preconditioning. Circulation 98:II, 1998.
13. Mindan JP, Panizo A: Pathology of heart transplant. Curr Top Pathol 92:137, 1999.
14. Orbaek Andersen H: Heart allograft vascular disease: An obliterative vascular disease in transplanted hearts. Atherosclerosis 142:243, 1999.
15. Pillai R, Bando K, Schueler S, et al: Leukocyte depletion results in excellent heart-lung function after 12 hours of storage. Ann Thorac Surg 50:211, 1990.
16. Reardon MJ, Letsou GV, Anderson JE, et al: Orthotopic cardiac transplantation after minimally invasive direct coronary artery bypass. J Thorac Cardiovasc Surg 117:390, 1999.
17. Spann JC, Van Meter C: Cardiac transplantation. Surg Clin North Am 78(5):679, 1998.

92. LUNG TRANSPLANTATION

Daniel R. Meldrum, M.D.

1. What are the general types of lung transplants?

Single, double (bilateral), and heart-lung.

2. Which human organ transplant was performed first, the heart or the lung?

Although heart transplantation progressed more rapidly at first and therefore seems to outdate lung transplantation, the first lung transplant actually preceded the first heart transplant.

3. Who performed the first human lung transplant? When?

James Hardy performed the first human lung transplant in 1963; however, more than 20 years passed before lung transplantation was performed routinely in clinical practice (during that 20-year period only 1 patient did well enough to leave the hospital). This delay was due to initial graft failure secondary to inadequate organ preservation, long ischemic times, lack of good immunosuppressants, and technical difficulties.

4. Who is a candidate for a lung transplant?

Patients with no other medical or surgical alternative who are likely to die of pulmonary disease within 12–18 months, are younger than 65 years, are not ventilator-dependent, and do not have a history of malignancy.

5. What are the most common indications for single lung transplant?

Emphysema (40%)

Idiopathic pulmonary fibrosis (20%)

Alpha-1 antitrypsin deficiency (11%)

Primary pulmonary hypertension and pulmonary hypertension secondary to correctable congenital heart disease (10%)

6. What are the most common indications for a double-lung transplant?

Cystic fibrosis (35%)

Emphysema (20%)

Alpha-1 antitrypsin deficiency (11%)

Primary pulmonary hypertension and pulmonary hypertension secondary to correctable congenital heart disease (20%)

Idiopathic pulmonary fibrosis (8%)

7. What are the most common indications for heart-lung transplant?

Primary pulmonary hypertension (30%) and cystic fibrosis (16%) are instances in which bad lungs have ruined a good heart. Conversely, with congenital heart disease (27%), a bad heart has destroyed good lungs.

8. What is sewn to what during a single lung transplant? A double lung transplant?

During a single lung transplant, recipient-to-graft bronchial, pulmonary artery, and pulmonary vein (atrial cuff) anastomoses are required. Anastomoses for double transplant are the same; however, cardiopulmonary bypass is required more often during double lung transplant. During implantation of the second lung, diversion of the entire cardiac output to the freshly ischemic lung often results in reperfusion lung edema and hypoxemia.

9. Which diagnoses carry the best results for single lung transplants?

Indeed, it makes a difference. Patients with emphysema and alpha-1 antitrypsin deficiency do significantly better with 1-year survival rates of 80%.

10. Why is the number of combined heart-lung transplants performed annually decreasing?

Approximately 250 heart-lung transplants were performed in 1990; the number has decreased to approximately 150 in 1999. As the results of single and double lung transplants have improved, the need to perform heart-lung transplants in patients with isolated pulmonary disease has been obviated.

11. What are the most common complications after lung transplant?

Airway surgical healing defects (early)
Rejection (early)
Bacterial and cytomegalovirus infections (weeks to months)
Bronchiolitis obliterans (months to years)

12. What is bronchiolitis obliterans?

Bronchiolitis obliterans, a major cause of long-term morbidity after lung transplantation, is a process in which membranous and respiratory bronchioles demonstrate histologic evidence of subepithelial scarring that eventually progresses to occlusion of the bronchiolar lumen. Clinically, it is characterized by dyspnea and airflow obstruction.

13. How is lung transplant rejection diagnosed?

Unlike hearts, the diagnosis of rejection in the transplanted lung is imprecise and based on a collection of symptoms and signs. Decreased oxygen saturation, fever, decreased exercise tolerance, and radiologic infiltrate suggest rejection. Sequential quantitative lung perfusion scans that demonstrate a decrease in perfusion are helpful in the diagnosis of rejection after single lung transplants. Transbronchial biopsy is useful after single and double lung transplants.

14. Describe the phenomenon of chimerism in transplantation.

Chimerism is leukocyte sharing between the graft and the recipient so that the graft becomes a genetic composite of both donor and recipient. Chimerism enhances the host's tolerance of the graft. The first evidence of chimerism was observed in 1969 when female recipients of male livers developed entirely female Kupffer cell (liver macrophage) systems (as demonstrated by the Barr bodies in the macrophage). In 1992 the concept of *sharing* became clinically evident when it was discovered that leukocytes from donor kidneys occupied remote lymph nodes.

15. Do resident macrophages exist in the heart and lungs?

Absolutely. Resident myocardial macrophage and resident alveolar macrophage are incredibly active cellular components of the heart and lungs.

16. Does chimerism develop in the heart and the lungs?

Yes. Because the heart and lungs each have leukocytes to share, they participate in chimerism.

17. Why is chimerism exciting?

Nature is trying to teach us how to perform transplantation without the use of immunosuppression. Our job is to learn why chimerism is induced in some recipients and not in others, i.e., to dissect the mechanisms of chimerism induction so that we may pharmacologically induce chimerism in all recipients.

18. What are the major types of preservation solutions for heart and lung grafts?

Euro-Collins (EC) solution and University of Wisconsin (UW) solution for lung and crystalloid cardioplegia and UW solution for hearts.

19. What percent of pulmonary blood flow goes to the transplanted lung after single lung transplant?

Usually, much more than one-half (predictably almost all) of the pulmonary blood flow passes through the lower resistance circuit of the transplanted lung (depending on the pulmonary vascular resistance of the contralateral native lung). If a preoperative perfusion scan exists, other factors being equal, the lung with the best perfusion is preserved and the other is replaced.

20. Is cardiopulmonary bypass required for lung transplantation?

No. However, for patients with pulmonary hypertension (primary or secondary), cardiopulmonary bypass is routinely used before removal of the recipient's lung. Cardiopulmonary bypass is always on standby.

21. Is living-related lung transplant possible?

Yes. Living-related lung transplants are an innovative approach to increasing the donor pool.

22. What is lung volume reduction surgery? How may it be important to patients on the lung transplant waiting list?

Lung volume reduction surgery offers a therapeutic option for patients who are either (1) not candidates to receive a lung transplant or (2) on a long waiting list. Lung volume reduction surgery removes nonfunctional/destroyed lung. Removal of defunctionalized lung makes more room for airflow in the functional lung, thereby treating the distended chest, flattened diaphragms, and dyspnea associated with cigarette smoking (destroyed upper lobes) and alpha-1 antitrypsin deficiency (destroyed lower lobes).

23. Who is the best candidate for lung volume reduction surgery?

The patient without contraindication who has absent or reduced perfusion of approximately 30–40% of the lung, with the remainder showing homogeneous flow distribution. Thus, quantitative lung perfusion scans provide essential information for patient selection.

24. What are the contraindications to lung reduction surgery?

Pulmonary hypertension (mean pulmonary artery pressure [PAP] > 35 mmHg or systolic PAP > 45 mmHG)

Significant coronary artery disease

Previous thoracotomy or pleurodesis

Long-standing history of asthma, bronchiectasis, or chronic bronchitis with purulent sputum

Severe kyphoscoliosis

25. What are the main differences in composition between Euro-Collins solution and University of Wisconsin solution?

Euro-Collins solution is a glucose-based solution with an ionic composition that approximates that of the intracellular environment.

University of Wisconsin solution does not contain glucose but does contain the following components not found in EC solution: hydroxy-ethyl starch (prevents expansion of the interstitial space), lactobionate and raffinose (suppress hypothermia-induced cell swelling), glutathione and allopurinol (reduce cytotoxic injury from oxygen free radicals), and adenosine (substrate for adenosine triphosphate formation, vasodilator, and activates the protective mechanisms of preconditioning).

26. How many lung transplants are performed annually? Is the number increasing or decreasing?

Of interest, although the first human lung transplant was performed in 1963, significant numbers were not performed until the late 1980s (in 1986, 1 lung transplant; in 1989, 132 lung transplants). This number rapidly increased to 700/year in 1994 and has since declined to approximately 625/year.

27. Are the survival rates different for single and double lung transplants?
No. The 3-year actuarial survival rate is about 50% for each.

28. What are the 1-year, 2-year, and 3-year actuarial survival rates for single lung retransplants?
Actuarial survival rates are 45%, 40%, and 30%, respectively. Predictably, such patients do significantly worse.

BIBLIOGRAPHY

 1. Baumgartner WA: Myocardial and pulmonary protection: Long-distance transport. Prog Cardiovasc Dis 33:85, 1990.
 2. Christie JD, Bavaria JE, Palevsky HI, et al: Primary graft failure following lung transplantation. Chest 114:51, 1998.
 3. Cooper JD, Patterson GA: Lung Transplantation. In Sabiston D, Spencer F (eds): Surgery of the Chest. Philadelphia, W.B. Saunders, 1995, pp 2117–2134.
 4. Gaynor JW, Bridges ND, Clark BJ, et al: Update on lung transplantation in children. Curr Opin Pediatr 10:256, 1998.
 5. Henke JA, Golden JA, Yelin EH, et al: Persistent increases of BAL neutrophils as a predictor of mortality following lung transplant. Chest 115:403, 1999.
 6. Hosenpud JD, Bennett LE, Keck BM, et al: The Registry of the International Society for Heart and Lung Transplantation: Fifteenth official report—1998. J Heart Lung Transplant 17:656, 1998.
 7. Keller CA: The donor lung: Conservation of a precious resource. Thorax 53:506, 1998.
 8. Meyers BF, Patterson GA: Technical aspects of adult lung transplantation. Semin Thorac Cardiovasc Surg 10:213, 1998.
 9. Nunley DR, Grgurich W, Iacono AT, et al: Allograft colonization and infections with pseudomonas in cystic fibrosis lung transplant recipients. Chest 113:1235, 1998.
10. Prince HM: Gene transfer: A review of methods and applications. Pathology 30:335, 1998.
11. Rich S, McLaughlin VV: Lung transplantation for pulmonary hypertension: Patient selection and maintenance therapy while awaiting transplantation. Semin Thorac Cardiovasc Surg 10:135, 1998.
12. Sundaresan S: The impact of bronchiolitis obliterans on late morbidity and mortality after single and bilateral lung transplantation for pulmonary hypertension. Semin Thorac Cardiovasc Surg 10:152, 1998.
13. Vongpatanasin W, Brickner ME, Hillis LD, et al: The Eisenmenger syndrome in adults. Ann Intern Med 128:745, 1998.
14. Waddell TK, Keshavjee S: Lung transplantation for chronic obstructive pulmonary disease. Semin Thorac Cardiovasc Surg 10:191, 1998.
15. Zenati M, Keenan RJ, Courcoulas AP, et al: Lung volume reduction or lung transplanation for end-stage pulmonary emphysema? Eur J Cardiothorac Surg 14(1):27, 1998.

XI. Urology

93. INFERTILITY

Randall B. Meacham, M.D., and Gwendolyn J. Hewitt, M.D.

1. How common a problem is infertility?

Infertility, defined as the inability to establish a pregnancy during 1 year of well-timed intercourse, affects 15% of all couples in the United States. In 50% of such couples, a female fertility problem is responsible; in 30% of couples, a male factor prevents pregnancy; and in 20% of couples a combination of female and male factors is responsible for the inability to conceive.

2. What are the odds that a fertile couple will become pregnant after a single episode of well-timed intercourse?

During a given ovulatory cycle, approximately 18% of fertile couples become pregnant after well-timed intercourse.

3. What is the best timing for intercourse if a couple is trying to conceive?

Sperm can survive in the cervical mucus for 48 hours. To achieve pregnancy, therefore, the most effective timing of intercourse is every other day, starting a few days before ovulation is anticipated.

4. What environmental factors may play a role in male infertility?

Although reproductive function is relatively durable, various toxins have a negative impact on male fertility. Cigarette smoke and alcohol have been implicated as dose-dependent gonadotoxins, as have recreational drugs, including marijuana, cocaine, and heroin. Radiation (in amounts as low as 200 rads) can have a significant effect on spermatogenesis, as can a variety of chemotherapeutic agents. Calcium channel blockers may interfere with the ability of sperm to fertilize eggs.

5. Can a vasectomy be successfully reversed?

Although vasectomy reversal is a relatively common surgical procedure, the success rate is affected by the amount of time since the original vasectomy. Among patients who are less than 3 years from vasectomy, the conception rate after reversal is roughly 75%. This success rate declines to about 50% when the reversal is performed 3–8 years after vasectomy and further declines to 30% when 15 or more years have passed.

6. What is in vitro fertilization (IVF)?

IVF is a process in which eggs are harvested from a female and combined with sperm in a laboratory setting. The resulting embryos are then transferred to the uterine cavity, where they mature into a fetus. In a specialized version of this technology (intracytoplasmic sperm injection), an individual sperm is injected into each egg, thus facilitating fertilization and allowing pregnancy even in the presence of small numbers of motile sperm.

7. What is the role of IVF in male infertility?

Because use of IVF greatly reduces the number of motile sperm needed to generate a pregnancy, it can be quite helpful in men with poor semen quality. The IVF team needs only as many motile sperm as there are oocytes (eggs) to be fertilized.

8. Can sperm obtained directly from the testicle be used to generate a pregnancy?

For the past several years, it has been recognized that incubation of testicular tissue generally yields small numbers of motile sperm. Through the use of in vitro fertilization, such sperm can be used to generate pregnancies. Even among men suffering from severe testicular failure, it may be possible to retrieve adequate sperm for use in IVF.

9. What is the role of sperm freezing in the treatment of infertility?

Sperm can be frozen (termed cryopreservation) with relative ease. Once cryopreserved, sperm remain viable for extended periods. Cryopreservation can be helpful among men planning to undergo treatment with chemotherapy or radiation therapy.

10. Does wearing boxer shorts versus tight underwear affect male fertility?

The type of underwear that a man wears has minimal if any effect on semen quality or fertility.

11. Since normal levels of testosterone are necessary for sperm production, is it helpful to give subfertile men additional testosterone?

Although decreased levels of testosterone can cause impaired male fertility, giving additional testosterone to men with normal testosterone levels can actually cause a dramatic decline in semen quality. Administration of exogenous testosterone causes the patient to cease production of native testosterone within the testes. The resultant decrease in intratesticular testosterone causes a decline in sperm production.

12. What is the most common cause of male fertility?

Varicocele, a collection of dilated veins above one or both testes, is the most common cause of male infertility. Among men presenting for treatment of infertility, 40% have a varicocele. Correction of varicocele leads to improvement in semen quality in 70% of patients.

13. If we can clone Dolly (a sheep derived from cloning a fully differentiated mammary cell), can we clone Dallas cheerleaders?

Although for a number of critical ethical reasons cloning technology is not currently used in human reproduction, it theoretically allows the cloning of any individual, creating a genetic duplicate. Cloning probably will not play a role in the treatment of human infertility.

BIBLIOGRAPHY

1. Hargreave T, Ghosh C: Male fertility disorders. Endocrinol Metab Clin North Am 27:765–782, 1998.
2. Ismail MT, Sedor J, Hirsch IH: Are sperm motion parameters influenced by varicocele ligation? Fertil Steril 71:886–890, 1999.
3. Johnson MD: Genetic risks of intracytoplasmic sperm injection in the treatment of male infertility: Recommendations for genetic counseling and screening. Fertil Steril 70:397–411, 1998.
4. Kim ED, Winkel E, Orejuela F, et al: Pathological epididymal obstruction unrelated to vasectomy: Results with microsurgical reconstruction. J Urol 160(6 Pt 1):2078–2080, 1998.
5. Naysmith TE, Blake DA, Harvey VJ, et al: Do men undergoing sterilizing cancer treatments have a fertile future? Hum Reprod 13:3250–3255, 1998.
6. Palermo GD, Schlegel PN, Hariprashad JJ, et al: Fertilization and pregnancy outcome with intracytoplasmic sperm injection for azoospermic men. Human Reprod 14:741–748, 1999.
7. Rutkowski SB, Geraghty TJ, Hagen DL, et al: A comprehensive approach to the management of male infertility following spinal cord injury. Spinal Cord 37:508–514, 1999.
8. Scherr D, Goldstein M: Comparison of bilateral versus unilateral varicocelectomy in men with palpable bilateral varicoceles. J Urol 162:85–88,1999.
9. Wilmut I: Cloning for medicine. Sci Am 279:58–63, 1998.

94. URINARY CALCULUS DISEASE

Brett B. Abernathy, M.D.

1. What are the most common types of urinary stones found in North America?

1. Calcium stones (calcium oxalate, calcium phosphate, or mixed calcium stones): 70%.
2. Struvite or magnesium ammonium phosphate stones, often associated with infection: 20%.
3. Uric acid stones (radiolucent): 5%
4. Cystine stones, often with a genetic association: 5%

2. What are the typical presenting symptoms of a patient with an obstructing stone?

1. Pain, usually colicky in the flank or radiating to the groin. Patients are usually agitated and cannot get in a comfortable position.
2. Hematuria, gross or microscopic.
3. Nausea and vomiting due to obstruction and pressure on the renal capsule.

3. What studies are best to diagnose stones?

1. The standard test has always been the excretory urogram, or intravenous pyelogram (IVP). Ninety percent of stones are radiopaque and can be seen on a plain film of the kidney, ureter, and bladder. The IVP serves as a functional study to determine the degree of obstruction, level of obstruction, and presence of a contralateral kidney.
2. Rapid-sequence helical computed tomography scan also can accurately identify both renal and ureteral stones. Its advantages include no need for contrast, rapid study, and identification of calcium-containing, as well as uric acid and cystine, stones.
3. Ultrasound is particularly advantageous in pregnant women.

4. What are the indications for admitting a patient to the hospital with an obstructing stone?

1. Any sign of infection (fever, leukocytosis, bacteriuria). Infection behind an obstructing stone may result in urosepsis and death.
2. Intractable vomiting requiring IV fluids.
3. Pain requiring parenteral analgesics.
4. Bilateral obstructing stones or obstruction in a solitary kidney.

5. What are the treatment options for ureteral calculi?

1. Expectant management consists of controlling pain, fluid hydration therapy, controlling nausea, and straining the urine to identify any stone that passes. Approximately 90% of stones, 3 mm in size in the distal ureter, will pass. Approximately 50% of 5-mm stones will pass, and approximately 20% of stones larger than 6 mm will pass.
2. Ureteroscopy and stone basketing or intraureteral lithotripsy (stone blasting) with a laser (holmium, pulsed dye) or electrohydraulic lithotripsy (EHL).
3. Extracorporeal lithotripsy (ESWL), or shock waves directed at the stone to break it into small pieces that will then pass spontaneously.
4. Open ureterolithotomy, now rarely used because of the success of the less invasive techniques listed above.

6. What are the treatment options for renal calculi?

1. Expectant management in asymptomatic noninfectious stones
2. ESWL
3. Percutaneous nephrostolithotomy (particularly for stone burden larger than 2 cm)

4. Combination of ESWL and percutaneous nephrostolithotomy
5. Open lithotomy (less common because of the success of less invasive treatment options)

7. What is a steinstrasse?
Steinstrasse (German for stone street) is a collection of small calculi that pile up together in the ureter and cause obstruction or symptoms. This problem may occur after lithotripsy treatment.

8. What is a stent?
A stent is a small plastic catheter that coils in the renal pelvis, traverses the ureter, and coils in the bladder. Stents are useful to relieve ureteral obstruction temporarily and possibly to facilitate stone passage once the stent is removed. Stents often cause some degree of ureteral dilatation after they have been removed.

9. What is a metabolic evaluation? Who needs one?
A metabolic evaluation involves examining serum and a 24-hour urine specimen for factors that contribute to stone formation. The goals are to identify an abnormality and to treat it medically to prevent further stone formation. Indications for metabolic evaluation include recurrent stones, multiple stones, bilateral stones, stones in children, and non–calcium-containing stones.

10. Can stones be dissolved?
• Uric acid stones often can be dissolved by alkalinizing the urine and with hydration therapy.
• Cystine, struvite, and appetite stones sometimes can be dissolved.
• Calcium stones cannot be dissolved.

BONUS QUESTIONS

11. What mammal other than humans is at risk for uric acid stone disease?
The dalmatian dog excretes uric acid and therefore is at risk for developing uric acid stones.

12. What toxic substance can be produced by using the holmium:YAG laser on uric acid stones?
Cyanide can be created from the uric acid. The clinical significance appears negligible.

BIBLIOGRAPHY

1. Drach GW: Urinary lithiasis: Etiology, diagnosis and medical management. In Walsh PC, Retik AB, Vaughan ED, et al (eds): Campbell's Urology, 7th ed. Philadelphia, W.B. Saunders, 1998, pp 2083–2146.
2. Teichman JM, Vassar GJ, Glickman RD: Holmium:YAG lithotripsy photothermal mechanism converts uric acid calculi to cyanide. J Urol 160:320–324, 1998.

95. RENAL CELL CARCINOMA
Brett B. Abernathy, M.D.

1. How common is renal cell carcinoma?
In the United States, approximately 30,000 new cases of renal cell carcinoma are predicted for 1999. It represents about 3% of all adult malignancies.

2. How is kidney cancer detected?
Renal cell carcinoma may present with hematuria, flank pain, or abdominal mass. This classic triad is found in only about 10% of cases. Many solid renal tumors are found when computed

tomography scanning of the abdomen is performed for other reasons and tumors are detected incidentally.

3. Are all solid masses in the kidney renal cell carcinoma?

No. Other solid masses include angiomyolipomas, oncocytomas, sarcomas, and metastatic lesions. However, all solid masses should be presumed to be renal cell carcinoma until proved otherwise.

4. What is the unique relationship between renal cell carcinoma and its vasculature?

Renal cell carcinoma has a tendency to invade its own venous drainage. Tumor thrombus may extend along the renal vein into the inferior vana cava and even to the right atrium.

5. How should suspected involvement of the vena cava be evaluated?

Magnetic resonance imaging or venacavography can identify the extent of the vena caval involvement with tumor.

6. How is renal cell carcinoma treated?

Surgery is usually the best treatment for localized renal cell carcinoma. The standard operation is a radical nephrectomy, including all the contents within Gerota's fascia.

7. Does the whole kidney have to be removed in all cases of renal cell carcinoma?

No. Nephron-sparing surgery can be performed in cases of bilateral renal cell carcinoma or renal cell carcinoma in a solitary kidney. Because of the risk of postoperative tumor recurrence, nephron-sparing surgery in the presence of a normal contralateral kidney is controversial.

8. How is metastatic renal cell carcinoma treated?

Chemotherapy has been disappointing. The most encouraging results to date are with interleukin-2 (IL-2) treatment; some evidence of definite durable responses has been noted. Research is ongoing using IL-2 with other forms of immune enhancing technology.

BONUS QUESTION

9. What is Stauffer's syndrome?

Elevated liver function tests (LFTs) in the presence of renal cell carcinoma that normalize after nephrectomy and tumor removal. It is thought to be a type of paraneoplastic syndrome.

BIBLIOGRAPHY

1. De Kernion JB, Belledegrun A: Urinary lithiasis. In Walsh RC, Retik AB, Vaughan ED, et al: Compbell's Urology, 7th ed. Philadelphia, W.B. Saunders, 1998, pp 1053–1087.
2. Figlin RA: Renal cell carcinoma: Management of advanced disease. J Urol 161:391, 1999.
3. Landis SH, Murray T, Bolden S, Wingo PA: Cancer statistics 1999. Cancer J Clin 49:12, 1999.
4. Resnick MI, Novick AC: Urology Secrets, 2nd ed. Philadelphia, Hanley & Belfus, 1999.

96. BLADDER CANCER

Brett B. Abernathy, M.D.

1. How common is bladder cancer?

About 54,000 new cases of bladder cancer will be diagnosed in 1999 in the United States. The male-to-female ratio is almost 3:1.

2. What are the risk factors for bladder cancer?

Cigarette smoking, exposure to aniline dyes or aromatic amines, phenacetin abuse, and treatment with chemotherapy (cyclophosphamide).

3. How does bladder cancer present?

Bladder cancer usually presents with painless hematuria (gross or microscopic). Irritative voiding symptoms such as frequency, urgency, and dysuria, also may be presenting symptoms, especially for carcinoma in situ.

4. What is the most common histologic type of bladder cancer?

Transitional cell carcinoma (TCC) makes up more than 90% of bladder cancers. Other histologic types include adenocarcinoma, squamous cell carcinoma, and urachal carcinoma.

5. How is TCC of the bladder treated?

Initially, the tumor is resected through a transurethral resection of the bladder tumor. Further treatment is determined by the pathologic evaluation of the specimen (i.e., if carcinoma in situ or muscle invasive disease is present).

6. Is carcinoma in situ (CIS) a less aggressive type of bladder cancer?

No. TCC in situ is a flat but poorly differentiated tumor. It can progress to metastatic disease and should be treated as an aggressive form of bladder cancer.

7. How is CIS treated?

Immunotherapy with intravesical bacillus Calmette-Guerin (BCG) is currently the first-line treatment. Response rates to BCG approach 70%. Other intravesical agents such as mitomycin C also may be used but are generally less effective than BCG.

8. What are the side effects of BCG?

Mild symptoms of urinary frequency, urgency, and dysuria are common. Myalgias and low-grade fever (flu-like symptoms) also occur. High or persistent fever suggests a more serious problem requiring antituberculous therapy. Death from BCG has been reported. Deaths usually have followed administration of BCG after traumatic catheterization.

9. How is muscle-invasive bladder cancer treated?

Muscle-invasive disease usually is treated with radical cystectomy (or cystoprostatectomy in males) with some form of urinary diversion.

10. What types of urinary diversion are used with radical cystectomy?

Urinary diversion is usually classified as a conduit or a continent reservoir. The most common example is an ileal conduit. An external collection device must be worn with a conduit. Continent reservoirs are made of combinations of large and small bowel and may be emptied via the urethra or a continent stoma.

11. How is metastatic bladder cancer treated?
Metastatic bladder cancer is usually treated with chemotherapy. Most regimens include a platinum-based agent.

12. Can invasive bladder cancer be cured without removal of the entire bladder?
Controversial. Some cancers may be suitable for partial cystectomy (i.e., tumors isolated in the dome of the bladder). Investigations are ongoing to evaluate transurethral resection of bladder tumor plus radiation and chemotherapy to try to preserve the bladder in invasive TCC.

BONUS QUESTIONS

13. In certain countries TCC is not the predominant form of bladder cancer. What is the predominant histologic type? Why?
Some countries such as Egypt have a high rate of schistosomiasis, which predisposes to squamous cell carcinoma of the bladder. Squamous cell is more common than TCC in these areas.

14. Can any markers be used to help predict the prognosis of TCC?
The p53 tumor suppressor protein is a marker that may be helpful in assessing both the biologic behavior of the tumor and possibly in assisting with treatment option decisions for the patient. Work evaluating the utility of the p53 marker is ongoing.

BIBLIOGRAPHY

1. Catalona W: Urothelial tumors of the urinary tract. In Walsh PC, Retik AB, Vaughan ED, et al (eds): Campbell's Urology, 7th ed. Philadelphia, W.B. Saunders, 1998, pp 1094–1146.
2. Herr HW, Bajorn DF, Scher HL: Can p53 help select patients with invasive bladder cancer for bladder preservation? J Urol 161:20, 1999.
3. Landis SH, Murray T, Bolden S, Wingo PA: Cancer statistics 1999. Cancer J Clin 49:12, 1999.
4. Resnick MI, Novick AC: Urology Secrets, 2nd ed. Philadelphia, Hanley & Belfus, 1999.

97. PROSTATE CANCER

Brett B. Abernathy, M.D.

1. How common is prostate cancer?
Prostate cancer is the most common malignancy diagnosed in men in the United States; 179,000 new cases are predicted for 1999.

2. Do most men die "with" prostate cancer, rather than "from" it?
Yes, but approximately 37,000 men will die of prostate cancer in 1999 in the United States. Thus it should not be treated as a benign process in all cases.

3. What are the early symptoms of prostate cancer?
None. By the time significant symptoms develop, the disease is likely to be advanced. This is an argument for screening to detect prostate cancer.

4. What is the best screening method for prostate cancer?
Digital rectal examination (DRE) combined with serum prostate-specific antigen (PSA).

5. How is prostate cancer diagnosed?

Prostate cancer is diagnosed by tissue biopsy, which usually is done by needle biopsy of the prostate using transrectal ultrasound for guidance. Some cancers are diagnosed with transurethral resection of the prostate (TURP), which is performed for benign prostatic hyperplasia (BPH).

6. When is prostate biopsy indicated?

When either the PSA or DRE is abnormal.

7. Does an elevated PSA mean a man has prostate cancer?

No. PSA can be elevated with BPH, prostatitis, or after prostate trauma. It is prostate-specific, not prostate cancer-specific.

8. What is a free PSA?

Free PSA is a measure of the percentage of PSA that is not bound to a serum protein carrier. The ratio of free to total PSA may be helpful in determining when to do a prostate biopsy. "Free" is good, because a higher ratio of free to total PSA is less likely to represent a prostate cancer.

9. Are there any known risk factors for prostate cancer?

Yes. African-American men and men with a family history of prostate cancer are at an increased risk.

10. What is Gleason's sum?

Gleason's sum is the score that the pathologist gives prostate cancer to estimate its aggressiveness. The two predominant patterns of cancer are scored 1 to 5, and the sum is therefore between 2 and 10. Tumors can be well differentiated (2, 3, 4), moderately differentiated (5, 6, 7), or poorly differentiated (8, 9, 10).

11. How is clinically localized prostate cancer treated?

Treatment options for localized prostate cancer include surgery (radical prostatectomy), radiation therapy by external beam or interstitial seed implant, cryotherapy, or watchful waiting.

12. How is advanced metastatic prostate cancer treated?

Advanced prostate cancer can be treated with hormonal ablation therapy (orchiectomy or luteinizing hormone-releasing hormone agonist drugs) or chemotherapy, but these treatments are generally palliative and not curative.

13. What is the best treatment for prostate cancer?

The answer is currently highly controversial. Patients must weigh factors such as age, overall health, grade and stage of the disease, and risk of side effects versus complications from the various treatment options. Each patient must decide what is best with appropriate consultation from his physician.

BIBLIOGRAPHY

1. Catalona WJ: Clinical utility of free and total prostate specific antigen. Rev Prostate 7(Suppl): 64–69, 1996.
2. D'Amico AV, Whittington R, Malkowicz SB, et al: Biochemical outcome after radical prostatectomy, external beam radiation therapy, or interstitial radiation therapy for clinically localized prostate cancer. JAMA 280:969, 1998.
3. Keetch DW, Humphrey PA, et al: Clinical and pathological features of hereditary prostate cancer. J Urol 155:1841–1842, 1996.
4. Landis SH, Murray T, Bolden S, Wingo PA: Cancer statistics 1999. Cancer J Clin 49:12, 1999.
5. Polascik TJ, Pound CR, et al: Comparison of radical prostatectomy and iodine-125 interstitial radiotherapy for the treatment of clinically localized prostate cancer: A 7-year biochemical (PSA) progression analysis. Urology 51:884–890, 1998.
6. Resnick MI, Novick AC: Urology Secrets, 2nd ed. Philadelphia, Hanley & Belfus, 1999.
7. Stamey TA, McNeal JE: Adenocarcinoma of the prostate. In Walsh PC, Retik AB, Vaughan ED, et al (eds): Campbell's Urology, 7th ed. Philadelphia, W.B. Saunders, 1998, pp 1159–1214

98. URODYNAMICS AND VOIDING DYSFUNCTION

Firouz Daneshgari, M.D.

1. What is urodynamics?

Urodynamic studies assess the functional aspects of the storage and emptying ability of the lower urinary tract (LUT). The principles of urodynamic studies originated from hydrodynamics. The components of urodynamic studies are cystometrogram, leak point pressures, urethral profile pressures, pressure-flow studies, uroflowmetry, and electromyography. These studies have evolved into videourodynamics with the addition of fluoroscopy/video.

2. What is uroflowmetry?

Uroflowmetry is the measurement of voided urine (ml) per unit of time (second). The important elements of the test are voided volume (should be > 150 ml), maximum flow rate (Q_{max}), and the curve of the flow, which should be bell-shaped. The normal Q_{max} is > 20 ml/sec in men and > 25 ml/sec in women.

3. What is BPH?

Benign prostatic hyperplasia (BPH) is benign enlargement of the prostate gland, which may lead to bladder outlet obstructive symptoms in men. These symptoms have recently been termed lower urinary tract symptoms (LUTS).

4. What is an AUA symptom score?

The self-reported questionnaire developed and popularized by the American Urological Association (AUA) for the assessment of bothersome LUTS in men. This questionnaire has 7 questions with a maximum score of 35. The higher the score, the more severe and bothersome the symptoms. The AUA symptom score has become an index for both the diagnosis and evaluation of treatment outcome in patients with LUTS.

5. What are the main functions of the LUT?

Storage and emptying of urine. For practical purposes, all symptoms of LUT dysfunction can be categorized into the malfunction of either storing or emptying ability.

6. What are the control mechanisms for LUT function?

The control mechanisms for LUT function are recognized as central and peripheral. The central control mechanisms consist of the cortical portion of the frontal lobe of the brain and pontine micturition center. The peripheral control mechanisms include the thoracic sympathetic and lumbar parasympathetic innervation and neuromuscular apparatus of the LUT organs.

7. What is the role of the autonomic nervous system in the function of the LUT?

Sympathetic fibers, which originate from the T10–L2 portion of the spinal cord, innervate the bladder neck and proximal urethra. These fibers mostly control the contraction of the proximal urethra/bladder neck and relaxation of the bladder, which results in storage of urine. The parasympathetic fibers, which originate primarily from the S2–S4 portion of the spinal cord, innervate the bladder body. The parasympathetic innervation allows contraction of the bladder smooth muscle, leading to emptying of the bladder.

8. What is the role of the somatic nervous system in the function of the LUT?

Voluntary control of the striated muscle of the external urinary sphincter is controlled by the somatic nervous system. Somatic fibers are conveyed to the sphincter by the pudendal nerve.

9. What is bulbocavernosal reflex?

Bulbocavernosal reflex tests the integrity of peripheral neurologic control of the LUT. This reflex is elicited by stimulation of the glans penis in men or the clitoris in women, which causes contraction of the external anal sphincter or bulbocavernosus muscle. Alternatively, the reflex may be stimulated by pulling the balloon of a Foley catheter against the bladder neck. This reflex is present in all normal men and in approximately 70% of normal women. Absence of this reflex in a man is strongly suggestive of a sacral neurologic lesion.

10. What is the most common cause of incontinence in the geriatric population?

Transient causes, mostly external, which disrupt the fragile balance of LUT function in elderly patients and cause urinary incontinence. These causes can be recalled with the mnemonic **DIAPPERS**:

Delirium
Infections
Atrophic urethritis/vaginitis
Pharmaceuticals
Psychological (depression)
Endocrine (hypercalcemia, hyperglycemia)
Restricted mobility
Stool impaction

11. What is spinal shock? What type of urinary dysfunction does it cause?

Spinal shock refers to the loss of contractility of the smooth muscle below the level of spinal cord injury, leading to difficulty in bladder emptying or urinary retention. This phenomenon may last from hours to several months with a high chance of reversibility if the spinal cord injury is not permanent.

12. What is autonomic dysreflexia? How is it treated?

Autonomic dysreflexia results from systematic outpouring of sympathetic discharge, as in patients with spinal cord lesions at or above the T6 level. This dysreflexia is triggered by distention of the bladder or other stimulus of the bowel or LUT. It is manifested by hypertension, bradycardia, hot flush, sweating, and headache. Initial treatment consists of removal of the stimulus, such as emptying the bladder and placing the patient in a sitting position. Nifedipine or nitroprusside may be used as either prophylaxis or treatment of severe episodes. This condition may lead to significant cerebrovascular complication if untreated.

13. What type of bladder dysfunction is seen in diabetic patients?

Diabetic cystopathy is manifested primarily as atonic bladder with difficulty in emptying due to impaired contractility of the bladder/detrusor muscle.

14. What type of bladder dysfunction is seen in patients with multiple sclerosis (MS)?

Urgency (83%), urge incontinence (75%), detrusor hyperreflexia (62%), and detrusor sphincter dyssynergia (25%) are among the most common LUT symptoms in patients with MS. Variation in symptoms depends on the site of involvement by MS. Involvement of pontine pathways (tegmentum) is associated with a much higher rate of urinary symptoms.

15. Which sacral roots control the micturition physiology?

S2–S4.

16. What is the cause of urinary retention after abdominal or pelvic surgery?

Injuries and/or disruption of pelvic plexus innervation to the LUT.

17. What is Ogilvie's syndrome?

Acute massive dilation of the cecum and ascending and transverse colon without organic obstruction is known as Ogilvie's syndrome. This syndrome can be seen in pelvic urologic surgeries, possibly as a result of an imbalance in parasympathetic stimulation of the colon.

18. What is reflex vs. psychic erection?

Erection after local stimulation is termed reflex erection. The afferent nerves for reflex erection run in the pudendal nerves, and the efferent fibers are found in the S2–S4 parasympathetic outflow. The psychic erection is caused by stimulation of cerebral erotic centers. The afferent stimuli for psychic erection travel through the thoracolumbar sympathetic outflow and sacral parasympathetic fibers.

BIBLIOGRAPHY

1. Barry KJ, Fowler FJ Jr, O'Leary MP, et al: The American Urological Association symptom index for benign prostatic hyperplasia. The Measurement Committee of the American Urological Association. J Urol 148:1549, 1992.
2. Holtgrewe HL: Current trends in management of men with lower urinary tract symptoms and benign prostatic hyperplasia. Urology 51(Suppl 4A):1–7, 1998.
3. Litwiller SE, Forhman EM, Zimmern PE: Multiple sclerosis and the urologist. J Urol 161:743–757, 1999.
4. McConnell JD, Berry MJ, Bruskewitz RC: Benign Prostatic Hyperplasia: Diagnosis and Treatment. Publication No. 94-0582. Rockville, MD, Agency for Health Care Policy and Research, U.S. Department of Health and Human Services, 1994.
5. McVary KT, Dalton DP, Blum MD: Acute intestinal pseudo-obstruction (Ogilvie's syndrome) complicating radical retropubic prostatectomy. J Urol 141:1210, 1989.
6. Resnick NM, Yalla SV: Geriatric incontinence and voiding dysfunction. In Walsh PC, Retik AB, Vaughan ED, et al: Campbell's Urology, 7th ed. Philadelphia, W.B. Saunders, 1998.
7. Steers WD, Barrett DM, Wein AJ: Voiding dysfunction, diagnosis, classification and management. In Gillenwater JY, Grayhack JT, Howards SS, Duckett JW (eds): Adult and Pediatric Urology, 3rd ed. St. Louis, Mosby, 1996.

99. PEDIATRIC UROLOGY

Kirstan K. Donnahoo, M.D., and Mark P. Cain, M.D.

1. A healthy 3-year-old girl develops a urinary tract infection (UTI). How should she be evaluated?

After treatment of the infection, the patient should undergo urinary tract evaluation with a renal-bladder sonogram and voiding cystourethrogram (VCUG). Approximately 50% of children under 12 presenting with UTI are found to have abnormalities of the genitourinary tract, the most common of which are vesicoureteral reflux, obstructive uropathies, and neurogenic bladder.

2. What is vesicoureteral reflux (VUR) disease?

VUR is a condition in which urine refluxes from the bladder into the upper urinary tract. Primary VUR is caused by an inadequate valvular mechanism at the ureterovesical junction, presumably related to a shortened submucosal ureteral tunnel. Approximately one-third of children with culture-documented UTIs have VUR.

3. Is VUR harmful to the kidney?

Sterile reflux is unlikely to cause renal damage; however, persistent reflux of infected urine may cause pyelonephritis and progressive renal scarring. Currently, renal scarring is the fourth leading cause for renal transplantation in children. The combination of VUR and elevated bladder storage pressure (e.g., neuropathic bladder or bladder outlet obstruction) is also harmful to the kidney.

4. What are the indications for surgical correction of VUR?

Reflux disappears spontaneously in many children; however, high-grade reflux, especially when bilateral, is unlikely to resolve spontaneously. In general, children with high-grade reflux or breakthrough UTIs despite antibiotic prophylaxis should be managed surgically. Surgical management also should be considered in children with reflux persisting into late childhood or adolescence.

5. What is the most common cause of antenatal hydronephrosis?

Ureteropelvic junction (UPJ) obstruction. Hydronephrosis is the most common abnormality detected on prenatal ultrasound and accounts for approximately 50% of all prenatally detected lesions. Fifty percent of prenatal hydronephrosis, in turn, is caused by UPJ obstruction. UPJ obstruction is bilateral in approximately 20% of cases and associated with VUR in 10–15% of cases.

6. What is the most common cause of UPJ obstruction?

Intrinsic stenosis, which occurs in approximately 75% of all UPJ obstructions. Less common causes include lower pole crossing vessels, anomalous ureteral insertions, and peripelvic fibrosis.

7. Can UPJ obstruction resolve spontaneously? What are the indications for pyeloplasty?

Yes. Ultimately, only about 25% of children with UPJ obstruction require pyeloplasty. The indications for surgical intervention include worsening hydronephrosis, poor or declining renal function, pain, and presence of a solitary kidney or bilateral hydronephrosis.

8. What is the Meyer-Weigert law?

This law refers to the position of the ureteral orifices in patients with complete ureteral duplication. Occasionally, two ureteral buds develop independently from the mesonephric duct. As the ureteral buds are absorbed into the developing bladder, the bud located in a lower position along the duct (draining the lower pole of the kidney) is carried to a more cranial and lateral position. The ureteral bud located in a higher position along the duct (draining the upper pole of the kidney) is carried to a more caudal and medial position within the bladder. Lower pole ureters are more likely to reflux because of their lateral position within the bladder, whereas upper pole ureters are more frequently obstructed.

9. What is a ureterocele?

A ureterocele is a cystic dilatation of the distal portion of the ureter. Ureteroceles usually are associated with the upper pole ureter of a duplicated collecting system; however, they also may develop from single ureters. They are most commonly ectopic (i.e., some portion of the ureterocele is positioned at the bladder neck or urethra) and usually cause ureteral obstruction.

10. What is the most common presenting symptom of a girl with an ectopic ureter?

Incontinence. In girls ectopic ureters usually drain into the bladder neck, proximal urethra, or vestibule. The orifice also may be located in the vagina (25%) and occasionally the uterus. When the ectopic ureteral orifice is positioned below the external sphincter or within the female genital tract, incontinence may develop.

11. Do boys with ectopic ureters present with incontinence?

No. The ectopic pathway in boys extends from the bladder neck through the posterior urethra to the mesonephric duct derivatives (i.e., vas deferens, epididymis, and seminal vesicle). Therefore, the ectopic ureteral orifice is not positioned below the continence mechanism.

12. What percentage of full-term male infants have an undescended testicle?

Three percent. This number decreases to 0.8% by 1 year of age.

13. What is the most common location of an undescended testicle?

The inguinal canal (72% of undescended testicles). The testicle also may be located in the abdomen (8%) or prescrotal area (20%). Twenty percent of undescended testicles are nonpalpable at presentation; of these, 50% are absent.

14. Why should the testicle be brought back into the scrotum?

Patients with cryptorchidism have a 20–50-fold increased risk of germ cell cancer compared with the normal population. Although positioning of the testicle within the scrotum does not alleviate this risk, it does permit routine, thorough, testicular examination. Patients with cryptorchidism also are at risk for infertility. Histologic studies have demonstrated progressive germ cell loss in the undescended testicle beginning at 6 months of age. It is thought that early orchiopexy can minimize the extent of germ cell loss and thereby decrease the chance of future infertility. In general, the higher the testicle (i.e., abdomen), the greater the risk of cancer and infertility.

15. Who described the most common current technique for orchiopexy?

C. Everett Koop.

16. What is the most common cause of bladder outlet obstruction in boys? In girls?

Posterior urethral valves and ureterocele, respectively.

17. What are the urinary manifestations of posterior urethral valves?

Posterior urethral valves are congenital leaflets of tissue, which extend from the verumontanum to the anterior urethra in boys. They occur at an incidence of 1/5000–1/8000 live male births. Posterior urethral valves cause bladder outlet obstruction, which in turn leads to variable degrees of bladder and renal injury. Severe obstruction may result in oligohydramnios and pulmonary hypoplasia, bladder hypertrophy, vesicoureteral reflux, hydroureteronephrosis, and renal dysplasia. Approximately 50% of affected children have reflux, and 25–40% progress to end-stage renal disease.

18. What is a myelomeningocele? What are its urologic consequences?

A myelomeningocele is a hernial protrusion of the spinal cord and its meninges through a defect in the vertebral column. The resulting neurologic injury causes, among other problems, bladder dysfunction. Patients with myelomeningocele are usually incontinent because of detrusor hyperactivity, detrusor hypoactivity, poor bladder compliance, inadequate outlet resistance, detrusor-outlet dyssynergy, or a combination of these factors. More importantly, patients with hyperactive, high-pressure bladders may develop upper urinary tract deterioration. Life-long follow-up is necessary because the neurologic lesion can change with time. Treatment goals include maintenance of a low-pressure urinary reservoir, prevention of urinary tract infections, and achievement of continence.

19. What is the most common cause of ambiguous genitalia in the newborn?

Congenital adrenal hyperplasia, most commonly due to a 21-hydroxylase deficiency.

20. What diagnostic evaluation should be performed in any male infant presenting with hypospadias and cryptorchidism?

The presence of cryptorchidism and hypospadias should alert the physician to the possibility of an androgenized female. A karyotype should always be obtained before reconstruction.

21. What are the two most important prognostic factors in Wilms' tumor?

Wilms' tumor is the most common malignant renal tumor of childhood with an incidence of 1 in 10,000 children. Wilms' tumor is associated with congenital anomalies, including sporadic aniridia, hemihypertrophy, and congenital urinary tract malformations. The two most important prognostic factors in Wilms' tumor are histology and stage.

BIBLIOGRAPHY

1. Coplen DE: Current management of ureteroceles. AUA Update Series 17:234–239, 1998.
2. Dinneen MD, Duffy PG: Posterior urethral valves. Br J Urol 78:275–281, 1996.
3. Elder JS, Peters CA, Arant BS Jr, et al: Pediatric vesicoureteral reflux guidelines panel summary report on the management of primary vesicoureteral reflux in children. J Urol 157:1846–1851, 1997.
4. Gill B, Kogan S: Cryptorchidism. Current concepts. Pediatr Clin North Am 44:1211–1227, 1997.
5. Gunther DF, Bukowski TP: Congenital adrenal hyperplasia: A spectrum of disorders. Contemp Urol 11:52–69, 1999.
6. Kirsch AJ, Escala J, Duckett JW, et al: Surgical management of the nonpalpable testis: The Children's Hospital of Philadelphia experience. J Urol 159:1340–1343, 1998.
7. Kirsch AJ, Snyder HM: What's new and important in pediatric urologic oncology. AUA Update Series 17:82–87, 1998.
8. Koop CE: Technique of herniorraphy and orchidopexy. Birth Defects Orig Artic Ser 13:293–303, 1977.
9. Pohl HG, Rushton HG: The diagnosis and management of urinary tract infection in children. AUA Update Series 17:242–247, 1998.
10. Poppas DP, Bauer SB: Urologic evaluation of the myelodysplastic child. AUA Update Series 16:282–287, 1997.
11. Reddy PR, Mandell J: Ureteropelvic junction obstruction: Prenatal diagnosis; therapeutic implications. Urol Clin North Am 25:171–195, 1998.
12. Snyder HM: Anomalies of the ureter. In Gillenwater JY, Grayhack JT, Howards SS, Duckett JW (eds): Adult and Pediatric Urology, 3rd ed. St. Louis, Mosby, 1996, pp 2197–2228.

XII. Health Care

100. HEALTH CARE REFORM

Alden H. Harken, M.D.

1. Is health care reform an oxymoron?
Yes.

2. What is fee for service?
The doctor establishes the price, and the patient agrees to pay it. This traditional system of exchange has great merit if both parties understand the value of the service provided. If either (usually the patient) cannot estimate the service value, it is possible (even likely) that the doctor will honestly escalate the service value in a fashion unchecked by the patient's perceptions. Thus, in a fee-for-service system medical prices tend to rise.

3. What is discounted fee for service?
The patient gets together with a group of friends, and they come to the doctor with the following proposition: "Hey, Doc, you can dazzle us with your fancy medical talk, but we still think that your prices are too high. How about me and my pals will pay you 80% of what you charge us?"

4. Is there a difference between hospital costs and hospital charges?
Absolutely. Hospital cost is the sum of the expenses (sutures, nurses' salaries, electricity, instrumentation sterilization, and band-aids) that are expended in suturing a laceration. The hospital typically charges about twice the cost (100% mark-up) for repairing a cut finger. This mark-up is highly industry-specific. Thus, intensely competitive food chains may make a profit of only 1 penny on a loaf of bread, whereas hospitals and liquor stores usually charge twice the cost.

5. What are fixed costs?
After accounting for light, heat, and staff (nurses, housekeepers, administrators) at a hospital but before seeing a single patient, the doctor has already spent a huge amount of money. Doctors must pay fixed costs whether or not they provide medical services.

6. What are actual costs?
The incremental costs of actually providing a service in a hospital (in addition to the fixed costs of light and heat). Thus, the patient shows up in the emergency department at midnight complaining of a lump on the tip of his nose. The doctor, with characteristic erudition, says, "Yep, you have a wart on your nose," and sends the patient home with a bill for $500. The actual cost of this encounter is obviously negligible. The patient is really paying for the fixed costs of nurses and emergency resuscitative equipment should he have a cardiac arrest (when he sees the bill).

7. Is hospital accounting a precisely scientific and objective analysis of financial data?
Obviously it is not.

8. What is health insurance?
Traditionally, people can purchase insurance that may pay either all or a portion of their hospital and physician charges if they become ill. Insurance companies make a profit, therefore, only

if the patient stays healthy. Insurance companies have elaborate tables to predict who will get sick, and they prefer to sell policies exclusively to young decathlon champions. This practice is termed "skimming." The insurance company takes all of the risk—and they like to keep it low. Conversely, hospitals must cover fixed costs—and the more expensive the health care that physicians provide, the better for them.

9. So along came the HMOs. What are they?

Health maintenance organizations (HMOs) are complex systems composed, in their most comprehensive form, of a hospital(s), doctors plus offices, and an insurance company. HMOs contract with large groups of people (potential patients) to maintain their health. The enrollee pays a monthly fee (just like health insurance) so that all hospital and physician charges are covered if the enrollee becomes ill. Unlike health insurance, however, in the HMO model hospitals and physicians get paid whether or not the enrollee gets sick. So it is better for everyone if enrollees stay healthy—and out of the hospital.

10. Initially, a lot of physicians did not like HMOs. Why?

Because physicians are fiercely independent. They did not want a bunch of business managers telling them how to manage patients.

11. Why are physicians fiercely independent?

Probably they were born that way.

12. Is that good?

Probably not. Eventually everyone will need to work together and not hit each other when they are mad.

13. Do HMO administrators really dictate how physicians manage their patients?

Yes and no. Physicians have developed medically effective and optimally efficient strategies—termed clinical pathways—for caring for many common illnesses. Although physicians must treat each patient individually, when they adhere to predetermined treatment guidelines (as encouraged by HMO administrators), patients usually get better faster and cheaper.

14. Do physicians follow these clinical pathways?

Traditionally, they have not.

15. So where do the HMO managers come in?

They evaluate each physician's utilization of expenive resources (within the predetermined clinical pathways) relative to the health of the physician's patients.

16. Do physicians welcome this kind of scrutiny?

No.

17. What is a PPO?

A preferred provider organization (PPO) is a group of doctors who have elected to remain legally independent of a hospital and insurance company (if they joined together, they would be an HMO)—and, most of all, patients. But PPOs maintain their independence as physicians, even though most PPOs require administrators to coordinate programs, keep the books, and keep the doctors from hitting each other. PPOs have the perception of independence, however.

18. Is health care expensive?

Unfortunately, yes. Physicians argue that patients pay a lot but also get a lot. In the United States, patients expect unlimited access to liver transplantation and an MRI for every headache. Americans believe that fancy, expensive health care is not just a privilege—it is a right.

19. So what is the problem?

The chief executive officers (CEOs) of big American corporations argue that the mandatory expense of health care is driving up the cost of U.S. products and making American companies less competitive in the global market— "there is more health care than steel in a new Chevrolet."

20. Does big business have a solution?

They think so. The CEOs still want unlimited access to the most modern health care for themselves and their families. Without sounding cynical, the CEOs want to save health care dollars spent on their employees and "other people's families." They want to limit access to health care, but they do not want to wield the ax personally. So they developed the idea of capitation.

21. What is capitation?

The CEOs of large businesses come to hospitals, HMOs, or PPOs and say: "Why don't you provide *all* health care for *all* my employees at a fixed price (say, $180 per month per head)?" Hence, capitation. In this model, physicians make the decisions about who gets how much medical care (satisfying their urge for independence), but they also promise to provide *all* necessary medical care for a prearranged price. Thus they take *all* of the risk. CEOs like this model because they can still offer health care as an employee benefit and budget the cost in advance.

22. Why do physicians not like capitation?

All of a sudden physicians may have acquired a little more independence than they bargained for. Now they are paid in advance so that all costs of patients' health care are subtracted from the bag of money that they negotiated upfront. Now they must advise against an MRI for every headache and break the news to Granny that she will not think better if they dialyze her blood urea nitrogen down to 50. This is the reverse of the good old days when physicians were rewarded if their patients got sick and stayed sick. Physicians could ply them with a smorgasbord of drugs and technologies. Now physicians are trying to control health care costs.

23. Is all this change good?

Absolutely. Medicine has always changed—and the faster the better. Physicians were initially attracted to medicine as an intellectually stimulating discipline because medicine and surgery evolve rapidly.

24. Can physicians keep up with all this change?

Absolutely.

25. Despite all of the medical Chicken Littles who sonorously declare that the sky is falling, is medicine (and even more clearly, surgery) still the most gratifying, stimulating, and rewarding profession?

Absolutely.

BIBLIOGRAPHY

1. Berliner H: U.S. healthcare. Boom or bust? Health Serv J 109:32, 1999.
2. Blumenthal D: Health care reform at the close of the 20th century. N Engl J Med 340:1916–1920, 1999.
3. Josten B: Bad medicine for health care. Healthplan 40:11–12, 1999.
4. Young O: Making a case for a single-payer system. Manag Care 8:47–52, 1999.

101. RISKS OF BLOOD-BORNE DISEASE

Doru I.E. Georgescu, M.D., FACS

1. Which blood-borne pathogens have major significance for the surgeon?

Although the epidemic of human immunodeficiency virus (HIV) increased general concern about blood-borne pathogens, the prevalence of hepatitis C virus (HCV) throughout North America led to a shift of emphasis from HIV to hepatitis as the greatest risk. Hepatitis B, an occupational infection, has been recognized for nearly 50 years in surgery, but the increased number of surgeons who are vaccinated and a relatively efficient protocol after exposure have helped to lower the consequences of contamination with hepatitis B virus (HBV).

2. What is the relative risk of exposure to HIV, HBV, and HCV?

HIV. At present approximately 1 million U.S. residents are infected with HIV. The current evidence shows that transmission of HIV in health care settings is an infrequent event. Only 5% of cases of AIDS thus far reported have occurred in health care workers, and the majority of these workers had nonoccupational risk factors that were presumed to be responsible. Nurses and laboratory technicians have the highest occupational risk. As of January 1, 1998, there is no documented transmission of HIV infection from a patient to a surgeon secondary to occupational exposure.

HBV. Without doubt all surgeons are exposed to HBV during the course of a normal career. At present it is estimated that 1.25 million U.S. residents have chronic hepatitis B. Approximately 30% of percutaneous hollow needle exposures are followed by acute infection. Seventy-five percent of hepatitis B cases are clinically occult, and 10% of infected people remain carriers of the virus for life. Many carriers are asymptomatic and seem to have minimal or no progression of active liver disease, although they are potentially infectious to others. About 40% have a steady progression of disease that leads to cirrhosis, end-stage liver disease, and even hepatocellular carcinoma.

HCV. Hepatitis C has become the greatest concern for surgeons. It is estimated that approximately 4 million U.S. residents have chronic hepatitis C. The risk of seroconversion from a percutaneous hollow needle injury is approximately 10%, but 50% of acute infections result in the chronic carrier state. The natural history of hepatitis C infection is still controversial, but up to 40% of patients may develop cirrhosis from chronic hepatitis C infection. Of those, a high number develop hepatoma, with the proportion reaching 50% over 15 years.

3. Does hepatitis B vaccination offer absolute protection against the disease?

Effective hepatitis B vaccination is currently available for all surgeons and health care providers working in the operating room. The hepatitis B vaccine is produced by recombinant technology and does not represent the denatured particles from infected people. Three doses of vaccine are given, and after the complete series surface antibody titer should be determined to ensure that vaccination has been successful. Approximately 5% of people who are vaccinated do not develop an antibody response and should have a repeat vaccination. Some people remain refractory to the vaccination and thus are at risk for contracting acute hepatitis B infection. Vaccination does not equal immunity. According to some studies, 50% of practicing surgeons may not have adequate immunity to HBV for various reasons: lack of vaccination in older surgeons, vaccination more than 5 years ago, inadequate amount of recombinant vaccine or improper vaccination, and, finally, failure to mount an appropriate immunologic response.

4. Are patients at risk of infection from surgeons who are infected with HBV?

Transmission of hepatitis B infection from surgeons to patients has been documented. Surgeons who are at risk for transmitting infection to patients are generally positive for the e-antigen of

318

hepatitis B. The e-antigen is a degradation product of the nucleocapsid of the virus and represents active viral replication within the liver. People who test positive for the e-antigen have high viral titers and are quite infectious. The large number of documented transmissions of hepatitis B to patients by surgical providers is particularly troublesome and may require restriction of clinical privileges for clinicians who have been documented to transmit hepatitis infection. Furthermore, a recent report from England documented transmission of hepatitis B infection from surgeons to patients even when the surgeon was negative for the e-antigen. Recently, one national organization called for the restriction of privileges of e-antigen–positive surgeons. Whether surgeons with chronic hepatitis B should continue to practice will be debated in upcoming years.

5. What is the proper response after percutaneous exposure to a patient with known hepatitis B?

The response depends on the provider's vaccination status. If the provider has been vaccinated and has a positive antibody titer, no additional response is necessary. If the provider has not been vaccinated and is negative for antibodies to HBV, he or she should receive a dose of hepatitis B immunoglobulin and begin the hepatitis B vaccination series. Providers who previously have been vaccinated successfully but have an absent or weakly positive antibody titer should receive a dose of hepatitis B immunoglobulin and a booster dose of the hepatitis B vaccine. Because in most cases of exposure the status of the patient is unknown, it generally is prudent for surgeons to know their antibody status and to have periodic booster doses of hepatitis B vaccine. Booster dosing should be given every 7 years.

6. How does HCV differ from HBV? Which is more dangerous?

Prevalence in U.S.
  HBV: estimated 1.25 million patients
  HCV: estimated 4 million patients
Route and consequences of transmission
  HBV: blood-borne DNA virus with 10% rate of chronic infection after acute disease
  HCV: blood-borne RNA virus with 50% rate of chronic infection after acute disease
Prevention
  HBV: effective vaccine produced by recombinant technology
  HCV: no vaccine currently available
Postexposure protection
  HBV: hepatitis B immunoglobulin is useful in people who have not been vaccinated and
    do not have antibodies to HBV
  HCV: immunoglobulin for hepatitis C has not been proved to be of clinical value
Surgeons in the U.S. care for a larger population with chronic hepatitis C than with chronic hepatitis B, and no vaccine is available for HCV infection. Although the rate of seroconversion for hepatitis C is 10% vs. 30% for hepatitis B, when acute infection occurs, there is a much higher chance of developing chronic hepatitis (50% vs. 10%) after HCV infection. Thus, HCV infection is a far greater threat for surgeons.

7. Are health care workers at significant risk for acquiring HIV infection?

The first HIV seroconversion in a health care worker was reported in 1984. As of December 1997, the Centers for Disease Control and Prevention (CDC) had received approximately 200 reports of occupational infection. Case studies showed that 132 of the workers had nonoccupational risk factors, and only 54 had a documented transmission. In cases of documented transmission, the health care worker had a documented exposure to the blood or body fluids of an infected patient and HIV seroconversion was subsequently identified. Nurses and clinical laboratory technicians are by far at greatest risk for occupational exposure. The total number of transmissions is quite small compared with the large number of exposures that probably have occurred since the onset of the epidemic in the early 1980s. Only 6 surgeons have been identified as possible occupational transmissions from the analysis of the 640,000 AIDS cases reported to the CDC since the beginning of the epidemic; none of them fulfilled criteria for documented HIV infection.

8. Does laparoscopic surgery minimize the risk of HIV contamination?

Laparoscopic surgery recently has been encouraged as an alternative to open procedures in patients infected with HIV. The laparoscopic technique reduces exposure to blood products and sharp instruments; however, it exposes the surgical team to the HIV-infected patient in a manner not encountered during open procedures. The evacuation of the pneumoperitoneum during laparoscopic procedures releases aerosolized HIV-infected blood and peritoneal fluid into the operative suite. Evacuation of the pneumoperitoneum into a closed system and appropriate precautions during instrument changes diminish this exposure.

9. Is double gloving an effective method of protection?

The potential for blood contact with nonintact skin puts operating room personnel at increased risk of exposure to hepatitis or HIV. Although double gloving may not prevent percutaneous injury, it clearly has been demonstrated to reduce blood exposure. Studies of blood exposure in the operating room indicate that 90% of all blood contact with the surgeon's skin occurs from the elbow distally, including the gloves. In one study the contact rates between blood and the surgeon's skin were decreased by 70% when the surgeon wore two pairs of gloves. Outer glove perforation occurred in 25% of cases, whereas inner glove perforation occurred in only 10% of cases (surgeons, 8.7%; assistants, 3.7%). The inner glove perforations occurred during procedures that lasted longer than 3 hours, and in no case was there an inner glove defect without a corresponding outer glove defect. The nondominant index finger was the most common location.

10. Are eye splash injuries a major threat for surgeons?

A CDC study demonstrated that approximately 13% of documented HIV transmissions occurred by mucocutaneous contact. Eye splash injuries during surgery are often underestimated, although they are the easiest type of contact to prevent. A recent study examined 160 eye shields used by surgeons and assistants. All operations lasted 30 minutes or longer. The shields were inspected for macroscopic splashes and then tested for microscopic splashes. Forty-four percent of the shields tested positive for blood. The surgeon was aware of a spray in only 8% of cases. The splashes were macroscopically visible in only 16% of cases. The risk of eye splashes was higher for the surgeon than for the assistant and increased with the length of the operation. The type of operation also proved to be a determining factor; vascular surgery and orthopedic surgery had the higher risks for eye splash injuries. Eye protection should be mandatory for all personnel in the operating room, particularly those directly involved with the operation.

11. What is the surgeon's rate of exposure to blood and body fluids?

Surgeons are exposed to blood by percutaneous injuries (needlesticks, cuts) and mucocutaneous contact (perforated glove, nonintact skin, eye splashes). Percutaneous blood exposure occurs in 1.2–5.6% of surgical cases and mucocutaneous blood contact in 6.4–50.4%. The discrepancy among reported rates reflects differences in data collection, procedures performed, surgical technique, and degree of precautions. For example, surgeons at San Francisco General Hospital take extra precautions by using waterproof gowns and double gloving. There is no evidence of any health care worker becoming infected through exposure of intact skin to infected blood and body fluids. However, transmission of HIV after mucocutaneous contact with HIV-infected blood has been reported in health care workers without other risk factors. The risk of transmission after such exposure remains unknown because no serconversion has been detected in prospective studies of health care workers after mucous membrane and skin contact with HIV-infected blood.

The risk of contamination is real for all personnel in the operating room, but it is much higher for surgeons and first assistants, who account for 80% of all body contamination and 65% of injuries.

12. Are skin contaminations determined only by surgical technique?

Exposure of nonintact skin to blood or body fluids may occur even when all available precautionary guidelines are followed. Unfortunately, not all protective garments are equally protective. In one study 2% of sterile surgical gloves had perforations when they were examined immediately after removal from the package.

13. What are the seroconversion rates for HIV and HBV exposure?

Seroconversion rates from a hollow needle stick are 0.3% for HIV and 30% for HBV.

14. What is the lifetime occupational risk of HIV infection for surgeons?

The risk of HIV infection for a surgeon can be calculated by obtaining the product of HIV seroprevalence in surgical patients (0.32–50%), percutaneous injury rate (1.2–6%), and seroconversion rate (0.29–0.50%). The calculated risk per case of acquiring HIV ranges from 0.11 per million to 66 per million. Assuming that a surgeon performs 350 operations per year over a 30-year career, the estimated lifetime cumulative risk ranges from 0.12% to 50.0%, depending on the variables. Several assumptions are inherent in this calculation:

1. The formula assumes a constant HIV prevalence, but it is estimated that the prevalence increases by 4.0–8.6% annually in the United States.

2. The formula assumes that exposure to HIV-infected blood occurs only through percutaneous injuries, disregarding the risk due to mucocutaneous exposure.

3. The formula assumes that every operation carries the same risk, whereas the risk varies with length and urgency of the procedure and amount of blood loss.

Clearly these assumptions are imprecise, and the calculated risk is merely a rough estimate based on currently available data.

15. Are surgeons aware of their professional risk?

Most are not.

16. Are there effective methods to reduce the risk of transmission of blood-borne diseases to surgeons?

For HBV infection, in addition to universal precautions, a highly effective vaccine is available, but it is not used as much as it should be. Most surgeons who are 45 years or older have not been vaccinated. A precisely defined postexposure protocol is also available. For HCV and HIV infections the most pragmatic approach is to lower the rate of percutaneous and mucocutaneous injuries with use of optimal techniques and precautions.

Finally, prompt response to blood exposure is required. Contamination of the hands or arms is best dealt with by immediate rescrubbing. If this is not practical, the area should be irrigated with povidone iodine, and rescrubbing should be done at a convenient point in the procedure.

BIBLIOGRAPHY

1. Barrie PS, Patchen Dellinger E, Dougherty SH, Fink MP: Assessment of hepatitis B virus immunization status among North American surgeons. Arch Surg 129:27–32, 1994.
2. Eubanks S, Newman L, Lucas G: Reduction of HIV transmission during laparoscopic procedures. Surg Laparosc Endosc 3:2–5, 1993.
3. Fry DE: Blood-borne diseases in 1998. Bull Am Coll Surg 83:13–18, 1998.
4. Gerberding JL: Reducing occupational risk of HIV infection. Hosp Pract 113–110, 115–118, 1991.
5. Lin EY, Brumcardi C: HIV infection and surgeons. World J Surg Sept-Oct:753–757, 1994.
6. Marasco S, Woods S: The risk of eye splash injuries in surgery. Aust N Z J Surg Nov:785–787, 1998.
7. Megan J, Patterson M, Novak CB, et al: Surgeons' concern and practices of protection against bloodborne pathogens. Ann Surg 228:266–272, 1998.
8. Pietrabissa A, Merigliano S, Montorsi M, et al: Reducing the occupational risk of infections for the surgeons: Multicentric national survey on more than 15,000 surgical procedures. World J Surg July-Aug:573–578, 1997.

102. ETHICS IN THE SURGICAL INTENSIVE CARE UNIT

Ricardo J. Gonzalez, M.D., and Patrick J. Offner, M.D., M.P.H.

1. What are the four principles of medical ethics?

1. **Beneficence** describes the active role of doing good by intervention.
2. **Nonmaleficence** is equivalent to saying, "First do no harm."
3. **Autonomy** accounts for informed consent, competence, and the patient's right to refuse treatment.
4. **Justice** means that all patients should receive fair and equal care.

2. What is a do-not-resuscitate (DNR) order?

A DNR order instructs the surgeon not to resuscitate the patient if cardiopulmonary arrest occurs; however, a DNR order is much more involved and complicated than the acronym would have you believe.

The Joint Commission for the Accreditation of Healthcare Organizations mandates that hospitals have written guidelines that promote accountability for the DNR order. All DNR orders must be documented in writing, like all other orders, in the appropriate section of the patient's chart. They should specify the treatments to be withheld and treatments that the patient wishes to have implemented. Patients and families must participate in the DNR decision. Moreover, the DNR status should be discussed and reviewed with the other members of the health care team. Finally, a DNR must not mean that the patient is medically abandoned.

3. What is the difference between withdrawing and withholding support?

A decision to withdraw should not be more problematic than a decision to withhold, because one cannot be sure that an intervention will work unless it is attempted. There is no moral or ethical distinction between withdrawal and withholding of support. Either of the two allows natural progression of disease without interface of medical technology. The decision to withdraw or withhold support does not equate with patient death, although the probability of death may be greater. Once the decision has been made, appropriate management should focus on the patient's comfort.

4. What is an advance directive?

An advance directive is a method of delineating a competent patient's wishes for application at a time when he or she is no longer competent. Medical management or the lack thereof can be based on the patient's wishes rather than a perceived sense of what is best for the patient. Advance directives may be an informal document, such as a living will, or a formal legal document, such as medical durable power of attorney.

5. What is durable power of attorney?

A durable power of attorney is a patient-appointed proxy decision-maker. The proxy decision-maker becomes active once the patient is no longer able to make competent medical decisions. Hence the durable power of attorney must have been established in advance of the cognitive decline of the patient.

6. What is a a living will?

A living will, much like a durable power of attorney, is a formal advanced directive in which the competent patient produces a preillness guideline for future care in accordance with his or her wishes.

7. What is included in informed consent?

Information about the patient's condition as well as risks and benefits of the recommended treatment. Moreover, the operative and nonoperative alternatives, including no treatment, should be discussed with the patient. The patient's understanding of the information and alternatives should be assessed as part of the informed consent. Finally, informed consent is a voluntary decision made by the patient or on behalf of the patient by a proxy decision-maker.

8. What are futile care and medical futility?

The definition of medically futile or inappropriate treatment is still debated. Nonetheless, there are four main concepts of medical futility:

1. Health care professionals are not required to provide **physiologically futile** treatment.

2. **Imminent demise** argues against treatment if the patient has no likelihood of survival to discharge.

3. Under the concept of **lethal condition**, medical care is considered futile if the patient will survive temporarily but ultimately expire as a result of the ongoing disease process.

4. Quality of life or **qualitative futility** argues against treatment if the patient's quality of life is so poor that it would be unreasonable to sustain life.

Care must be taken, however, in making medical decisions based on futility, because they may lead to a self-fulfilling prophecy.

9. What are the clinical determinants of brain death?

Many of the current concepts of brain death were based on the 1968 report from the ad hoc committee at Harvard Medical School, which called for a new neurologic definition of brain death. But it was not until 1981 that Bernat justified the neurologic criteria of brain death by stressing the need for intact brainstem integrative function in order for a person to function as a whole. By definition, brain death requires loss of brainstem reflexes in an irreversibly comatose patient.

Brain death includes loss of the pupillary, corneal, oculovestibular, oculocephalic, oropharyngeal, and respiratory reflexes for at least 6 hours. The patient also should undergo an apnea test, in which the pCO_2 is allowed to rise to at least 60 mmHg without coexistent hypoxia. The patient should be observed for spontaneous breathing. Other ancillary tests are not essential; for example, it is not necessary to perform an intravenous radioisotope cerebral angiogram or a four-vessel contrast cerebral angiogram or to document an isoelectric ("flat") electroencephalogram.

Of note, all of the above criteria for brain death require the absence of central nervous system depression due to barbiturates, narcotics, or hypothermia.

10. What is a persistent vegetative state?

In a persistent vegetative state, typically seen after improvement of a comatose state, the patient lies motionless and without activity. The patient appears to be awake but without awareness of surroundings or higher mental activity. Other names for this entity are coma vigil and akinetic mutism.

11. What is euthanasia?

Euthanasia requires that the physician play an active role in assisting in the death of the patient. The concepts of physician-assisted suicide and active and passive euthanasia are highly controversial. In 1992, the Society of Critical Care Medicine published the results of a survey of critical care specialists; 87% had withdrawn life-prolonging support from patients. In addition, the most recent U.S. law pertaining to assisted suicide was passed in Oregon in 1994. This law makes it legal for a physician to prescribe medication to a terminally ill patient for the purpose of committing suicide.

12. Who should approach the family about organ donation?

Some claim that the physician who has established good rapport with the patient's family should raise the issue of organ donation. Others believe that the local organ procuremement personnel should approach the family, because they have greater interest and training in the process. The best approach is a combined approach.

13. What should the family be told when organ donation is feasible?

One should stress that the patient has died despite an actively beating heart. The family should be questioned about the patient's wishes regarding organ donation. All topics should be based on the concepts of informed consent. The family should be made aware of the likelihood that several patients will benefit from the donated organs. The family needs to understand that there is no guarantee that the organs will be suitable for donation. They should be assured that they are not responsible for the cost of care provided after brain death is determined and that they may refuse organ donation without fear of prejudice.

14. What is the role of the hospital ethics committee?

The hospital ethics committee serves three functions: (1) it educates hospital staff; (2) it creates policy; and (3) it provides a source of consultation.

The function of education is accomplished through grand rounds, seminars, special lectures, and journal clubs. The hospital ethics committee should be viewed as an intrinsic part of the hospital community. Developed policies should be reviewed by other committees and divisions of the hospital to foster a better sense of cohesiveness when ethical and moral dilemmas arise.

The consultative function of the ethics committee produces the greatest amount of controversy. In fact, many hospitals negate this function by stating that it interferes with the physician–patient relationship. The hospital ethics committee can provide an arena for collaboration and general ethical education of the hospital.

BIBLIOGRAPHY

1. Ad Hoc Committee of the Harvard Medical School to Examine the Definition of Brain Death: A definition of irreversible coma. JAMA 205:337–340, 1968.
2. Aminoff MJ: The central nervous system. In Medical Diagnosis and Treatment. Norwalk, CT, Appleton & Lange, 1996.
3. Arnold RM, Siminoff LA, Frader JE: Ethical issues in organ procurement: A review for intensivists. Crit Care Med 12:29–48, 1996.
4. Bernat JL, Culver CM, Gert B: On the definition and criterion of death. Ann Intern Med 94:389–394, 1981.
5. Harken AH: Enough is enough. Arch Surg 1999 [in press].
6. Kelley DF, Hoyt JW: Ethics consultation. Crit Care Med 12:49–70, 1996.
7. McCollough L, Jones J, Brody B: Surgical Ethics. Oxford, Oxford University Press, 1998.
8. Nyman DJ, Eidelman AL, Sprung CL: Euthanasia. Crit Care Clin 12:85–96, 1996.
9. Society of Critical Care Ethics Committee: Attitudes of critical care medicine professionals concerning foregoing life-sustaining treatments. Crit Care Med 20:320–326, 1992.
10. State of Oregon: ORS.251.215, The Oregon Death with Dignity Act. Official 1994 Oregon General Election Handbook, 1994, pp 121–124.
11. Younger SJ: Medical futility. Crit Care Clin 12:165–178, 1996.

INDEX

Page numbers in **boldface type** indicate complete chapters.